Color Atlas of Obstetric and Gynecologic Pathology

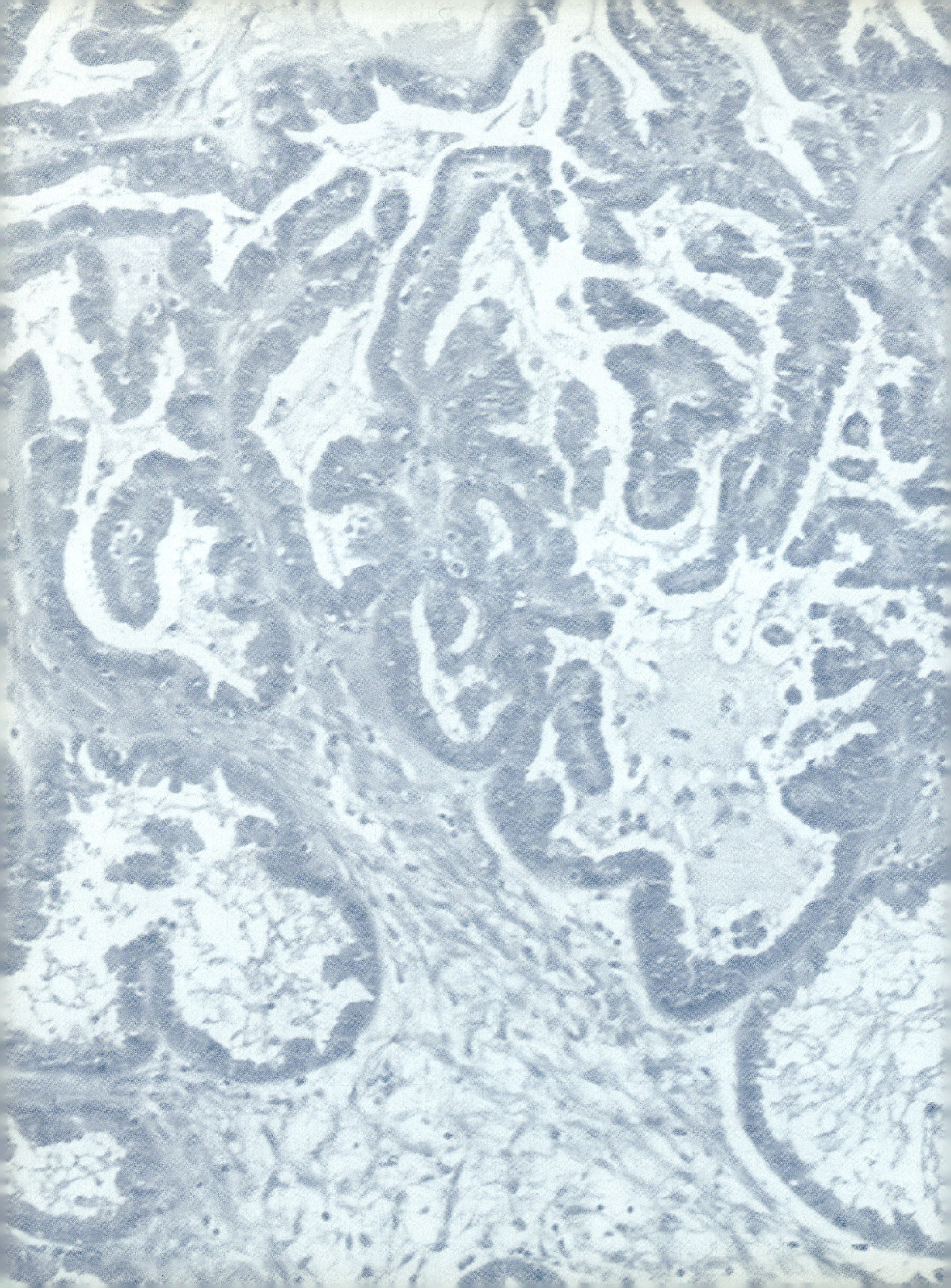

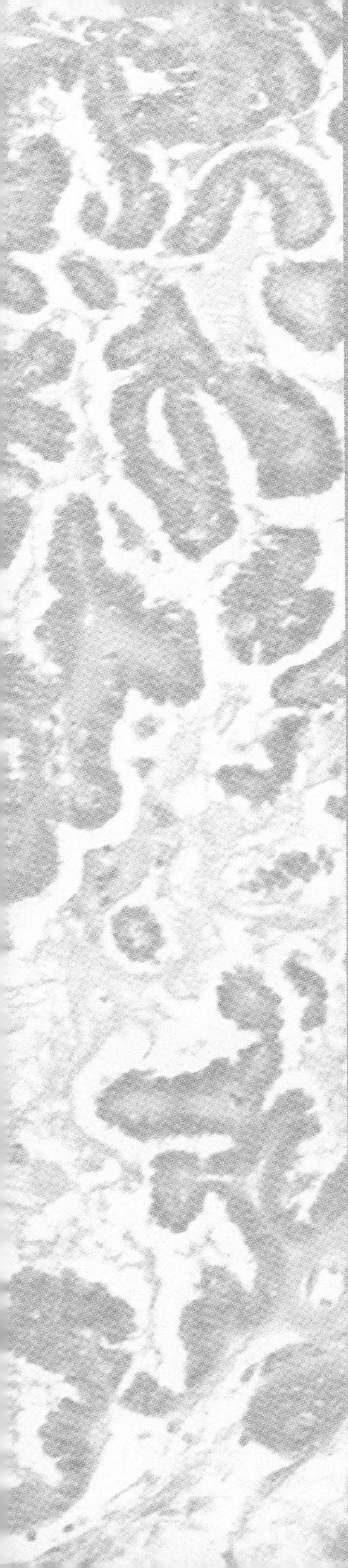

Color Atlas of Obstetric and Gynecologic Pathology

RICHARD L. VOET, M.D.
CLINICAL ASSOCIATE PROFESSOR OF PATHOLOGY
AND OBSTETRICS & GYNECOLOGY
UNIVERSITY OF TEXAS HEALTH SCIENCE CENTER AT DALLAS
DIRECTOR OF ANATOMIC PATHOLOGY
PRESBYTERIAN HOSPITAL
DALLAS, TEXAS

Mosby-Wolfe

St. Louis Baltimore Boston Carlsbad Chicago Naples New York Philadelphia Portland
London Madrid Mexico City Singapore Sydney Tokyo Toronto Wiesbaden

Mosby-Wolfe
Dedicated to Publishing Excellence

A Times Mirror
Company

Vice-President and Publisher: Anne S. Patterson
Senior Managing Editor: Lynne Gery
Project Manager: Linda Clarke
Production Editor: Jennifer Harper
Composition Specialist: Wendy Bellm
Manufacturing Manager: William A. Winneberger, Jr.
Design Manager: Nancy McDonald

Printed in Canada
Composition by Mosby Electronic Production, St. Louis
Printing/binding by Friesens—Altona, Manitoba
Lithography/color film by Colortronics

Mosby–Year Book, Inc.
11830 Westline Industrial Drive
St. Louis, Missouri 63146

Library of Congress Cataloging-in-Publication Data

Voet, Richard L.
Color atlas of obstetric and gynecologic pathology/Richard L. Voet. -- 1st ed.
p. cm.
Includes bibliographical references and index.
ISBN 0-8151-9048-4 (alk. paper)
1. Gynecologic pathology--Atlases. 2. Placenta--Diseases--Atlases. I. Title.
[DNLM: 1. Genital Diseases, Female--pathology--atlases. 2. Genitalia, Female--pathology--atlases. 3. Pregnancy Complications--pathology--atlases. WP 17 V876c 1997]
RG77.V64 1997
618'.047--dc20
DNLM/DLC 96-36128
for Library of Congress CIP

97 98 99 00 01 / 9 8 7 6 5 4 3 2 1

This book is dedicated to the three most important people in my life: my wife, Kathy, and my daughters, Amanda and Heidi. Without their love, support, and encouragement I would not have been able to complete this project.

Preface

Gynecologic pathology is a major subspecialty of surgical pathology. It often accounts for 30 to 50 percent of an average pathology practice. One of the rewarding aspects of this area is the interest in and understanding of the subject on the part of gynecologists. Some of this interest undoubtedly comes from their training and board requirements. Nevertheless, it results in well-informed clinicians who appreciate the importance as well as the limitations of pathology as it pertains to their patients. Unfortunately, time demands on OB/GYN residency programs are beginning to limit their exposure to pathology.

This book is intended to be used as a general reference and review of the field of obstetric and gynecologic pathology in a one-volume atlas. There are other more comprehensive books covering each specific topic in greater detail. The International Society of Gynecological Pathologists (ISGYP), under the direction of Dr. Robert Scully and in cooperation with the World Health Organization (WHO), developed nomenclature committees for histologic terminology in gynecologic pathology. This became the basis for the second revision of the WHO classification. The new WHO classifications for the ovary and fallopian tube were not yet published when this book went into production. The classification tables in these chapters were taken from preliminary ISGYP versions and may differ from the final WHO revision. Each chapter also includes the latest revision of the TNM staging classification. The American College of Surgeons now requires all accredited cancer centers to include the TNM stage on the chart of all patients with a diagnosis of cancer.

The illustrations were chosen to represent the major diagnoses for each section. Every attempt was made to include original photographs except where indicated. I apologize if I have inadvertently included someone's photograph from my files without acknowledgment. The text for each section is intended to be a guide through the topic and illustrations. The reader is reminded that this is an atlas and not a textbook. I had to constantly remind myself of this fact with each gentle nudge from the publisher. The references were also selected to be representative and not exhaustive.

It would be impractical to mention every person who contributed in some way to this book. However, there are some to whom I wish to extend a special acknowledgment. For the past 15 years it has been my privilege to work with two excellent gynecologic oncologists, Drs. Samuel Lifshitz and Steve Bernstein. A major portion of the case material in this book comes from their practice. The late Dr. Herbert Buchsbaum provided the opportunity for our association and stimulated much of my academic pursuits. Dr. Roger Bick was responsible for recommending me to the publisher. Dr. H. Richard Pascoe, Chairman of Pathology at Presbyterian Hospital of Dallas, encouraged me to take on this project and provided most of the support for the photographs. I would also like to thank my associates, Drs. Vance Bryan, Beverly Dickson, Aviva Hopkovitz, Pamela Jensen, W. Robert Laughlin, Mark Pollock, and Anne Vandersteenhoven, for their help in identifying interesting cases. Eileen Cahill, Cindy Goldman, and Danny Terrell helped with many of the gross photographs. The histotechnologists at Presbyterian Hospital, under the supervision of Maureen Hoops, were very helpful in cutting extra slides and restaining old slides to make them acceptable for photomicrography. Christy Nichol and Stacey Sullivan provided most of the typing.

It is my desire that this book will be used by residents and practicing physicians in both Pathology and Obstetrics and Gynecology as a tool for improved patient care. The diagnosis and treatment of diseases in women, especially cancer, require a multispecialty approach to health care. Uniform agreement in terminology and staging is the best way to improve information exchange. Ultimately, I hope those who suffer from these diseases will benefit the most from this book.

Richard L. Voet, M.D.

Contents

1. PATHOLOGY OF THE VULVA
   - Infectious Diseases 2
   - Squamous Lesions 5
   - Pigmented Lesions 11
   - Glandular Lesions 12
   - Bartholin Gland 13
   - Soft Tissue Lesions 16
   - Miscellaneous Lesions 18
   - Classification and Staging Tables 19

2. PATHOLOGY OF THE VAGINA
   - Classification and Staging Tables 36

3. PATHOLOGY OF THE UTERINE CERVIX
   - Epithelial Tumors and Related Lesions 42
   - Mesenchymal Tumors 58
   - Mixed Epithelial and Mesodermal Tumors 60
   - Miscellaneous Tumors 60
   - Secondary Tumors 61
   - Classification and Staging Tables 62

4. PATHOLOGY OF THE UTERINE CORPUS
   - Inflammation 72
   - Functional States of the Endometrium 73
   - Abnormal Proliferative States 77
   - Endometrial Carcinoma 79
   - Mesenchymal Tumors 84
   - Smooth Muscle Tumors 86
   - Mixed Epithelial and Mesenchymal Tumors 93
   - Classification and Staging Tables 96

5. PATHOLOGY OF THE FALLOPIAN TUBE, BROAD LIGAMENT AND PERITONEUM

Tumor-like Lesions 104

Inflammation 106

Tumors 110

Paratubal Cysts and Tumors. 113

Tumors and Tumor-like Lesions of the Peritoneum 115

Classification and Staging Tables 120

6. PATHOLOGY OF THE OVARY

Non-neoplastic Lesions. 128

Surface Epithelial Tumors. 132

Gonadal Stromal Tumors of the Ovary 144

Tumors of Germ Cell Origin 151

Miscellaneous Tumors of the Ovary 158

Classification and Staging Tables 160

7. PATHOLOGY OF THE PLACENTA AND TROPHOBLASTIC DISEASE

Placental Pathology 170

- Umbilical Cord 170
- Placental Membranes 173
- Placental Disk 176

Gestational Trophoblastic Disease 181

- Molar Trophoblastic Lesions 181
- Nonmolar Trophoblastic Lesions. 183
- Miscellaneous Trophoblastic Lesions 184

Classification and Staging Tables 185

8. PATHOLOGY OF THE BREAST

Reactive and Inflammatory Lesions 192
Proliferative Changes 193
Carcinoma in Situ 196
Papillary Lesions 198
Infiltrating Carcinoma 200
Mixed Epithelial and Mesenchymal Tumors 204
Diagnostic Procedures 206
Classification and Staging Tables 208

Color Atlas of Obstetric and Gynecologic Pathology

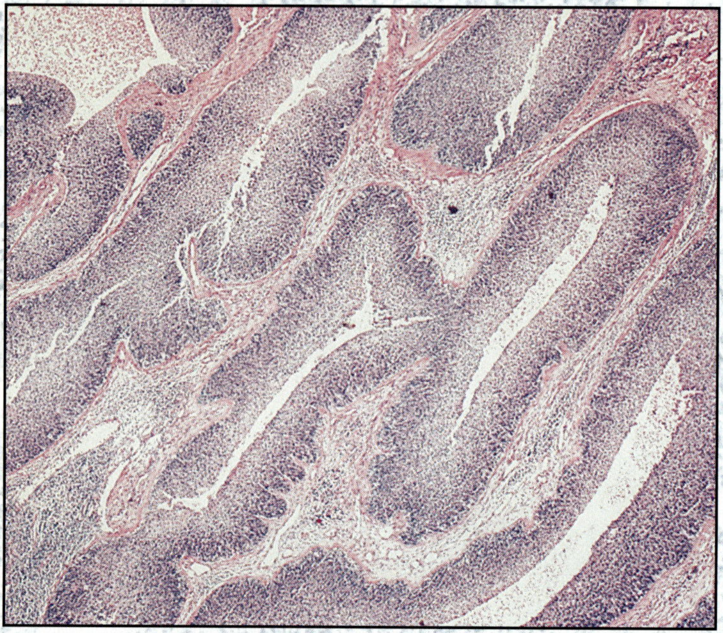

Chapter 1

Pathology of the Vulva

Since the major portion of the vulva is composed of squamous epithelium, a variety of dermatologic diseases may also affect the vulva. This chapter deals with the conditions that usually present in a gynecologic practice. Several excellent reviews of vulvar pathology are available for a more in-depth reading.[1–8]

INFECTIOUS DISEASES

A variety of infectious diseases may affect the vulva (Table 1-1). Herpes simplex is a viral infection that presents with ulcerated vesicles. Histologic examination of the lesions shows intranuclear viral inclusions that are best seen at the edge of the ulcer (Figures 1-1 and 1-2). Molluscum contagiosum is a DNA poxvirus infection that can affect the vulva. There appear to be unknown factors that make a person more predisposed to contracting this virus than others. Multiple papules are usually present that contain invaginated squamous epithelium with cytoplasmic inclusions (Figures 1-3 and 1-4). Primary syphilis, caused by the spirochete *Treponema pallidum*, presents as a painless, solitary chancre showing ulceration with acute and chronic inflammation. If untreated, syphilis may give rise to multiple secondary papular lesions known as condylomata lata. These lesions may clinically resemble condylomata acuminata. The inflammatory infiltrate contains increased numbers of plasma cells. Granuloma inguinale is caused by the bacteria *Calymmatobacterium granulomatis*. The organisms may be seen as intracytoplasmic Donovan bodies on direct smears (Figure 1-5). Condyloma acuminatum is caused by the human papillomavirus (HPV).[75, 80] The typical presentation on the vulva is the presence of multiple papillary lesions. Histologically, condyloma is characterized by a hyperplastic squamous proliferation with

TABLE 1-1 Infectious Diseases of the Vulva

Disease	Causative Microorganism	Salient Histopathologic Features	Diagnostic Methods
Condyloma acuminatum	Papillomavirus	Acanthosis, hyperkeratosis, parakeratosis, papillomatosis, perinuclear halo (koilocytosis)	Histopathology, immunohistochemistry, molecular hybridization
Herpes genitalis	Herpes simplex hominis Type II	Intranuclear inclusions	Cytopathology, culture serology
Syphilitic chancre	*Treponema pallidum*	Ulceration, chronic inflammation, vasculitis	Darkfield, fluorescence, silver, stain, serology
Condyloma latum	*Treponema pallidum*	Like chancre, with epithelial hyperplasia	Same as syphilitic chancre
Molluscum contagiosum	DNA poxvirus group	Intracytoplasmic inclusions	Cytopathology, histopathology
Granuloma inguinale	*Calymmatobacterium granulomatis*	Donovan bodies, granulomatous reaction without caseation, pseudoepitheliomatous hyperplasia	Giemsa stain, silver stain
Lymphogranuloma venereum	*Chlamydia* (TRIC agent)	Granulomatous reaction without caseation	Serology
Tuberculosis	*Mycobacterium tuberculosis*	Acid-fast bacilli (AFB), granulomatous reaction with caseation	AFB stain, AFB culture
Chancroid	*Haemophilus ducreyi*	Granulomatous reaction without caseation	Culture, Gram stain

Reproduced with permission. Wilkinson EJ: Benign diseases of the vulva. In Kurman RJ, (ed). New York Blaustein's Pathology of the Female Genital Tract, *1994, Springer-Verlag.*

TRIC, Trachema inclusion conjunctivitis.

parakeratosis and koilocytosis (Figures 1-6 and 1-7). HPV has been implicated in the development of squamous neoplasia of the vulva.[25,40,54,90] At times the diagnosis of HPV may be difficult to distinguish from reactive changes and vulvar intraepithelial neoplasia (VIN).[21,62,63] Vulvar vestibulitis is a clinical syndrome[9,36,37,59,61,73] characterized by chronic localized pain. The cause is unknown and attempts to associate it with HPV have been inconclusive.[72,101] Histologically (Figure 1-8), there is a nonspecific chronic inflammatory infiltrate; however, vestibular glands are often not present in a superficial biopsy. Hidradenitis suppurativa[89] is a chronic inflammatory disorder involving the apocrine glands of the vulva (Figure 1-9), axilla, and scalp. The treatment often requires surgical excision.

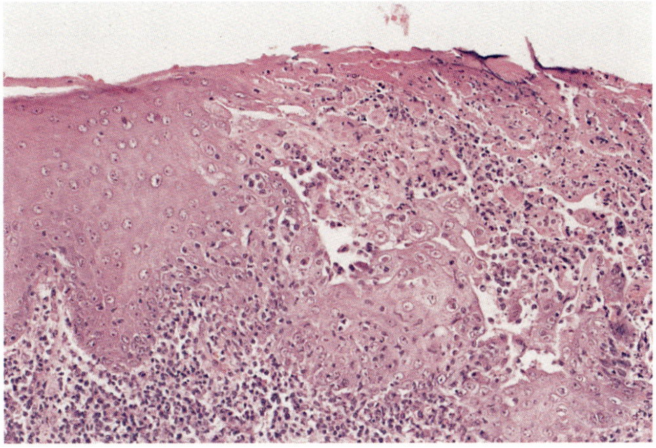

1.1 Ulcerated herpetic lesion of the vulva.

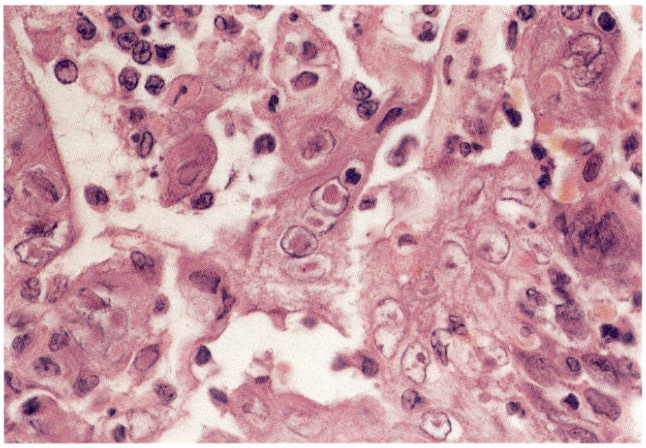

1.2 High-power view of the herpetic ulcer revealing nuclear inclusions.

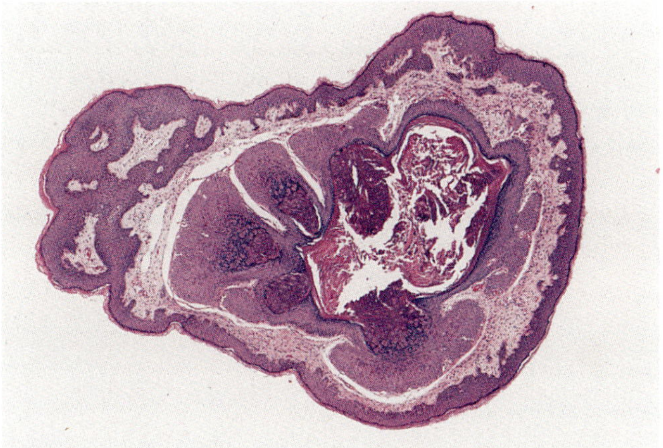

1.3 Molluscum contagiosum showing the central invaginated squamous proliferation.

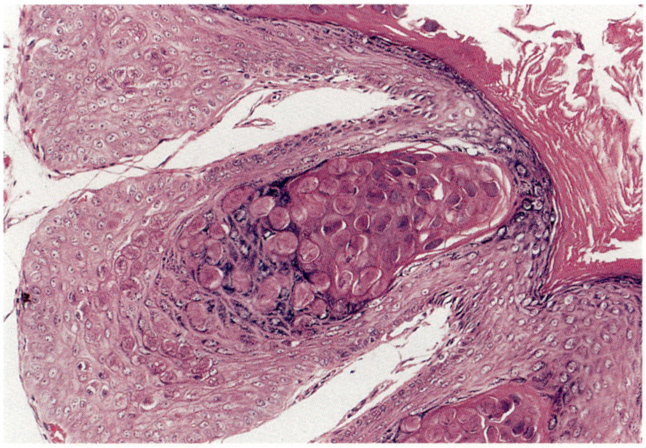

1.4 Higher-power view of molluscum contagiosum revealing cytoplasmic inclusions.

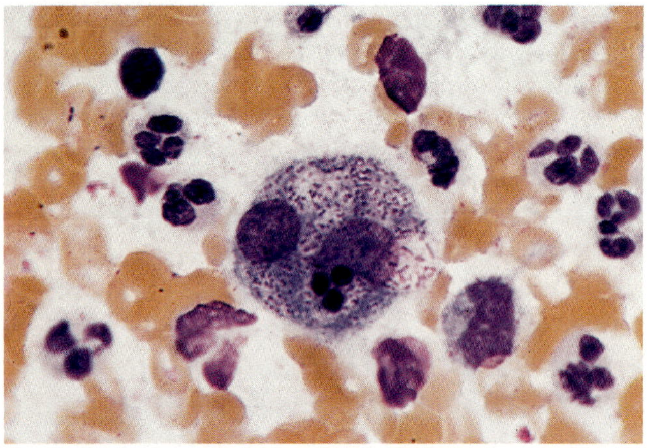

1.5 Wright-stained smear from a vulvar lesion in a patient with granuloma inguinale showing a histiocyte with intracytoplasmic Donovan bodies.

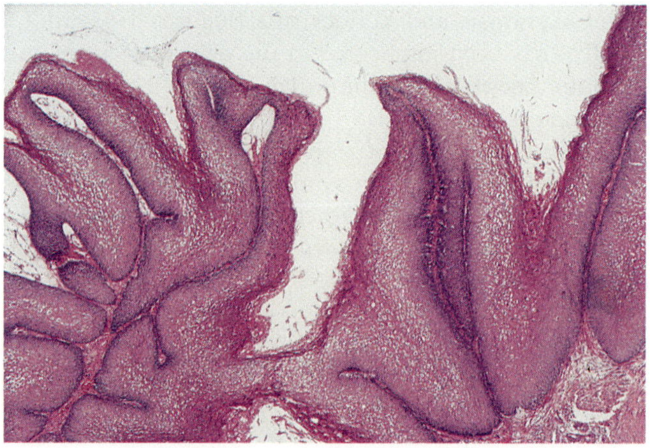

1.6 Low-power photograph of condyloma acuminatum revealing a papillary proliferation with a fibrovascular stalk.

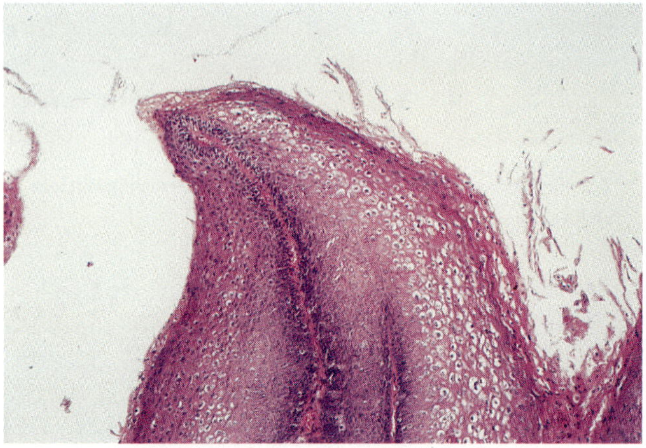

1.7 Higher-power view of condyloma acuminatum revealing koilocytotic atypia in the upper half of the epithelium.

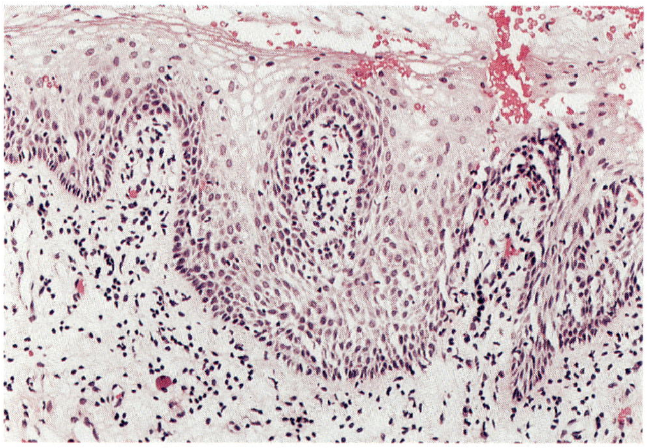

1.8 Biopsy from the vulva demonstrating a nonspecific chronic inflammatory infiltrate in a patient with vulvar vestibulitis.

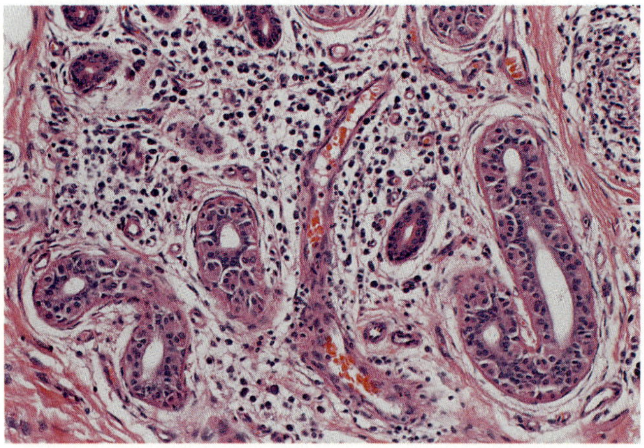

1.9 Hidradenitis suppurativa showing a chronic inflammatory infiltrate surrounding sweat glands.

SQUAMOUS LESIONS

Fibroepithelial polyps of the vulva[64,67] vary in size (Figure 1-10) and are lined with benign squamous epithelium. The stroma (Figure 1-11) contains a loose proliferation of fibroblasts and myofibroblasts. These lesions are sometimes confused with sarcoma botryoides. Keratinous epidermal inclusion cysts of the vulva are common. They are usually small and multiple but may form large cystic masses (Figure 1-12). The cyst wall is lined with benign squamous epithelium giving rise to the keratinous debris (Figures 1-13 and 1-14). Keratoacanthomas (Figure 1-15) form a cup-shaped invagination of squamous epithelium that may be difficult to distinguish from a well-differentiated squamous carcinoma. Keratoacanthomas are associated with a rapid clinical onset. Seborrheic keratosis (Figure 1-16) is a benign squamous epithelial proliferation that presents as a pigmented lesion.

The diagnosis and treatment of diseases of the vulva have undergone dramatic changes in the twentieth century.[93] The earliest terminology describing what is now referred to as vulvar dystrophies was based on the clinical appearance. The term "leukoplakia" (white plaque) was initially introduced in 1869 by Hulke in reference to oral lesions and in 1875 by Weir for vulvar lesions. Hallopeau, in 1887, described as "lichen planus atrophicus" what is now referred to as lichen sclerosus (Figure 1-17). The term "kraurosis vulvae" (brittle vulva) was introduced by Breiski in 1885.[77] In 1909, Berkeley and Bonney[14] described a condition known as "leukoplakic vulvitis" and associated it with kraurosis vulvae and carcinoma. In 1929, Taussig[86] also believed leukoplakia to be a premalignant condition. Lavery[55] and Lawrence[56] each provide excellent reviews of the historical perspectives of vulvar dystrophies. Kiryu and Ackerman[52] also critiqued the current classifications of vulvar diseases from a historical viewpoint.

Several attempts have been made to simplify the confusing array of clinical terms describing vulvar diseases.[35] The term "dystrophy" was introduced by Jeffcoate and Woodcock[47] in 1961. Jeffcoate replaced the term "chronic epithelial dystrophies" with "chronic vulvar dystrophies" in a subsequent article.[46] In 1976, the International Society for the Study of Vulvar Disease (ISSVD) adopted a new nomenclature for vulvar disease.[34] They recommended use of the terms "hyperplastic dystrophy" and "lichen sclerosus" and deletion of the terms "lichen sclerosus et atrophicus, leukoplakia, neurodermatitis, leukeratosis, Bowen's disease, erythroplasia of Queyrat, carcinoma simplex, leukoplakic vulvitis, hyperplastic vulvitis and kraurosis vulvae."

In 1983, the International Society of Gynecological Pathologists (ISGYP), under the direction of Dr. Robert Scully and in cooperation with the World Health Organization (WHO), developed nomenclature committees for histologic terminology in gynecologic pathology. Dr. Edward Wilkinson was named chairman of the committee on vulvar diseases. In 1986, the ISGYP committee recommended its classification to the ISSVD.[98,102] The ISSVD committee, under the direction of Dr. C. Marjorie Ridley, then adopted a new nomenclature (Table 1-2).[77,78] This included renaming hyperplastic dystrophy "squamous cell hyperplasia" and dropping the concept of a mixed dystrophy. The 1994 WHO terminology (see box on p. 19) uses the term "epithelial hyperplasia." This term is used only in the absence of epithelial atypia and when there is no significant inflammation (Figure 1-18). More specific dermatopathologic diagnoses should be used for lesions with inflammatory changes fulfilling other criteria.[60]

The classification of premalignant lesions of the vulva now follows the same terminology as that of the cervix. VIN has been introduced to replace the previous classification of atypia.[24,26,71,100] The lesions with atypia are called mild, moderate, or severe dysplasia or vulvar intraepithelial neoplasia (VIN I, II, or III). VIN III (Figure 1-19) encompasses severe dysplasia, carcinoma in situ, Bowen disease, and erythroplasia of Queyrat. The Bethesda System[28] for reporting cervical cytology introduced a new term, "squamous intraepithelial lesion" (SIL). Low-grade SIL combines HPV changes and CIN I. High-grade SIL combines CIN II and III.

TABLE 1-2 Nomenclature for Vulvar Disease International Society for the Study of Vulvar Disease, 1987[77]

NONNEOPLASTIC EPITHELIAL DISORDERS OF SKIN AND MUCOSA

1. Lichen sclerosis (lichen sclerosus et atrophicus)
2. Squamous cell hyperplasia (formerly hyperplastic dystrophy)
3. Other dermatoses

CLASSIFICATION OF VULVAR INTRAEPITHELIAL NEOPLASIA (VIN)

1. Squamous
   - VIN I Mild dysplasia (formerly mild atypia)
   - VIN II Moderate dysplasia (formerly moderate atypia)
   - VIN III Severe dysplasia (formerly severe atypia)
   - VIN III Carcinoma in situ
2. Nonsquamous
   - Paget disease (intraepithelial)
   - Melanoma in situ

Although the SIL terminology applies to cervical cytology, histologic extrapolation may follow.

VIN III may occur as either pigmented (Figure 1-20) or nonpigmented lesions, red lesions, or white lesions. These lesions may be multifocal[15,17] and have a history of preceding or concurrent condyloma acuminatum.[13] When HPV changes are associated with a VIN lesion, it is recommended that a phrase such as "with adjacent human papillomavirus changes" or "with adjacent condyloma acuminatum" be added. When only koilocytotic changes are seen without other diagnostic HPV changes, a phrase such as "with koilocytotic change" may be added. It is recommended that the term "bowenoid papulosis" not be used as a histopathologic term. Bowenoid papulosis is a clinical term that on biopsy shows the pathologic features of VIN.[51,68,91,95] A statement could be made such as "the pathologic findings are consistent with the clinical diagnosis of bowenoid papulosis." Some cases of VIN I (mild dysplasia) may be benign lesions related to viral infection. The presence or absence of skin appendage involvement should not alter the grading of the intraepithelial neoplasia.

Squamous cell carcinoma of the vulva[43,50,84,85] is the fourth most common female genital malignancy and accounts for approximately 5% of all gynecologic cancers. It is generally a disease of postmenopausal patients. Most of these tumors are squamous carcinoma. The staging of carcinoma of the vulva includes the size of the lesion as well as lymph node involvement and distant metastasis (see boxes on p. 20). A definition of microinvasive carcinoma of the vulva has not been established, but a proposal by the ISSVD is that superficially invasive carcinoma (stage Ia) represents 1 mm or less of invasion.* The measurement is taken from the epithelial stromal junction of the most superficial adjacent dermal papilla to the deepest point of invasion (Figures 1-21 to 1-23). The measurement from the most superficial level of the tumor to the deepest point of invasion is referred to as the "thickness of the tumor." It is recommended that the following information be included in the final pathology report: depth of invasion; tumor thickness; method of measurement; diameter of the invasive tumor; clinical measurement of the tumor diameter, when available; and the presence or absence of vascular space involvement by tumor. In difficult cases of questionable invasion, it is recommended that invasion *not* be diagnosed. Most squamous cell carcinomas of the vulva are keratinizing (Figures 1-24 and 1-25).

Verrucous carcinoma (Figures 1-26 to 1-29) is a highly differentiated variant of squamous carcinoma[23,44] that has a pushing margin at the base and rarely metastasizes. This term also replaces what was called the giant condyloma of Buschke and Löwenstein. It is important to distinguish this form of carcinoma from the more typical squamous carcinoma (Table 1-3). In cases in which squamous cell carcinoma is mixed with verrucous carcinoma, both diagnoses should be reported. Basal cell carcinomas (Figures 1-30 and 1-31) may arise on the vulva, but they rarely metastasize.[27,39,69] Verrucous carcinoma and basal carcinoma are usually treated by wide local excision without lymphadenectomy.

TABLE 1-3 Verrucous Carcinoma: Differential Diagnosis

Verrucous Carcinoma	Squamous Carcinoma
Pushing margin	Infiltrating margin
Rare keratin pearls	Keratin pearls
Minimal atypia	Moderate atypia

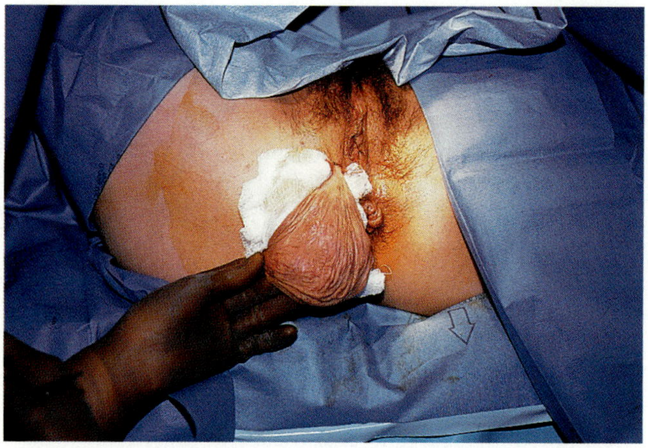

1.10 Patient with a large fibroepithelial polyp on a thin stalk.

*References 30, 42, 53, 97, 99, 103.

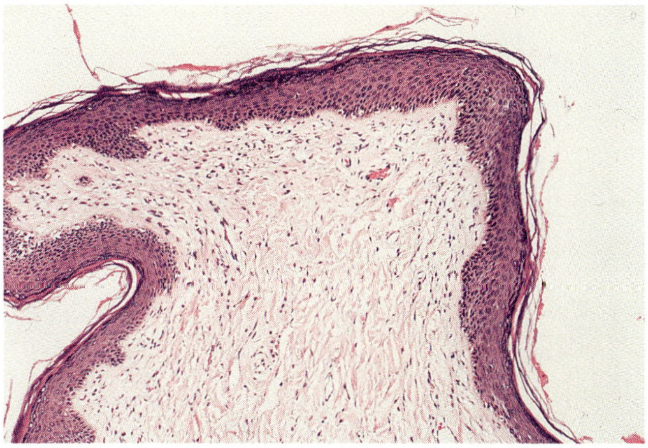

1.11 Photomicrograph of a fibroepithelial polyp showing bland squamous epithelium covering a loose fibrous stroma with scattered blood vessels.

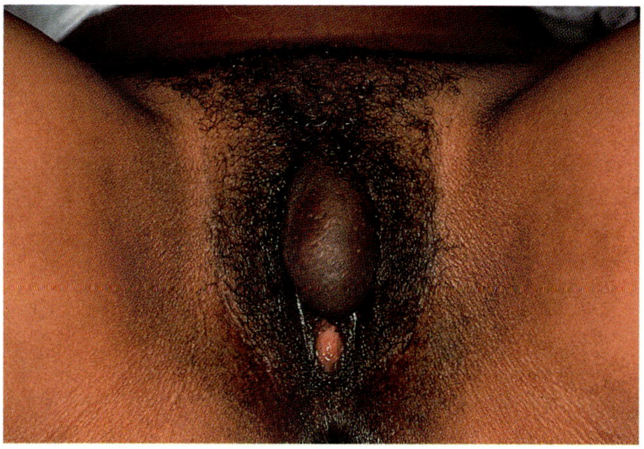

1.12 Large epidermal inclusion cyst of the vulva. (Courtesy Dr. Steven Bernstein.)

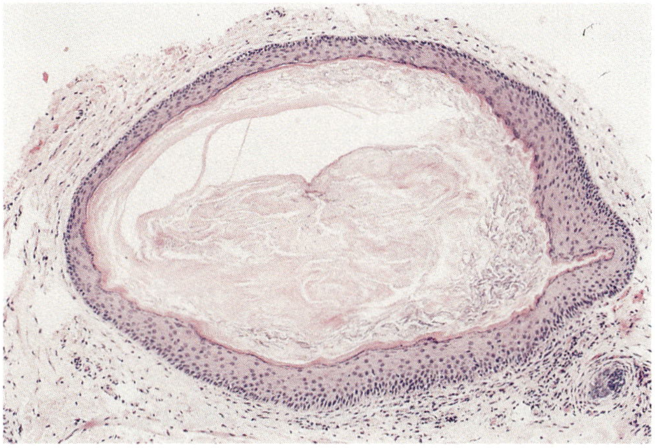

1.13 Low-power photomicrograph of an epidermal inclusion cyst containing an intact cyst lined with squamous epithelium and filled with keratinous debris.

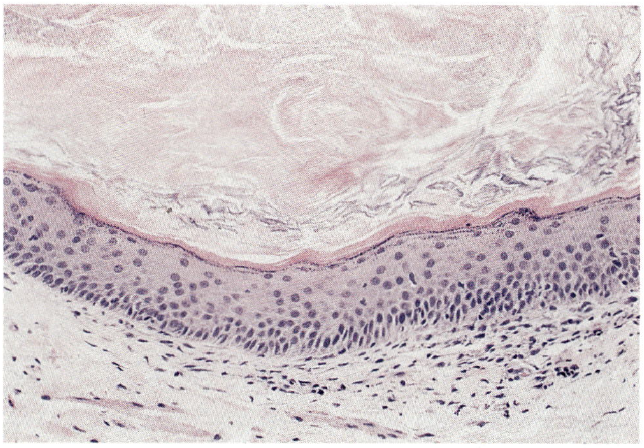

1.14 High-power view of an epidermal inclusion cyst revealing benign squamous epithelium with keratinous debris.

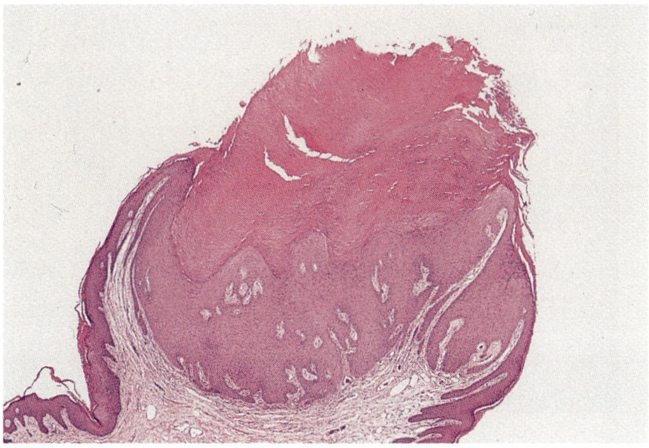

1.15 Keratoacanthoma revealing an invaginated cup-shaped squamous proliferation with hyperkeratosis.

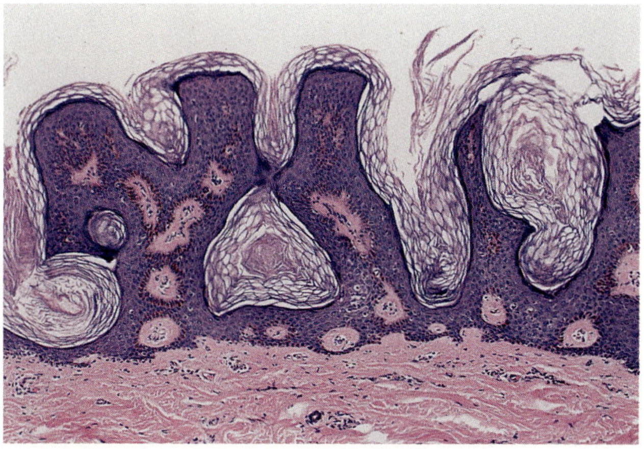

1.16 Seborrheic keratosis revealing epithelial hyperplasia with invaginated downward growth of the epithelium.

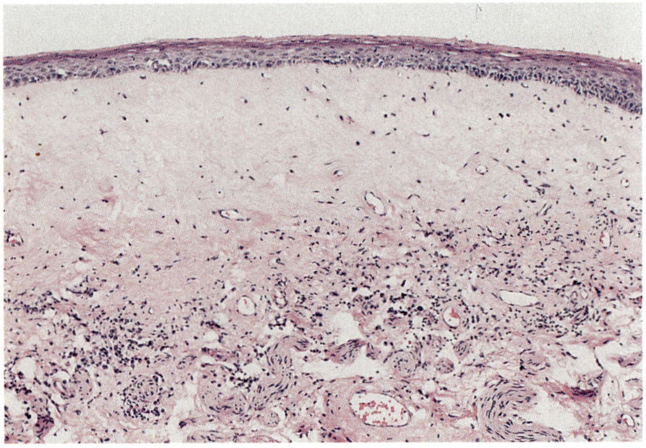

1.17 Lichen sclerosus revealing a characteristic thin epithelium with a subepithelial hypercellular zone beneath which is a band of scattered lymphocytes.

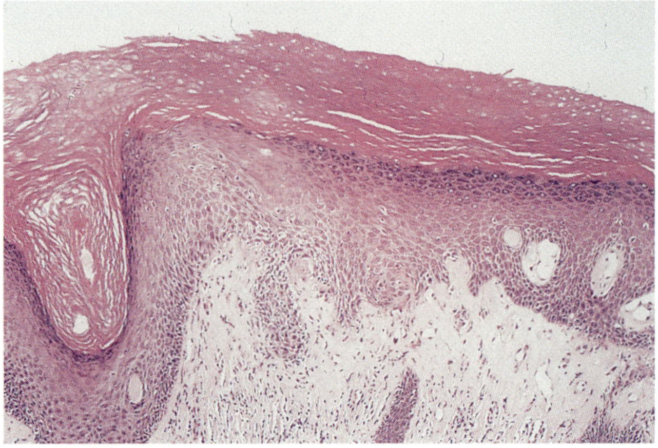

1.18 Epithelial hyperplasia with chronic inflammation (formerly hyperplastic dystrophy without atypia). The squamous epithelium shows increased thickness and hyperkeratosis without atypia.

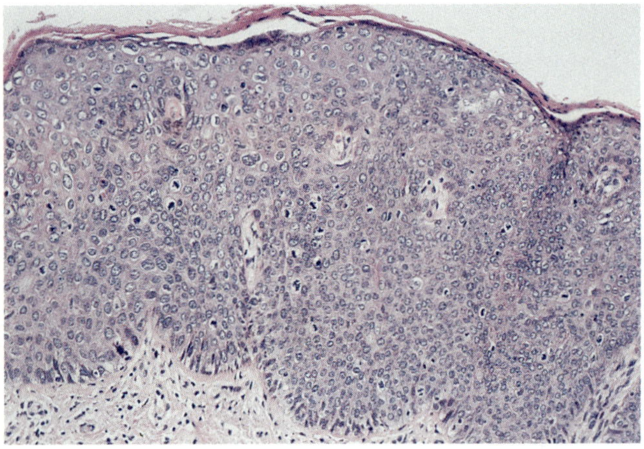

1.19 Squamous carcinoma in situ (VIN III) showing full-thickness atypia of the epithelium.

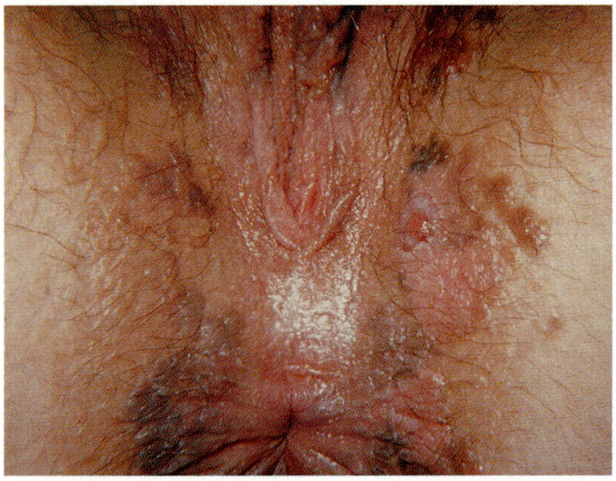

1.20 Patient with multifocal pigmented carcinoma in situ. (Courtesy Dr. Steven Bernstein.)

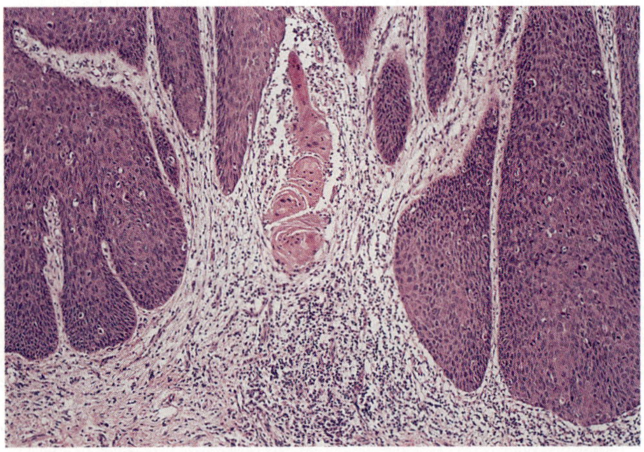

1.21 Low-power view of early stroma invasion. Notice that the adjacent squamous carcinoma in situ component is deeper in the stroma than in the invasive area.

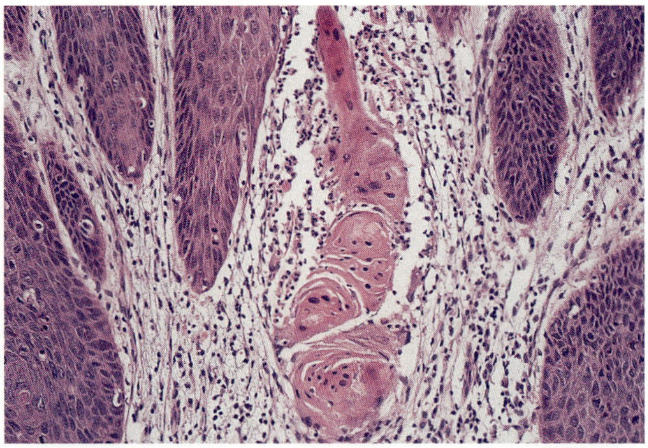

1.22 Early stromal invasion revealing increased eosinophilia in the invading cells.

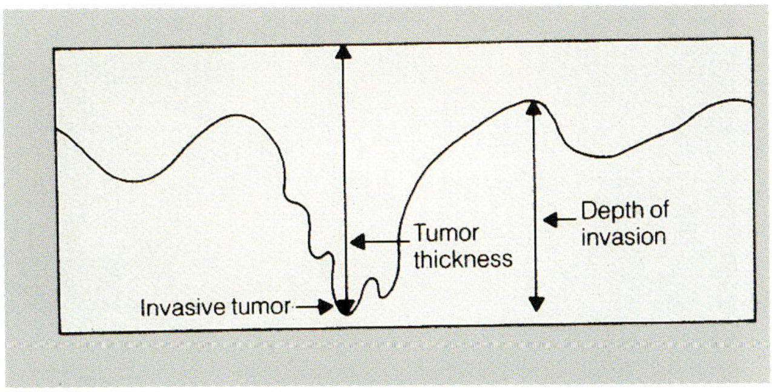

1.23 Diagram for the measurement of vulvar tumors. (From Scully RE, Bonfiglio TA, Kurman RJ, Silverberg SG, Wilkinson EJ: *World Health Organization. Histological classification of tumors of the female genital tract*, New York, 1994, Springer-Verlag, p 169, with permission.)

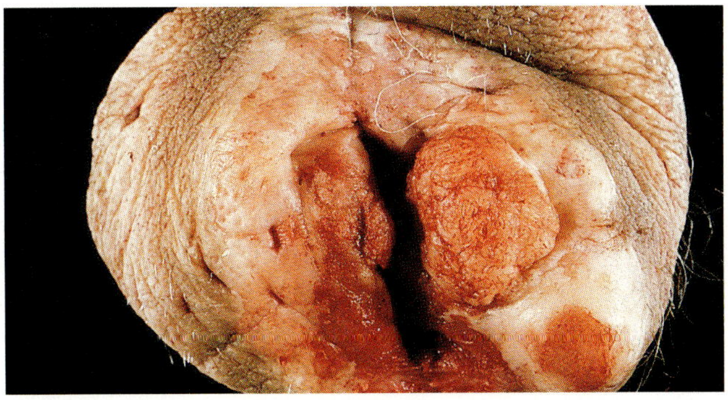

1.24 Radical vulvectomy specimen revealing invasive squamous cell carcinoma.

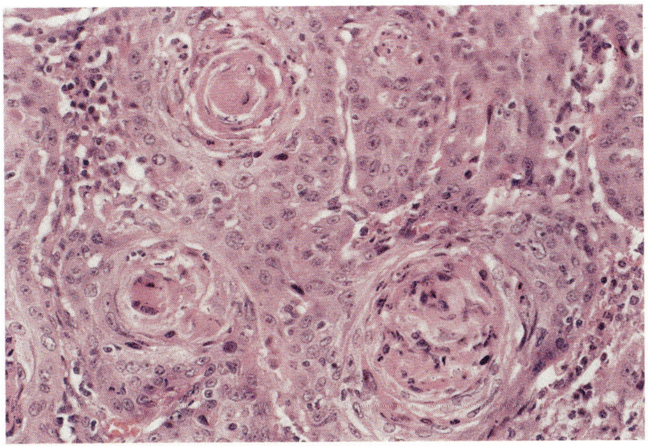

1.25 Moderately differentiated squamous cell carcinoma of the vulva with keratin pearls.

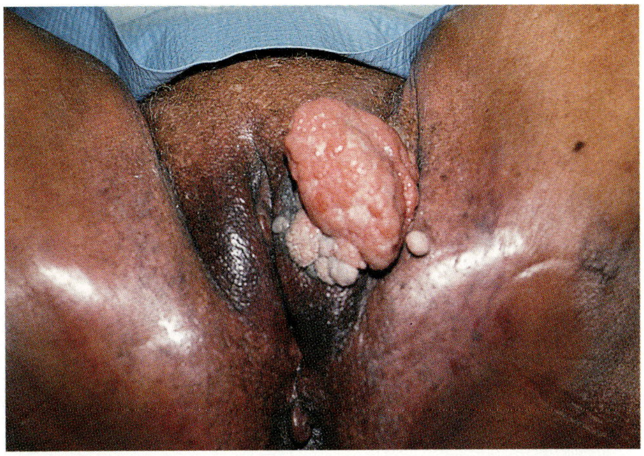

1.26 Patient with verrucous carcinoma of the vulva. (Courtesy Dr. Samuel Lifshitz.)

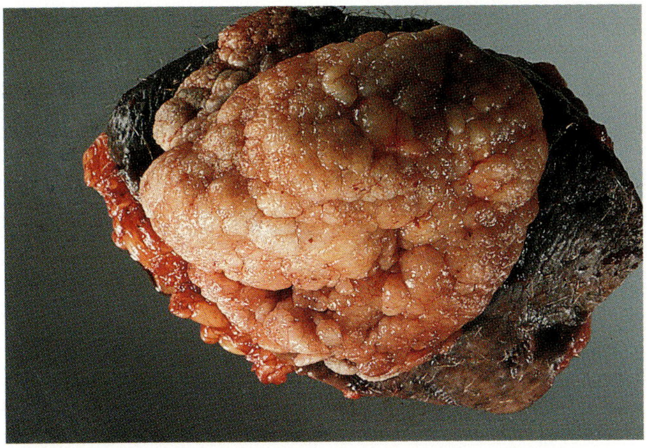

1.27 Wide excision of verrucous carcinoma of the vulva.

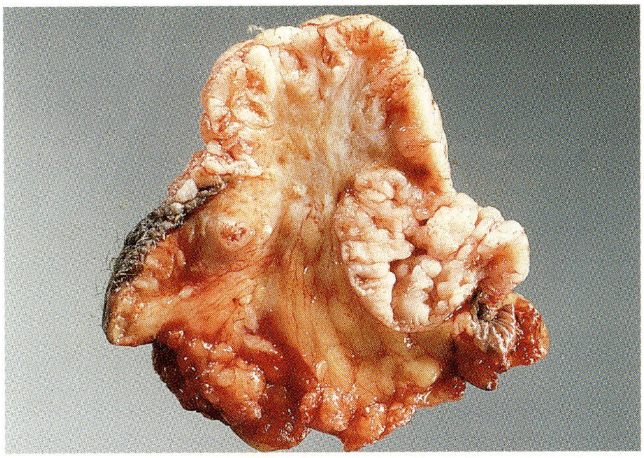

1.28 Cut surface of verrucous carcinoma revealing the pushing finger-like infiltration into the underlying stroma.

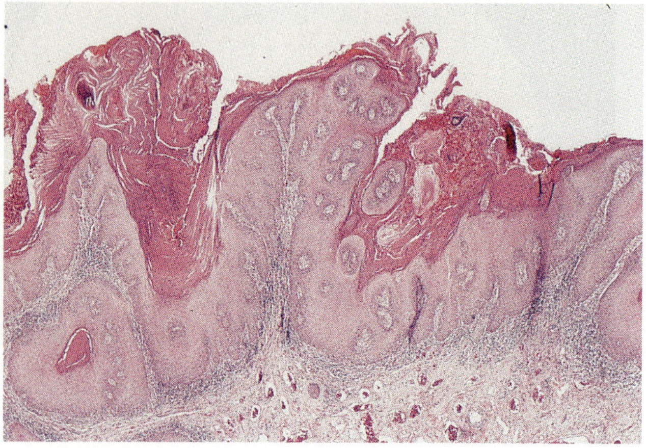

1.29 Photomicrograph of verrucous carcinoma revealing minimal atypia and a pushing margin at the epithelial stromal interface.

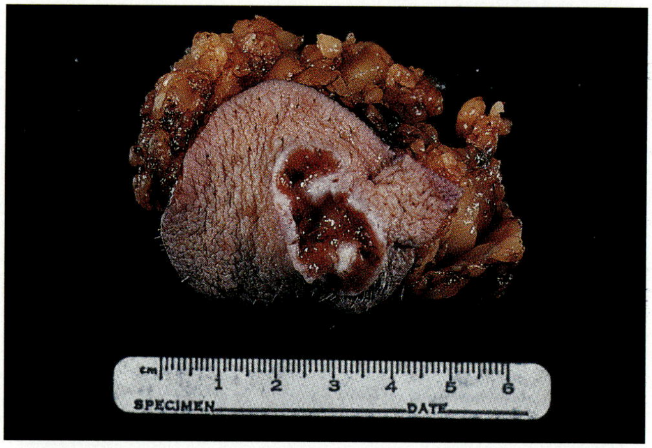

1.30 Wide excision of basal cell carcinoma showing central ulceration with a raised white rim around the ulcerated area.

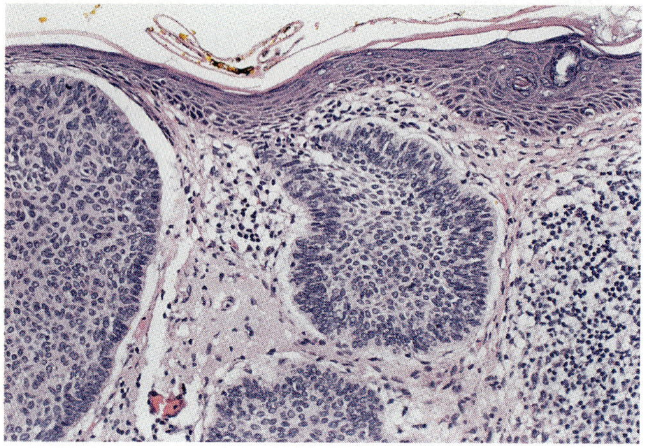

1.31 Photomicrograph of basal cell carcinoma revealing the characteristic peripheral palisading.

PIGMENTED LESIONS

Pigmentary disorders of the vulva can be categorized into hypopigmented and hyperpigmented lesions. The hypopigmented lesions include vitiligo, albinism, and postinflammatory depigmentation. Hyperpigmented lesions include freckles (ephelides), lentigo simplex (Figure 1-32), and nevi (Figure 1-33). Intraepithelial melanocytic neoplasia is lentigo maligna, or malignant melanoma in situ. This lesion occasionally needs to be differentiated from Paget disease, and immunoperoxidase stains for S-100 and HMB-45 are useful. Malignant melanoma of the vulva[12,18,45,48,70,74,81] (Figures 1-34 and 1-35) can occur on either the keratinizing epithelium (skin, labia majora) or nonkeratinizing mucous membranes (labia minora, urethra, vaginal introitus). The staging classification for malignant melanoma of the skin (see box on p. 21),[10] which includes Clark's levels, applies only to those lesions arising on the keratinizing epithelium of the vulva.

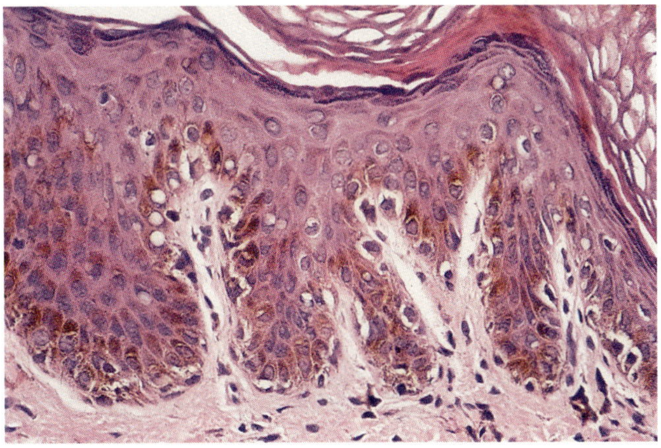

1.32 Lentigo simplex demonstrating melanocytic proliferation at the base.

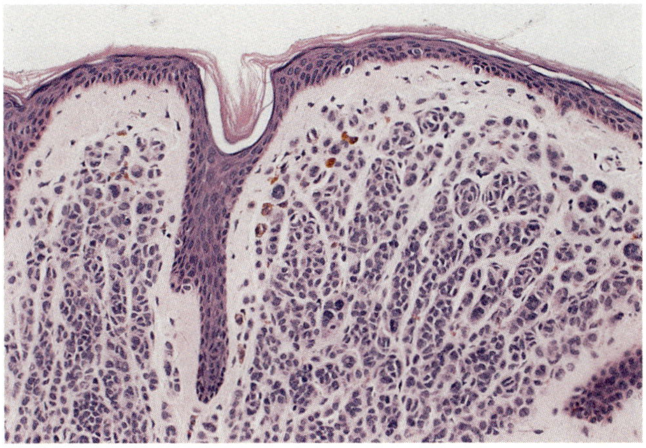

1.33 Intradermal nevus containing melanocytic cells in the dermis with scattered multinucleation.

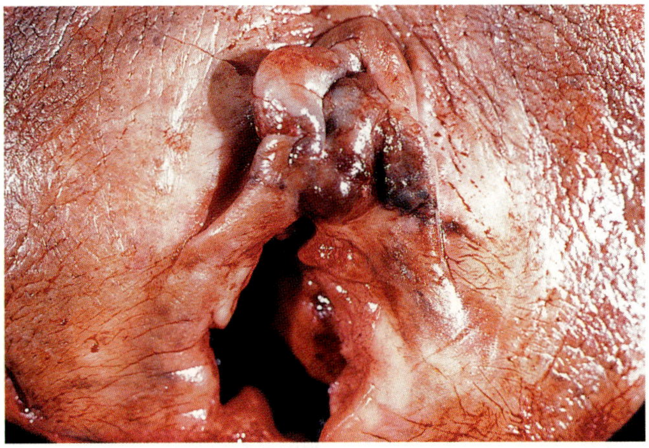

1.34 Wide excision of malignant melanoma of the vulva arising near the clitoris.

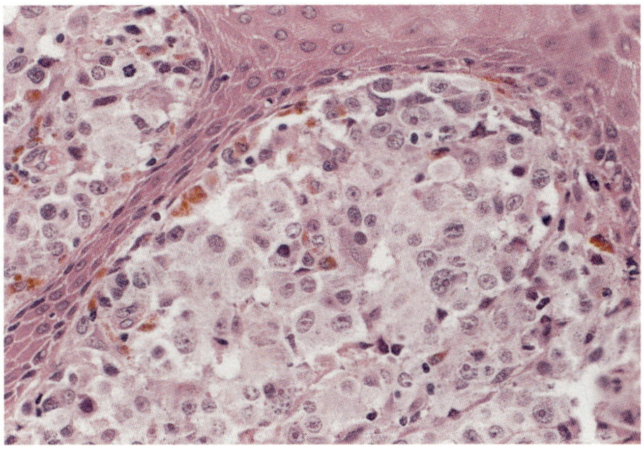

1.35 Photomicrograph of malignant melanoma showing large pale cells with pleomorphic nuclei beneath the overlying bland squamous epithelium.

GLANDULAR LESIONS

Mucinous cysts of the vulva[79] (Figure 1-36) arise in minor vestibular glands. Papillary hidradenoma (Figures 1-37 to 1-39) is a benign tumor arising in apocrine sweat glands.[105] Mammary glands and related tumors may occur on the vulva.[38,92]

Paget disease of the vulva[49,57,66] (Figures 1-40 to 1-42) is another form of intraepithelial carcinoma of the vulva. This is a rare intraepithelial proliferation of glandular cells, the origin of which is not clear. These lesions are usually not associated with an underlying adenocarcinoma, but a few case reports have been published. Paget disease of the vulva is difficult to treat, since the margins are difficult to evaluate clinically.

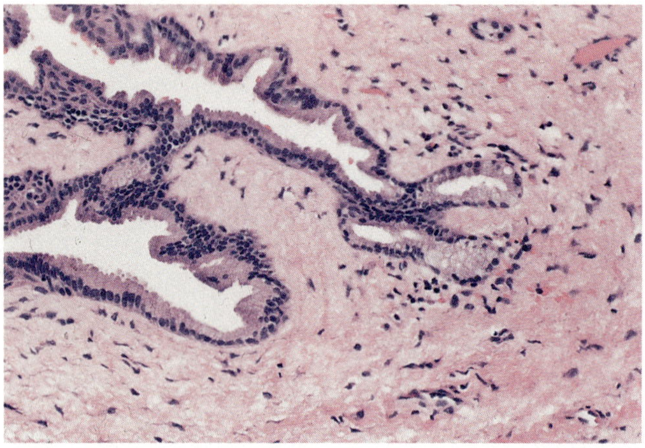

1.36 Mucinous cyst of the vulva arising in a minor vestibular gland.

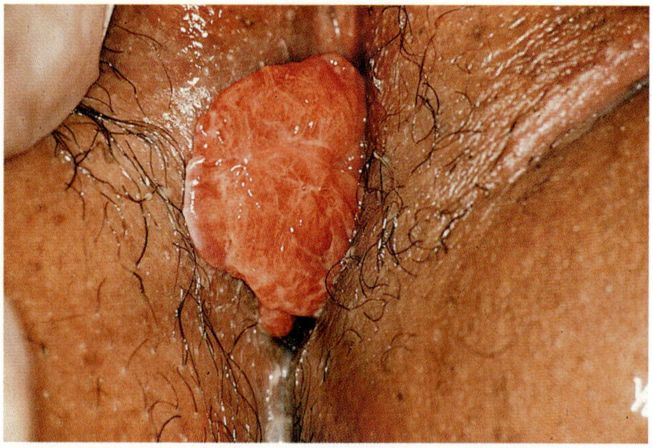

1.37 Patient with hidradenoma papilliferum showing a red polypoid nodule on the vulva. (Courtesy Dr. Jonathan Berek.)

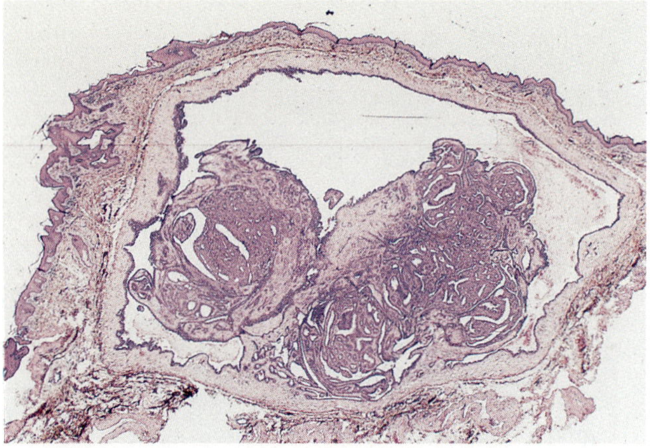

1.38 Low-power photomicrograph of papillary hidradenoma revealing a cystic space containing a complex papillary proliferation.

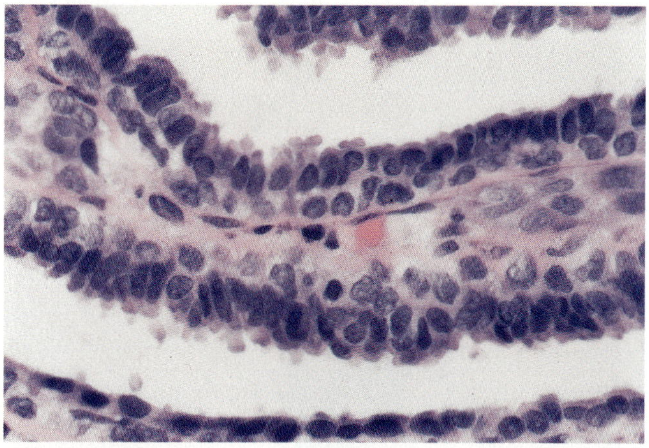

1.39 High-power view of papillary hidradenoma revealing a double cell layer with apocrine "snouts" on the cytoplasm.

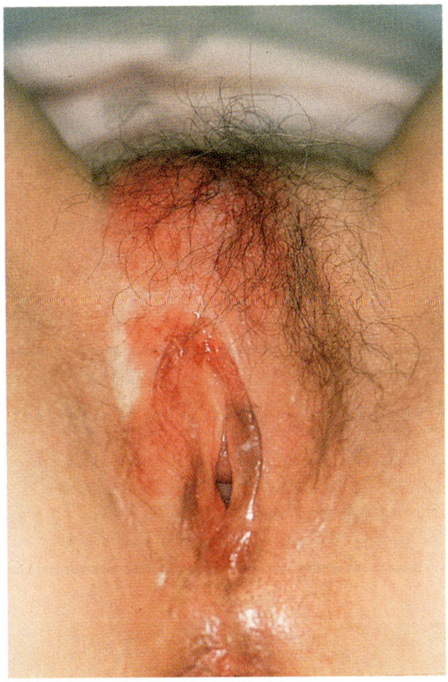

1.40 Patient with Paget disease of the vulva demonstrating red excoriated areas with involvement extending onto the mons pubis. (Courtesy Dr. Steven Bernstein.)

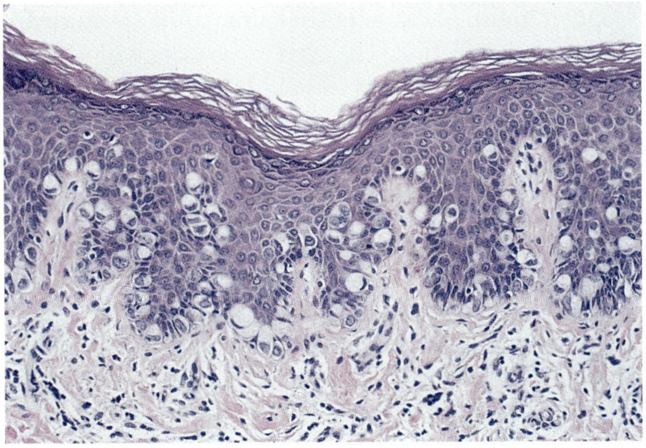

1.41 Low-power photomicrograph of Paget disease revealing the lack of invasion.

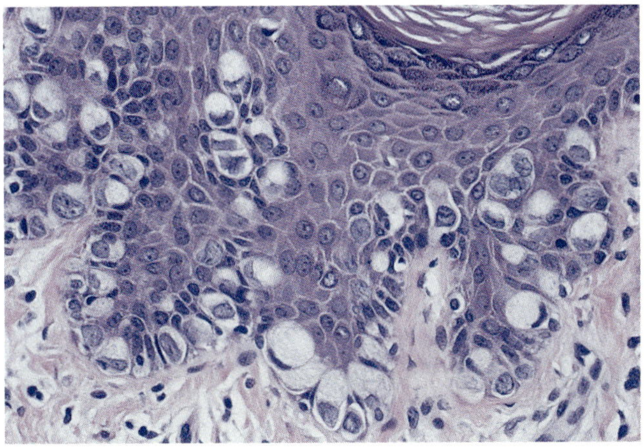

1.42 High-power view of Paget disease showing the two-cell population with the Paget cells extending upward in the epithelium.

BARTHOLIN GLAND

The Bartholin glands[31, 93] are homologous to the Cowper glands in the male. They are derived from the urogenital sinus, which forms a paired set of glands in the posterolateral aspect of the vestibule. Figure 1-43 illustrates the histologic pattern of the Bartholin gland with its various cell types. The acini are lined with an inner mucinous columnar epithelium. These smaller ducts empty into the main duct, which is lined with transitional epithelium until it reaches the most distal portion. At this point the duct merges with the squamous epithelium of the vagina and empties just outside the hymenal ring. The glands secrete a mucinous fluid in response to sexual stimulation, which lubricates the vagina.

Inflammatory disorders are common lesions of the Bartholin gland. A variety of organisms has been isolated, including aerobic and anaerobic bacteria, mycobacteria, fungi, parasites, *Chlamydia* organisms, and viruses. Most infections of the Bartholin gland culminate in an abscess. Abscesses often contain a mixed bacterial flora, with both aerobic and anaerobic bacteria recovered in culture. Although *Neisseria gonorrhoeae* may be responsible for the initial infection, it is usually not recovered from an abscess. Gram-negative rods and anaerobic organisms are more commonly found.

Cysts of the Bartholin gland are the result of an obstruction in the duct system with continued mucus production. The occlusion is usually in the main duct and is most likely a postinflammatory stricture from trauma or infection. The cysts are usually unilocular and may vary in size. The cyst wall can be lined with transitional epithelium, but squamous metaplasia often occurs (Figure 1-44), especially if there has been an inflammatory component. If the obstruction has occurred in the smaller ductule, the cyst may be lined with cuboidal or mucinous epithelium. Occasionally the inspissated mucus spills into the stroma and causes a fibrous reaction (Figure 1-45). These findings have been described as a solid adenoma, an adenofibroma, a hamartoma, and "mucocele-like changes."[32,33]

Malignant tumors of the Bartholin gland[22,58,96] are rare, accounting for 2% to 7% of all vulvar carcinomas and 0.001% of all female genital tract malignancies. Malignancy of the Bartholin gland was first reported by Klob in 1864, since when slightly over 200 cases have been reported in the world's literature. The criteria for the diagnosis of a primary malignancy of the Bartholin gland were originally described by Honan but were modified by Chamlian and Taylor[19] and are outlined in Table 1-4. The original criteria included intact overlying skin and a direct connection between benign and malignant elements. Most investigators believe that these requirements are too strict and eliminate many obvious Bartholin gland tumors. Malignant tumors of the Bartholin gland are more common in postmenopausal women. It is for this reason that all lesions in women in this age group, whether cystic or solid, should be excised.

Carcinoma is the most common form of malignancy of the Bartholin gland and is almost equally divided between squamous carcinoma and adenocarcinoma. Squamous carcinoma often occurs near the main duct (Figure 1-46) and may have adjacent squamous metaplasia (Figure 1-47). These tumors can be large cell keratinizing (Figure 1-48), nonkeratinizing, or small cell squamous carcinomas. Adenocarcinoma (Figures 1-49 and 1-50) is more likely to occur in the deeper glandular tissue. It is usually moderately differentiated and contains cytoplasmic mucin. Transitional cell carcinoma (Figure 1-51) has been rarely described but may occur more often than reported because it is difficult to distinguish from squamous carcinoma.

Adenoid cystic carcinoma[16] of the Bartholin gland (Figure 1-52) is rare but is the next most common cell type after squamous carcinoma and adenocarcinoma. This tumor has also been referred to as malignant cylindroma, adenomyoepithelioma, and pseudoadenomatous basal cell carcinoma. It is a malignant epithelial tumor that occurs most frequently in the salivary gland, but it has been described in the respiratory tract, breast, skin, and cervix. The histogenesis is uncertain, but it appears to have features of myoepithelium. The typical pattern has a cribriform structure (Figure 1-53) with acellular spaces containing redundant basal laminae. Adenoid cystic carcinoma tends to invade locally and may have prominent perineural invasion. The local infiltration can be deceptively extensive and most recurrences are local. Regional lymph node involvement is uncommon and a wide local excision has been recommended for this lesion.

TABLE 1-4 Criteria for a Primary Bartholin Gland Tumor

Appropriate vulvar site (± intact overlying skin)
Histologically compatible with Bartholin gland
Areas of apparent transition from normal to neoplastic elements
No other primary tumor

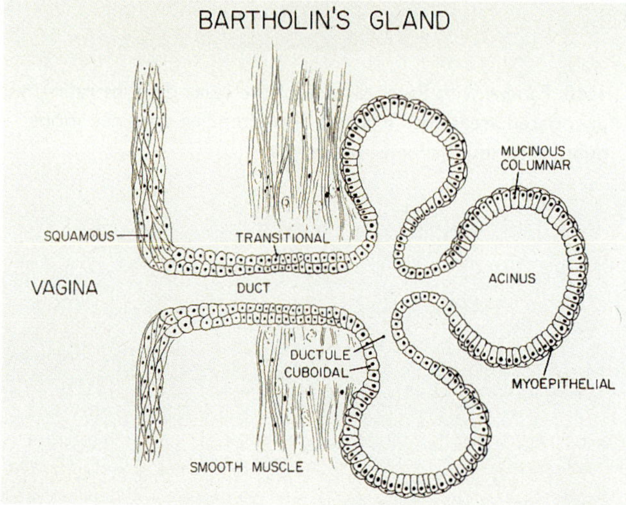

1.43 Diagram of the histologic components of the Bartholin gland. (From Bernstein SG, Voet RL, Lifshitz S, Buchsbaum HJ: Adenoid cystic carcinoma of Bartholin's gland, *Am J Obstet Gynecol* 147:385-390, 1983, with permission.)

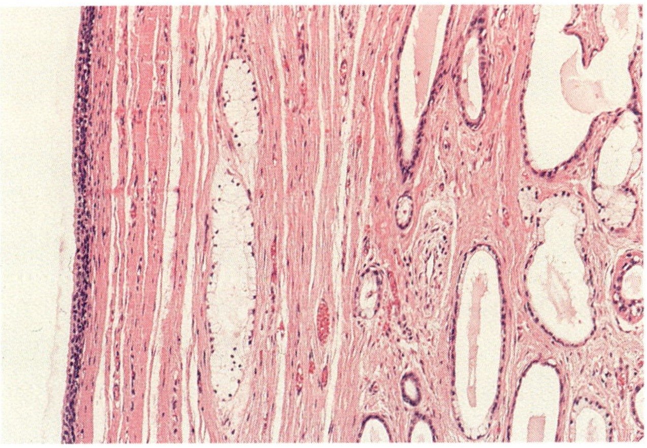

1.44 Bartholin gland cyst lined with bland squamous epithelium on the left and containing unremarkable mucinous glands.

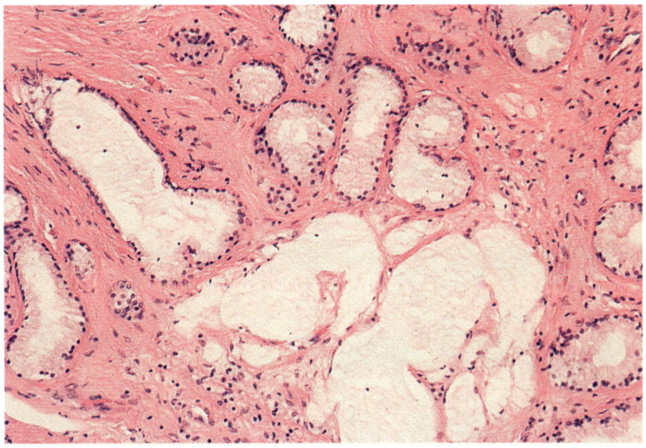

1.45 Inspissated mucin in a Bartholin gland forming mucocele-like changes.

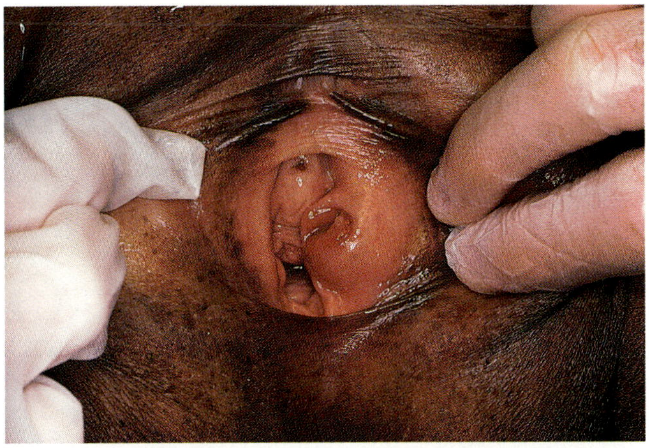

1.46 Patient with primary squamous cell carcinoma arising in the Bartholin gland. The duct is dilated with granulation tissue from a previous biopsy. The surrounding overlying skin is intact. (Courtesy Dr. Jonathan Berek.)

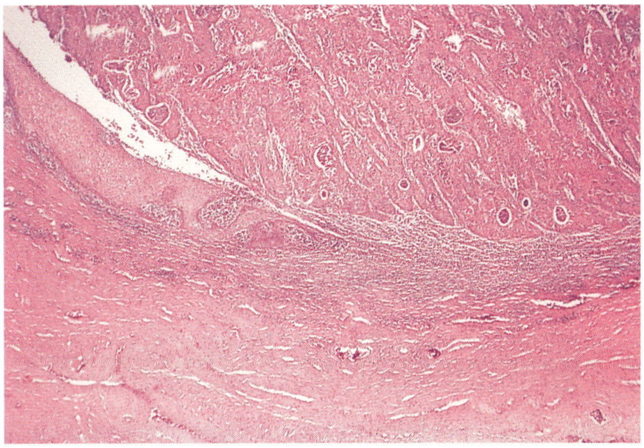

1.47 Low-power view of primary squamous cell carcinoma of the Bartholin gland with a transition to normal squamous epithelium.

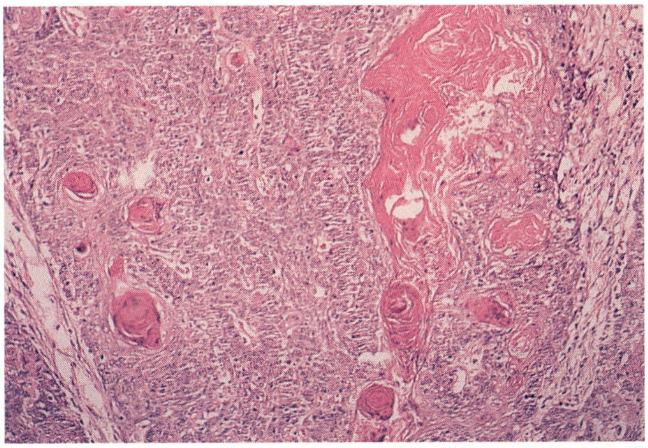

1.48 High-power view of squamous cell carcinoma showing a moderately differentiated tumor with keratinization.

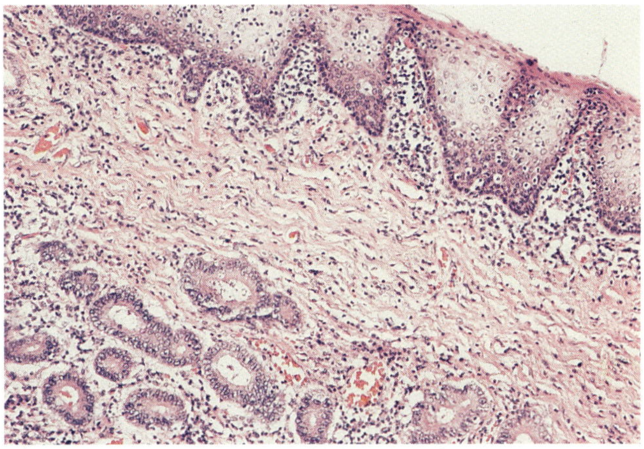

1.49 Low-power view of primary adenocarcinoma of the Bartholin gland with intact overlying squamous epithelium.

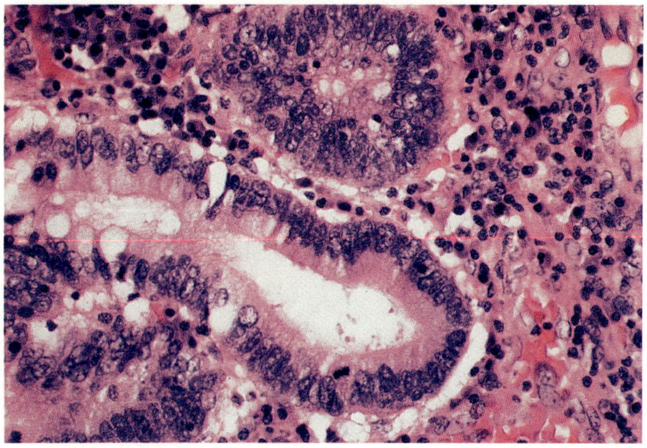

1.50 High-power view of adenocarcinoma of the Bartholin gland revealing a mucinous adenocarcinoma.

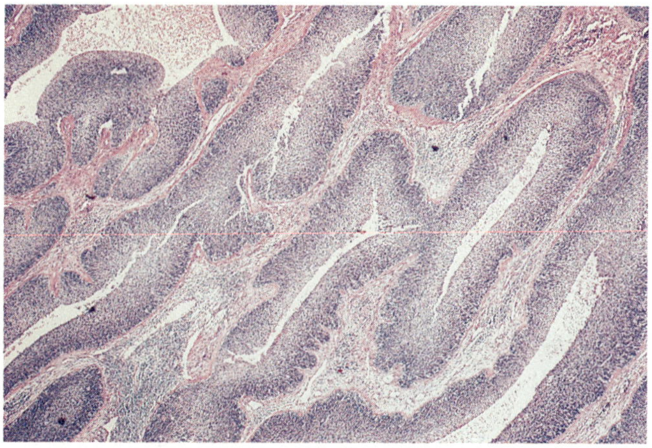

1.51 Primary transitional cell carcinoma of the Bartholin gland showing a pattern similar to that seen in the primary urothelial tumors.

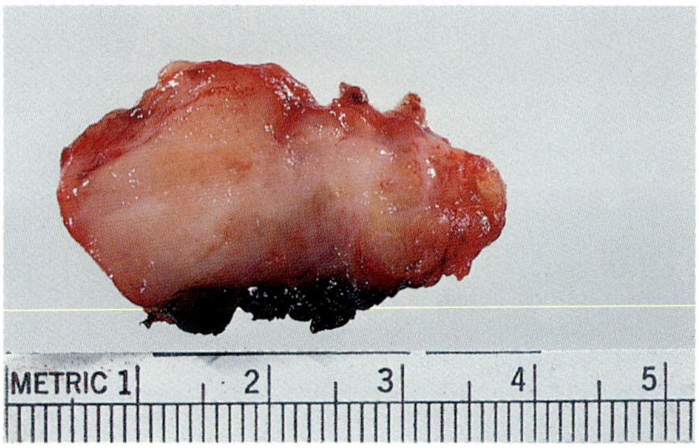

1.52 Gross view of primary adenoid cystic carcinoma of the Bartholin gland showing a solid tumor extending to the deep margin.

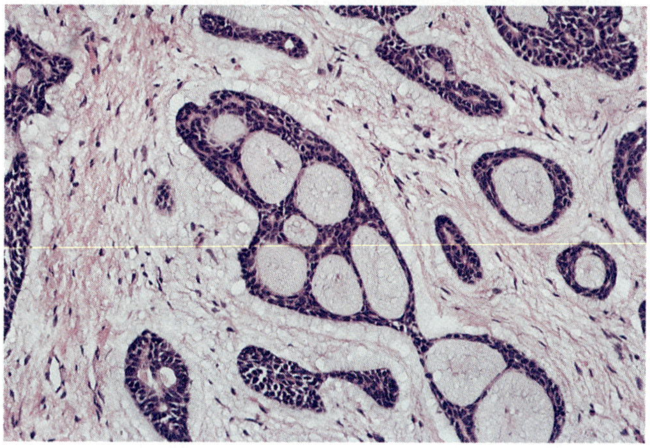

1.53 Photomicrograph of adenoid cystic carcinoma of the Bartholin gland revealing the typical cribriform pattern.

SOFT TISSUE LESIONS

A variety of benign and malignant[65] soft tissue tumors can occur in the vulva. The clinical behavior of smooth muscle tumors[87,88] of the vulva (Figures 1-54 and 1-55) is difficult to predict on histologic grounds alone. Tavassoli and Norris[87] identified three major features related to prognosis: (1) obvious aggressive behavior such as metastasis of infiltrating margins, (2) mitotic activity of greater than 5 mitoses per ten high-power fields, and (3) a size greater than 5 cm. If all three features are present, the lesion should be regarded as a leiomyosarcoma. If one or two features are present, the lesion is more likely to recur. Granular cell tumors (Figures 1-56 and 1-57) present as solid nodules and show the characteristic eosinophilic "granular" cytoplasm. They are thought to be derived from the Schwann cell. Aggressive angiomyxoma[11,41,82,83] (Figures 1-58 and 1-59) is a distinctive variant of myxoid tumors that occurs in the female pelvis. This tumor often recurs locally, since an adequate wide excision is difficult. Other soft tissue tumors that can be found in the vulva include hemangioma (Figures 1-60 and 1-61), pyogenic granuloma, and lipoma.

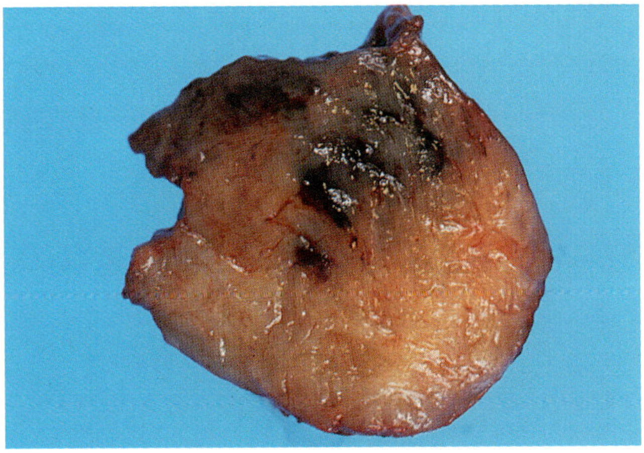

1.54 Primary arising leiomyoma of the vulva.

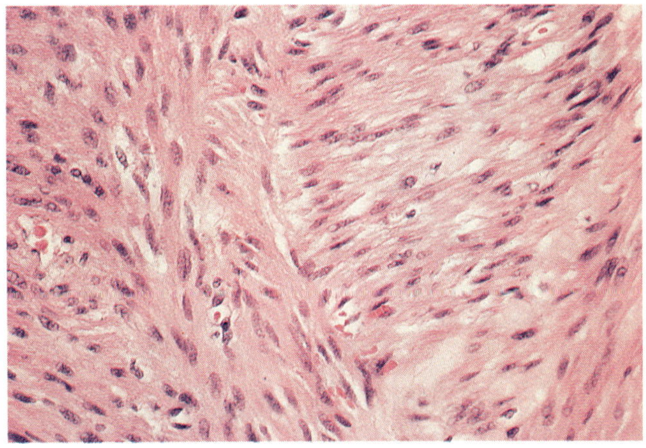

1.55 Photomicrograph of smooth muscle tumor showing a paucity of mitotic activity and minimal atypia.

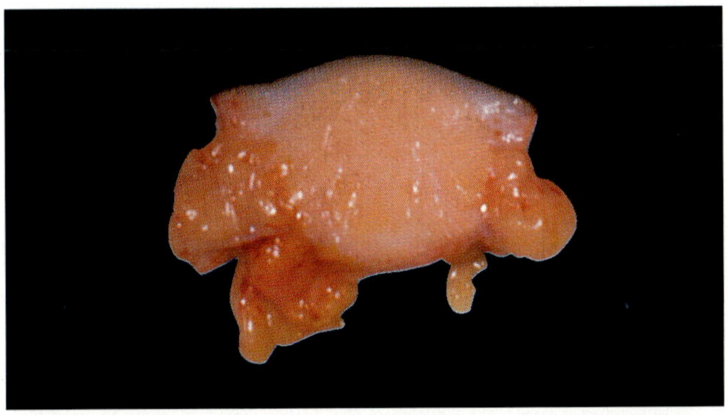

1.56 Gross photograph of the cut surface of a granular cell tumor of the vulva. The tumor is light tan and well circumscribed.

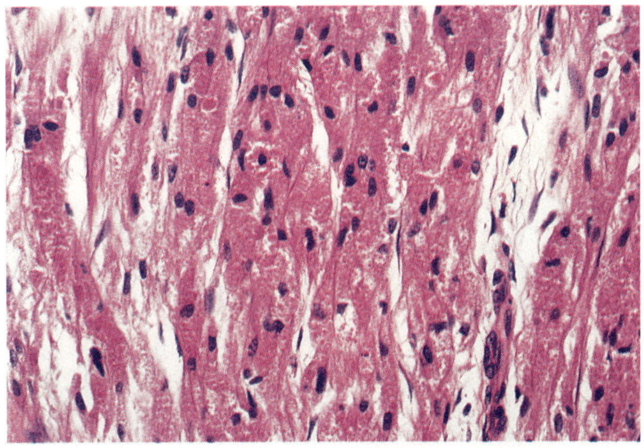

1.57 Photomicrograph of a granular cell tumor showing uniform small nuclei with eosinophilic granular cytoplasm.

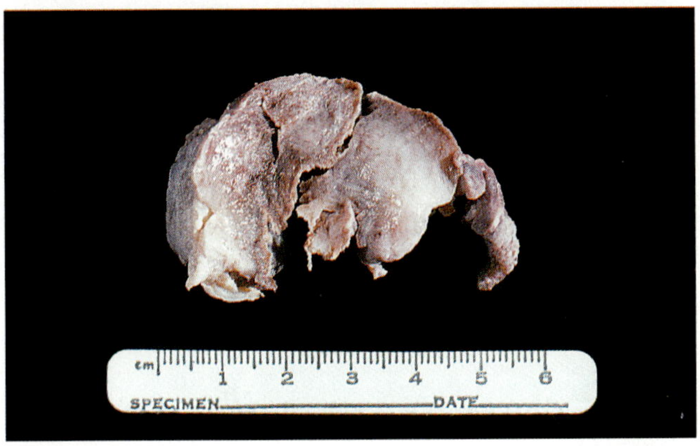

1.58 Gross view of aggressive angiomyxoma of the vulva. The tumor is soft and rubbery with ill-defined margins.

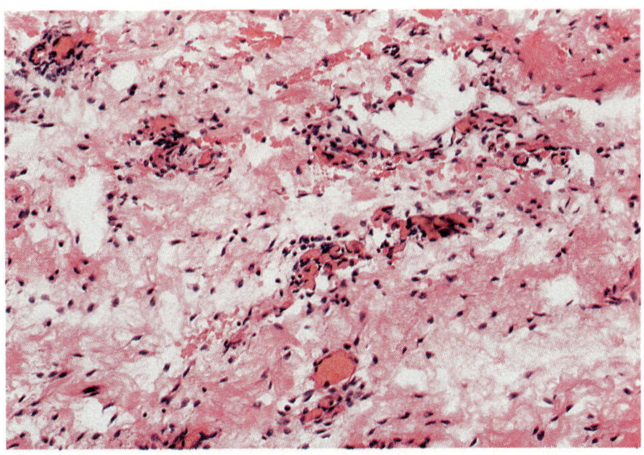

1.59 Photomicrograph of aggressive angiomyxoma demonstrating a loose myxoid stroma with marked vascular proliferation.

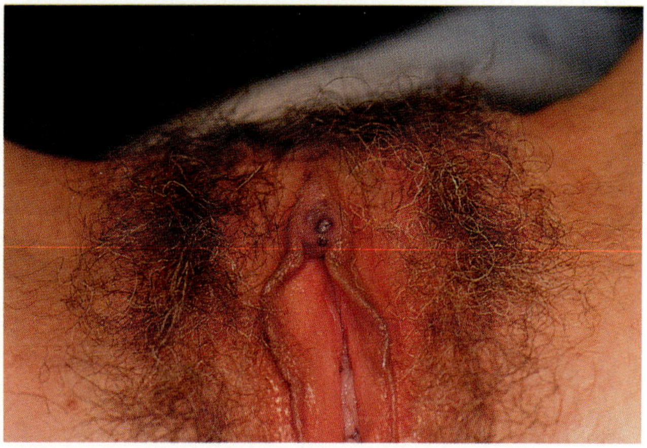

1.60 Patient with hemangioma of the clitoris. (Courtesy Dr. Steven Bernstein.)

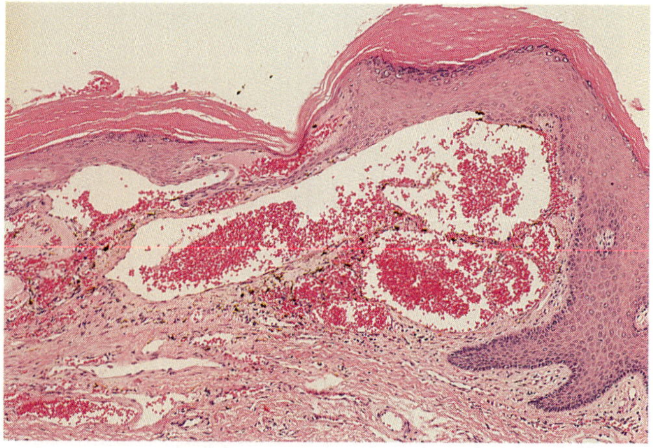

1.61 Photomicrograph of cavernous hemangioma revealing dilated vascular spaces filled with red blood cells.

MISCELLANEOUS LESIONS

Yolk sac carcinoma[29] (Figures 1-62 and 1-63) and other germ cell tumors occasionally arise in the vulva. Merkel cell carcinoma (Figure 1-64) is a skin tumor with neuroendocrine differentiation that may be seen in the vulva.[20]

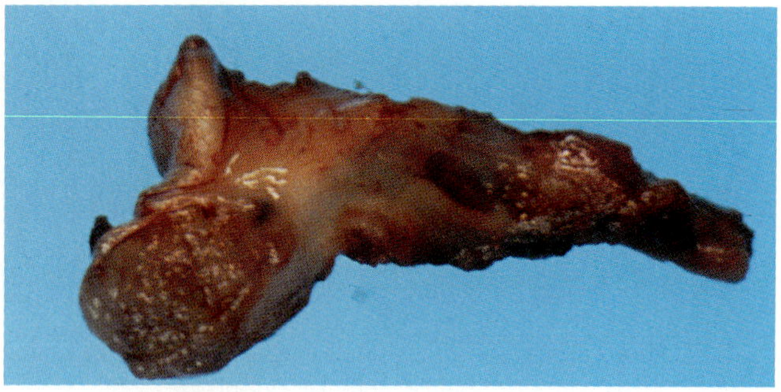

1.62 Primary endodermal sinus tumor arising in the clitoris of a 2-year-old infant.

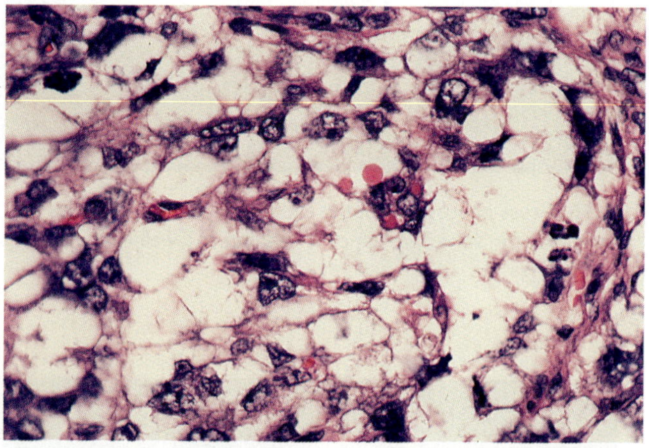

1.63 Endodermal sinus tumor showing marked nuclear pleomorphism and scattered hyaline droplets containing alpha-fetoprotein.

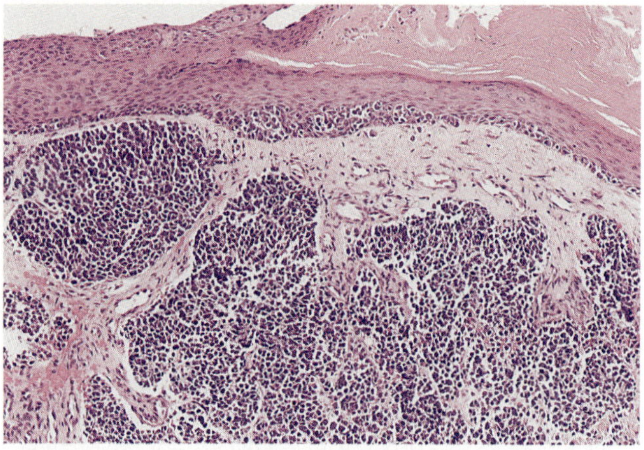

1.64 Merkel cell carcinoma showing an undifferentiated tumor with neuroendocrine differentiation.

World Health Organization (WHO) Histologic Classification of Tumors of the Vulva[5]

(with associated systematized nomenclature of medicine [SNOMED] codes)

I. Epithelial Tumors and Related Lesions	SNOMED
A. Squamous lesions	
1. Epithelial papillomas and polyps	
a. Vestibular squamous papilloma (vestibular papilloma)	80520
b. Fibroepithelial polyp	76810
3. Condyloma acuminatum	76760
4. Seborrheic keratosis	72750
5. Keratoacanthoma	72860
6. Squamous intraepithelial lesions (dysplasia–carcinoma in situ, vulvar intraepithelial neoplasia [VIN])	
a. Mild dysplasia (VIN I)	74006
b. Moderate dysplasia (VIN II)	74007
c. Severe dysplasia (VIN III)	74008
d. Carcinoma in situ (VIN III)	80702
7. Squamous cell carcinoma	80703
a. Keratinizing	80713
b. Nonkeratinizing	80723
c. Basaloid	
d. Verrucous	80513
e. Warty (condylomatous)	
f. Others	
8. Basal cell carcinoma	80903
B. Glandular lesions	
1. Papillary hidradenoma	84050
2. Clear cell hidradenoma	84020
3. Syringoma	84070
4. Trichoepithelioma	81000
5. Trichilemmoma	81020
6. Adenoma of minor vestibular glands	81400
7. Paget disease	85423
8. Bartholin gland carcinomas	
a. Adenocarcinoma	81403
b. Squamous cell carcinoma	80703
c. Adenoid cystic carcinoma	82003
d. Adenosquamous carcinoma	85603
e. Transitional cell carcinoma	81203
9. Tumors arising from ectopic breast tissue	
10. Carcinomas of sweat gland origin	
11. Adenocarcinomas of other types	
II. Soft Tissue Tumors	
A. Benign	
1. Lipoma and fibrolipoma	88500
2. Hemangiomas	91200
a. Capillary	91310
b. Cavernous	91210
c. Acquired	91200
3. Angiokeratoma	91410
4. Pyogenic granuloma	44440
5. Lymphangioma	91700
6. Fibroma	88100
7. Leiomyoma	88900
8. Granular cell tumor	95800
9. Neurofibroma	95400
10. Schwannoma (neurilemoma)	95600
11. Glomus tumor	87110
12. Benign fibrous histiocytoma	88320
13. Rhabdomyoma	89000
B. Malignant	
1. Embryonal rhabdomyosarcoma (sarcoma botryoides)	89103
2. Aggressive angiomyxoma	88411
3. Leiomyosarcoma	88903
4. Dermatofibrosarcoma protuberans	88323
5. Malignant fibrous histiocytoma	88303
6. Epithelioid sarcoma	88043
7. Malignant rhabdoid tumor	89633
8. Malignant nerve sheath tumors	95403
9. Angiosarcoma	91203
10. Kaposi sarcoma	91403
11. Hemangiopericytoma	91503
12. Liposarcoma	88503
13. Alveolar soft-part sarcoma	95813
III. Miscellaneous Tumors	
A. Melanocytic tumors	
1. Congenital melanocytic nevus	
2. Acquired melanocytic nevus	87200
3. Blue nevus	87800
4. Dysplastic melanocytic nevus	87270
5. Malignant melanoma	87203
B. Lymphoma and leukemia	95903
C. Yolk sac tumor (endodermal sinus tumor)	90713
D. Merkel cell tumor	82473
IV. Secondary Tumors	
V. Tumor-Like Lesions and Nonneoplastic Disorders	
A. Pseudoepitheliomatous hyperplasia	72090
B. Endometriosis	76500
C. Ectopic decidua	79510
D. Langerhans cell histiocytes (eosinophilic granuloma, histiocytosis X)	44050
E. Benign xanthogranuloma	44040
F. Verruciform xanthoma	
G. Desmoid tumor (fibromatosis)	88211
H. Sclerosing lipogranuloma	45690
I. Nodular fascitis	76130
J. Nevus lipomatosus superficialis	75760
K. Crohn disease	
L. Cysts	
1. Bartholin duct cyst	33400
2. Mucinous cyst	33790
3. Epidermal cyst	33410
4. Mesonephric cyst (wolffian duct cyst, Gartner duct cyst)	26370
5. Ciliated cyst	
6. Mesothelial cyst (cyst of the canal of Nuck)	33680
7. Periurethral cyst	33400
M. Other epithelial disorders	
1. Lichen sclerosus	58240
2. Squamous cell hyperplasia	72000
3. Other forms of dermatoses and dermatitis	

TNM Staging Classification of Vulvar Carcinoma

International Union against Cancer (UICC)

Primary Tumor (T)

- TX Primary tumor cannot be assessed
- T0 No evidence of primary tumor
- Tis Carcinoma in situ (preinvasive carcinoma)
- T1 Tumor confined to the vulva and/or perineum, 2 cm or less in greatest dimension
- T2 Tumor confined to the vulva and/or perineum, greater than 2 cm in greatest dimension
- T3 Tumor of any size with adjacent spread to the lower urethra and/or the vagina, or the anus, or invasion of the rectal wall or bladder wall (not mucosa)
- T4 Tumor of any size infiltrating the bladder mucosa and/or rectum mucosa including the upper part of the urethra mucosa and/or fixed to the bone.

Regional Lymph Nodes (N)

- NX Regional lymph nodes cannot be assessed
- N0 No regional lymph node metastasis
- N1 Unilateral regional lymph node netastasis
- N2 Bilateral regional lymph node metastasis

Distant Metastases (M)

- MX Presence of distant metastasis cannot be assessed
- M0 No distant metastases
- M1 Distant metastasis (including pelvic lymph node metastasis)

Grading (G)

1. Grading of the following tumors into well, moderately, and poorly differentiated categories, or grades 1, 2, and 3, is recommended: squamous cell carcinomas, adenocarcinomas, and transitional cell carcinomas.
2. Grading and mitotic activity may be of importance in some soft tissue sarcomas.

Stage Grouping of Vulvar Carcinoma

The International Federation of Gynecology and Obstetrics (FIGO)
International Union Against Cancer (UICC)
American Joint Committee on Cancer (AJCC)
International Society for the Study of Vulvar Disease (ISSVD)

STAGE	TNM	
Stage 0	Tis	Carcinoma in situ, intraepithelial carcinoma
Stage I	T1 N0 M0	Tumor confined to the vulva and/or perineum, 2 cm or less in greatest dimension. No nodal metastasis.
Stage IA*	T1 N0 M0	Solitary tumor ≤2 cm in diameter with a depth of invasion ≤1 mm (*microinvasion by ISSVD)
Stage II	T2 N0 M0	Tumor confined to the vulva and/or perineum, greater than 2 cm in great est dimension. No nodal metastasis.
Stage III		Tumor of any size with
	T3 N0 M0	1. Adjacent spread to the lower urethra and/or the vagina, or the anus, and/or
	T1 N1 M0	2. unilateral regional lymph node metastasis
	T2 N1 M0	
	T3 N1 M0	
Stage IVA		Tumor of any size with
	T4 any N M0	1. invasion of the upper urethra, bladder mucosa, rectal mucosa, pelvic bone, and/or
	T1 N2 M0	2. bilateral regional node metastasis
	T2 N2 M0	
	T3 N2 M0	
Stage IVB	Any T, any N, M1	Any distant metastasis including pelvic lymph nodes

TNM Staging Classification of Malignant Melanoma

International Union Against Cancer (UICC)

Primary Tumor (T)

- TX Primary tumor cannot be assessed
- T0 No evidence of primary tumor
- Tis Carcinoma in situ (Clark level I) (atypical melanocytic hyperplasia, severe melanocytic dysplasia, not an invasive malignant lesion)
- T1 Tumor 0.75 mm or less in thickness and invading the papillary dermis (Clark level II)
- T2 Tumor more than 0.75 mm but not more than 1.5 mm in thickness and/or invading the papillary-reticular dermal interface (Clark level III)
- T3 Tumor more than 1.5 mm but not more than 4.0 mm in thickness and/or invading the reticular dermis (Clark level IV)
  - T3a Tumor more than 1.5 mm but not more than 3.0 mm in thickness
  - T3b Tumor more than 3.0 mm but not more than 4.0 mm in thickness
- T4 Tumor more than 4.0 mm in thickness and/or invading subcutaneous tissue (Clark level V) and/or satellite(s) within 2 cm of the primary tumor
  - T4a Tumor more than 4.0 mm in thickness and/or invading subcutaneous tissue
  - T4b Satellite(s) within 2 cm of the primary tumor

Note: In case of discrepancy between tumor thickness and level, the T category is based on the less favorable finding.

Regional Lymph Nodes (N)

- NX Regional lymph nodes cannot be assessed
- N0 No lymph node metastasis
- N1 Metastasis 3 cm or less in greatest dimension in any regional lymph node(s)
- N2 Metastasis more than 3 cm in greatest dimension in any regional lymph node(s) and/or in-transit metastasis
  - N2a Metastasis more than 3 cm in greatest dimension in any regional lymph node(s)
  - N2b In-transit metastasis
  - N2c Both

Note: In-transit metastasis involves skin or subcutaneous tissue more than 2 cm from the primary tumor but not beyond the regional lymph node(s).

Distant Metastases (M)

- MX Presence of distant metastasis cannot be assessed
- M0 No clinical metastases
- M1 Distant metastasis
  - M1a Metastasis in skin or subcutaneous tissue or lymph node(s) beyond the regional lymph nodes
  - M1b Visceral metastasis

BIBLIOGRAPHY

General Reading

1. Friedrich E: *Vulvar disease*, ed 2, Philadelphia, 1983, WB Saunders.
2. Fu Y, Reagan J: *Pathology of the uterine cervix, vagina, and vulva*, Philadelphia, 1989, WB Saunders.
3. Kaufman RH, Faro S: *Benign diseases of the vulva and vagina*, ed 4, St. Louis, 1994, Mosby-Year Book.
4. Kurman RJ, Norris HJ, Wilkinson EJ: *Tumors of the cervix, vagina, and vulva. Atlas of tumor pathology*, 3rd series, fascicle 4, Washington, DC, 1992, Armed Forces Institute of Pathology.
5. Scully RE, Bonfiglio TA, Kurman RJ, Silverberg SG, Wilkinson EJ: *World Health Organization. Histological classification of tumors of the female genital tract*, New York, 1994, Springer-Verlag.
6. Wilkinson EJ, editor: *Pathology of the vulva and vagina*, New York, 1987, Churchill Livingstone.
7. Wilkinson EJ: *Benign diseases of the vulva*. In Kurman RJ, editor: *Blaustein's pathology of the female genital tract*, ed 4, New York, 1994, Springer-Verlag.
8. Woodruff JD, Angtuaco TL, Parmley TH: *Atlas of gynecologic pathology*, ed 2, New York, 1993, Raven Press.

References

9. Bazin S, Bouchard C, Brisson J, Morin C, Meisels A, Fortier M: Vulvar vestibulitis syndrome: an exploratory case-control study, *Obstet Gynecol* 83:47-50, 1994.
10. Bears OH, Henson DE, Hutter RVP, Kennedy BJ, editors: *AJCC manual for staging of cancer*, ed 4, Philadelphia, 1992, JB Lippincott.
11. Bégin LR, Clement PB, Kirk ME, Jothy S, McCaughey WTE, Ferenczy A: Aggressive angiomyxoma of pelvic soft parts: a clinicopathologic study of nine cases, *Hum Pathol* 16:621-628, 1985.
12. Benda JA, Platz CE, Anderson B: Malignant melanoma of the vulva: a clinical-pathologic review of 16 cases, *Int J Gynecol Pathol* 5:202-216, 1986.
13. Bergeron C, Naghashfar Z, Canaan C, Shah K, Fu Y, Ferenczy A: Human papillomavirus type 16 in intraepithelial neoplasia (bowenoid papulosis) and coexistent invasive carcinoma of the vulva, *Int J Gynecol Pathol* 6:1-11, 1987.
14. Berkeley CP, Bonney V: Leukoplakic vulvitis and its relation to kraurosis vulvae and carcinoma vulvae, *Br Med J* 2:1739-1745, 1909.
15. Bernstein SG, Kovacs BR, Townsend DE, Morrow CP: Vulvar carcinoma in situ, *Obstet Gynecol* 61:304-307, 1983.
16. Bernstein SG, Voet RL, Lifshitz S, Buchsbaum HJ: Adenoid cystic carcinoma of Bartholin's gland, *Am J Obstet Gynecol* 147:385-390, 1983.
17. Bornstein J, Kaufman RH, Adam E, Adler-Storthz K: Multicentric intraepithelial neoplasia involving the vulva, *Cancer* 62:1601-1604, 1988.
18. Bradgate MG, Rollason TP, McConkey CC, Powell J: Malignant melanoma of the vulva: a clinico-pathological study of 50 women, *Br J Obstet Gynaecol* 97:124-133, 1990.
19. Chamlian DL, Taylor HB: Primary carcinoma of Bartholin's gland: a report of 24 patients, *Obstet Gynecol* 39:489-494, 1972
20. Chen KTK: Merkel's cell (neuroendocrine) carcinoma of the vulva, *Cancer* 73:2186-2191, 1994.
21. Cone R, Beckmann A, Aho M, Wahlstrom T, Ek M, Corey L, Paavonen J: Subclinical manifestations of vulvar human papillomavirus infection, *Int J Gynecol Pathol* 10:26-35, 1991.
22. Copeland LJ, Sneige N, Gershenson DM, McGuffee VB, Abdul-Karim, F, Rutledge FN: Bartholin gland carcinoma, *Obstet Gynecol* 67:794-801, 1986.
23. Crowther ME, Lowe DG, Shepherd JH: Verrucous carcinoma of the female genital tract: a review, *Obstet Gynecol Surv* 43:263-280, 1988.
24. Crum CP: Vulvar intraepithelial neoplasia: the concept and its application, *Hum Pathol* 13:187-190, 1982.
25. Crum CP: Genital papillomaviruses and related neoplasms: causation, diagnosis and classification (Bethesda), *Mod Pathol* 7:138-145, 1994.
26. Crum CP, Liskow A, Petras P, Keng WC, Frick HC II: Vulvar intraepithelial neoplasia (severe atypia and carcinoma in situ). A clinicopathologic analysis of 41 cases, *Cancer* 54:1429-1434, 1984.
27. Cruz-Jimenez PR, Abell MR: Cutaneous basal cell carcinoma of vulva, *Cancer* 36:1860-1868, 1975.
28. Current Issues: The Bethesda System for reporting cervical/vaginal cytological diagnoses, *Diagn Cytopathol* 9:235-246, 1993.
29. Dudley AG, Young RH, Lawrence WD, Scully RE: Endodermal sinus tumor of the vulva in an infant, *Obstet Gynecol* 61:76S-79S, 1983.
30. Dvoretsky PM, Bonfiglio TA, Helm Kamp BF, Ramsey G, Chuang C, Beecham JB: The pathology of superficially invasive, thin vulvar squamous cell carcinoma, *Int J Gynecol Pathol* 3:331-342, 1984.
31. Editorial: The House of Bartholinus, *JAMA* 179:454-455, 1962

32. Foushee JHS, Reeves WJ, McCool JA: Benign masses of Bartholin's gland: solid adenomas, adenomas with cyst, and Bartholin's gland with varices and thrombosis or cavernous hemangioma, *Obstet Gynecol* 31:695-701, 1968.
33. Freedman SR, Goldman RL: Mucocele-like changes in Bartholin's glands, *Hum Pathol* 9:111-114, 1978.
34. Friedrich EG Jr: New nomenclature for vulvar disease, *Obstet Gynecol* 47:122-124, 1976.
35. Friedrich EG Jr: Vulvar dystrophy, *Clin Obstet Gynecol* 28:178-187, 1985.
36. Friedrich EG: Vulvar vestibulitis syndrome, *J Reprod Med* 32:110-114, 1987.
37. Furlonge CB, Thin RN, Evans BE, McKee PH: Vulvar vestibulitis syndrome: a clinicopathological study, *Br J Obstet Gynaecol* 98:703-706, 1991.
38. Garcia JJ, Verkauf BS, Hochberg CJ, Ingram JM: Aberrant breast tissue of the vulva, *Obstet Gynecol* 52:225-228, 1978.
39. Gleeson NC, Ruffolo EH, Hoffman MS, Cavanagh D: Basal cell carcinoma with groin node metastasis, *Gynecol Oncol* 53:366-368, 1994.
40. Gupta J, Pilotti S, Shah KV, De Palo G, Rilke F: Human papillomavirus-associated early vulvar neoplasia investigated by in situ hybridization, *Am J Surg Pathol* 11:430-434, 1987.
41. Hilgers RD, Pai R, Bartow SA, Aisenbrey G, Bowling MC: Aggressive angiomyxoma of the vulva, *Obstet Gynecol* 68:60S-62S, 1986.
42. Hoffman JS, Kumar NB, Morley GW: Microinvasive squamous carcinoma of the vulva: search for a definition, *Obstet Gynecol* 61:625-618, 1983.
43. Homesley HD: Lymph node findings and outcome in squamous cell carcinoma of the vulva, *Cancer* 74:2399-2402, 1994.
44. Japaze H, Dinh TV, Woodruff JD: Verrucous carcinoma of the vulva: study of 24 cases, *Obstet Gynecol* 60:462-466, 1982.
45. Jaramillo BA, Ganjei P, Averette HE, Sevin B, Lovecchio JL: Malignant melanoma of the vulva, *Obstet Gynecol* 66:398-401, 1985.
46. Jeffcoate TNA: Chronic vulvar dystrophies, *Am J Obstet Gynecol* 95:61-74, 1966.
47. Jeffcoate TNA, Woodcock AS: Premalignant conditions of the vulva with particular reference to chronic epithelial dystrophies, *Br Med J* 2:127-134, 1961.
48. Johnson TL, Kumar NB, White CD, Morley GW: Prognostic features of vulvar melanoma: a clinicopathologic analysis, *Int J Gynecol Pathol* 5:110-118, 1986.
49. Jones RE, Austin C, Ackerman AB: Extramammary Paget's disease. A critical reexamination, *Am J Dermatopathol* 1:101-132, 1979.
50. Jones RW, Rowan DM: Vulvar intraepithelial neoplasia III: a clinical study of the outcome in 113 cases with relation to the later development of invasive vulvar carcinoma, *Obstet Gynecol* 84:741-745, 1994.
51. Kao GF, Graham JH: Bowenoid papulosis, *Int J Dermatol* 21:445-446, 1982.
52. Kiryu H, Ackerman AB: A critique of current classifications of vulvar diseases, *Am J Dermatopathol* 12:377-392, 1990.
53. Kneale BL: Microinvasive cancer of the vulva. Report of the ISSVD task force, *J Reprod Med* 29:454-456, 1984.
54. Kurman RJ, Toki T, Schiffman MH: Basaloid and warty carcinomas of the vulva: distinctive types of squamous cell carcinoma frequently associated with human papillomaviruses, *Am J Surg Pathol* 17:133-145, 1993.
55. Lavery HA: Vulvar dystrophies: new approaches, *Clin Obstet Gynecol* 11:155-169, 1984.
56. Lawrence DW: Non-neoplastic epithelial disorders of the vulva (vulvar dystrophies): historical and current perspectives, *Pathol Annu* 28:23-51, 1993.
57. Lee SC, Roth LM, Ehrlich C, Hall JA: Extramammary Paget's disease of the vulva. A clinicopathologic study of 13 cases, *Cancer* 39:2540-2549, 1977.
58. Leuchter RS, Hacker NF, Voet RL, Berek JS, Townsend DE, Lagasse LD: Primary carcinoma of the Bartholin gland: a report of 14 cases and review of the literature, *Obstet Gynecol* 60:361-368, 1982.
59. Marinoff SC, Turner MLC: Vulvar vestibulitis syndrome, *Dermatol Clin* 10:435-444, 1992.
60. McKay M: Vulvar dermatoses, *Clin Obstet Gynecol* 34:614-629, 1991.
61. McKay M, Frankman O, Horowitz BJ, Lecart C, Micheletti L, Ridley CM, Chanco Turner ML, Woodruff JD: Vulvar vestibulitis and vestibular papillomatosis: report of the ISSVD committee on vulvodynia, *J Reprod Med* 36:413-415, 1991.
62. McLachlin CM, Kozakewich H, Craighill M, O'Connell B, Crum CP: Histologic correlates of vulvar human papillomavirus infection in children and young adults, *Am J Surg Pathol* 18:728-735, 1994.
63. McLachlin CM, Mutter GL, Crum CP: Multinucleated atypia of the vulva, *Am J Surg Pathol* 18:1233-1239, 1994.

64. Mucitelli DR, Charles EZ, Kraus FT: Vulvovaginal polyps: histologic appearance, ultrastructure, immunocytochemical characteristics, and clinicopathologic correlations, *Int J Gynecol Pathol* 9:20-40, 1990.
65. Nirenberg A, Östör AG, Slavin J, Riley CB, Rome RM: Primary vulvar sarcomas, *Int J Gynecol Pathol* 14:55-62, 1995.
66. Olson DJ, Fujimura M, Swanson P, Okagaki T: Immunohistochemical features of Paget's disease of the vulva with and without adenocarcinoma, *Int J Gynecol Pathol* 10:285-295, 1991.
67. Ostor AG, Fortune DW, Riley CB: Fibroepithelial polyps with atypical stromal cells (pseudosarcoma botryoides) of vulva and vagina. A report of 13 cases, *Int J Gynecol Pathol* 7:351-360, 1988.
68. Patterson JW, Kao GF, Graham JH, Helwig EB: Bowenoid papulosis. A clinicopathologic study with ultrastructural observations, *Cancer* 57:823-836, 1986.
69. Perrone T, Twiggs LB, Adcock LL, Dehner LP: Vulvar basal cell carcinoma: an infrequently metastasizing neoplasm, *Int J Gynecol Pathol* 6:152-165, 1987.
70. Phillips GL, Bundy BN, Okagaki T, Kucera PR, Stehman FB: Malignant melanoma of the vulva treated by radical hemivulvectomy. A prospective study of the Gynecologic Oncology Group, *Cancer* 73:2626-2632, 1994.
71. Prat J: Pathology of vulvar intraepithelial lesions and early invasive carcinoma, *Hum Pathol* 22:877-883, 1991.
72. Prayson RA, Stoler MH, Hart WR: Vulvar vestibulitis. A histopathologic study of 36 cases, including human papillomavirus in situ hybridization analysis, *Am J Surg Pathol* 19:154-160, 1995.
73. Pyka RE, Wilkinson EJ, Friedrich EG, Croker BP: The histopathology of vulvar vestibulitis syndrome, *Int J Gynecol Pathol* 7:249-257, 1988.
74. Ragnarsson-Olding B, Johansson H, Rutqvist L, Ringborg U: Malignant melanoma of the vulva and vagina, *Cancer* 71:1893-1897, 1993.
75. Reid R, Greenberg MD: Human papillomavirus-related diseases of the vulva, *Clin Obstet Gynecol* 34:630-650, 1991.
76. Ridley CM: Lichen sclerosus, *Dermatol Clin* 10:309-323, 1992.
77. Ridley CM, Frankman O, Jones ISC, Pincus SH, Wilkinson EJ: New nomenclature for vulvar disease: International Society for the Study of Vulvar Disease, *Hum Pathol* 20:495-496, 1989.
78. Ridley CM, Frankman O, Jones ISC, Pincus SH, Wilkinson EJ: New nomenclature for vulvar disease. Report of the committee on terminology of the International Society for the Study of Vulvar Disease, *J Reprod Med* 35:483-484, 1990.
79. Robboy SJ, Ross JS, Prat J, Keh PC, Welch WR: Urogenital sinus origin of mucinous and ciliated cysts of the vulva, *Obstet Gynecol* 51:347-351, 1978.
80. Sawchuk WS: Vulvar manifestations of human papillomavirus infection, *Dermatol Clin* 10: 405-414, 1992.
81. Scheistroen M, Trope C, Kaern J, Pettersen EO, Abeler VM, Kristensen GB: Malignant melanoma of the vulva. Evaluation of prognostic factors with emphasis on DNA ploidy in 75 patients, *Cancer* 75:72-80, 1995.
82. Simo M, Zapata C, Esquius J, Domingo J: Aggressive angiomyxoma of the female pelvis and perineum. Report of two cases and review of the literature, *Br J Obstet Gynaecol* 99:925-927, 1992.
83. Steeper TA, Rosai J: Aggressive angiomyxoma of the female pelvis and perineum, *Am J Surg Pathol* 7:463-475, 1983.
84. Stehman FB, Bundy BN, Dvoretsky PM, Creasman WT: Early stage I carcinoma of the vulva treated with ipsilateral superficial inguinal lymphadenectomy and modified radical hemivulvectomy: a prospective study of the Gynecologic Oncology Group, *Obstet Gynecol* 79:490-497, 1992.
85. Sturgeon SR, Brinton LA, Devesa SS, Kurman RJ: In situ and invasive vulvar cancer incidence trends (1973 to 1987), *Am J Obstet Gynecol* 166: 1482-1485, 1992.
86. Taussig YL: Leukoplakic vulvitis and cancer of the vulva, *Am J Obstet Gynecol* 18:472-503, 1929.
87. Tavassoli FA, Norris HJ: Smooth muscle tumors of the vulva, *Obstet Gynecol* 53:213-217, 1979.
88. Tawfik O, Huntrakoon M, Collins J, Owiety T, Seoud MAF, Weed J: Leiomyosarcoma of the vulva: report of a case, *Gynecol Oncol* 54:242-249, 1994.
89. Thomas R, Barnhill D, Bibro M, Hoskins W: Hidradenitis suppurativa: a case presentation and review of the literature, *Obstet Gynecol* 66: 592-595, 1985.
90. Toki T, Kurman RJ, Park JS, Kessis T, Daniel RW, Shah KV: Probable nonpapillomavirus etiology of squamous cell carcinoma of the vulva in older women: a clinocopathologic study using in situ hybridization and polymerase chain reaction, *Int J Gynecol Pathol* 10:107-125, 1991.

91. Ulbright TM, Ulbright TM, Stehman FB, Ruth LM, Ehrlich CE, Ransburg RC: Bowenoid dysplasia of the vulva, *Cancer* 12:2910-2919, 1982.
92. Van der Putte SCJ: Mammary-like glands of the vulva and their disorders, *Int J Gynecol Pathol* 13:150-160, 1994.
93. Voet RL, Buchsbaum HJ: Bartholin's gland, *Postgrad Obstet Gynecol* 5:1-6, 1985.
94. Voet RL: Classification of vulvar dystrophies and premalignant squamous lesions, *J Cutan Pathol* 21:86-90, 1994.
95. Wade TR, Kopf AW, Ackerman AB: Bowenoid papulosis of the genitalia, *Arch Dermatol* 115:306-308, 1979.
96. Wheelock JB, Goplerud DR, Dunn LJ, Oates JF: Primary carcinoma of the Bartholin gland: a report of ten cases, *Obstet Gynecol* 63:820-824, 1984
97. Wilkinson EJ: Superfically invasive carcinoma of the vulva, *Clin Obstet Gynecol* 28:188-195, 1985.
98. Wilkinson EJ: The 1989 presidential address. International Society for the Study of Vulvar Disease, *J Reprod Med* 35:981-991, 1990.
99. Wilkinson EJ: Superfically invasive carcinoma of the vulva, *Clin Obstet Gynecol* 34:651-661, 1991.
100. Wilkinson EJ: Normal histology and nomenclature of the vulva, and malignant neoplasms, including VIN, *Dermatol Clin* 10:283-296, 1992.
101. Wilkinson EJ, Guerrero E, Daniel R, Shah K, Stone K, Hardt NS, Friedrich EG: Vulvar vestibulitis is rarely associated with human papillomavirus infection types 6, 11, 16, or 18, *Int J Gynecol Pathol* 12:344-349, 1993.
102. Wilkinson EJ, Kneale B, Lynch PJ: Report of the ISSVD terminology committee, *J Reprod Med* 31:973-974, 1986.
103. Wilkinson EJ, Rico MJ, Pierson KK: Microinvasive carcinoma of the vulva, *Int J Gynecol Pathol* 1:29-39, 1982.
104. Woodworth H Jr, Dockerty MB, Wilson RB, Prat JH: Papillary hidradenoma of the vulva: a clinicopathologic study of 69 cases, *Am J Obstet Gynecol* 110:501-508, 1971.

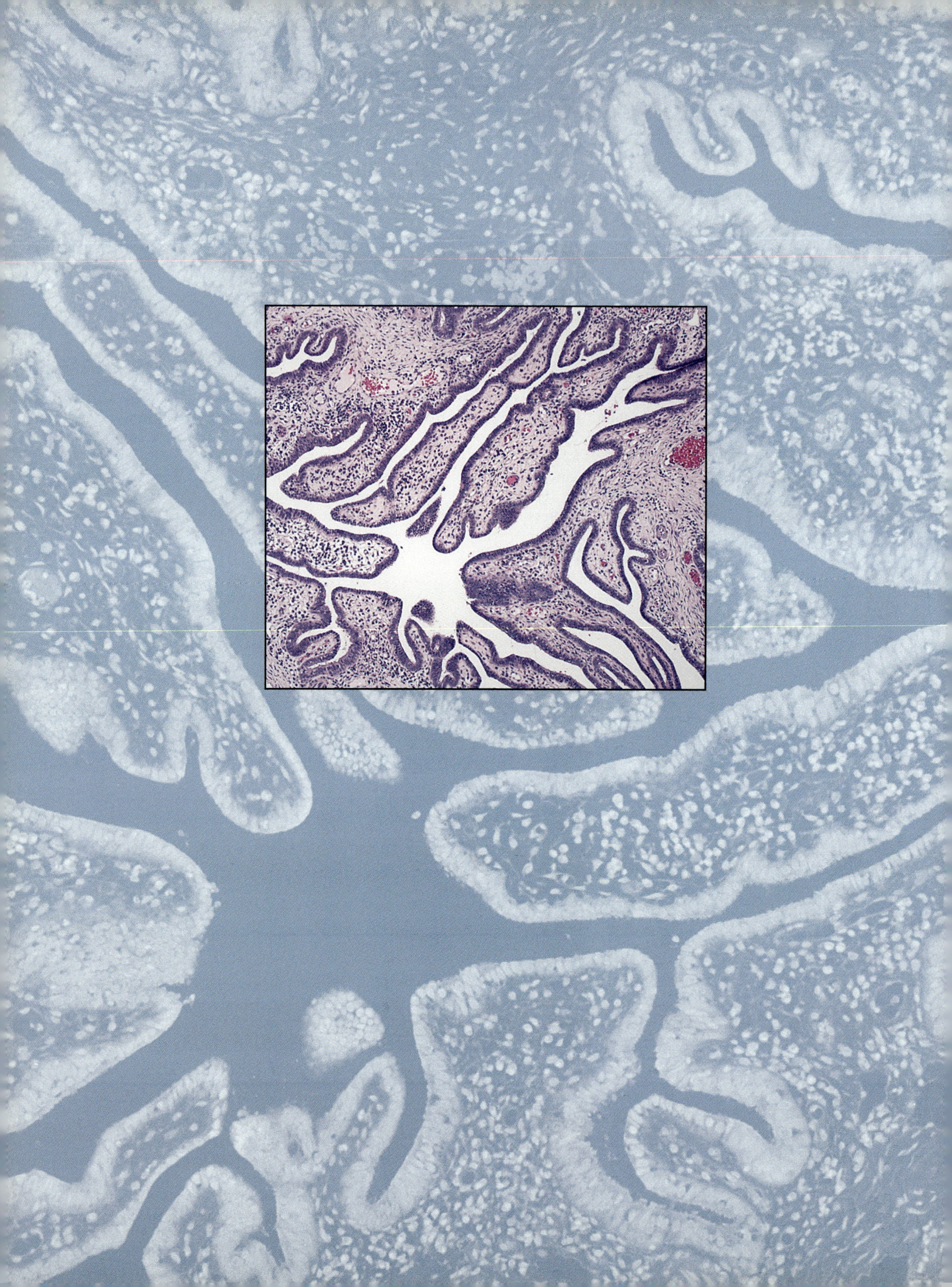

Chapter 2

Pathology of the Vagina

The upper portion of the vagina begins at the cervix and is formed from fusion of the müllerian ducts. The lower portion of the vagina begins at the hymenal ring and is formed from the urogenital sinus. Developmental abnormalities of the vagina include agenesis, hypoplasia, septa, and adenosis. Adenosis is the presence of glandular epithelium (Figures 2-1 to 2-3) or its mucinous products in the vagina. There is a high incidence of this condition among diethylstilbestrol (DES)-exposed offspring, and it is postulated that in utero exposure to DES[19,20,26] interferes with the urogenital sinus covering the glandular epithelium with squamous epithelium. The residual areas of glandular epithelium are referred to as adenosis. Adenosis is usually endocervical like but may also be endometrioid or tubelike in appearance. An ectropion (ectopy or eversion) consists of the presence of glandular epithelium or its mucinous products on the ectocervix. A summary of the effects of DES exposure is presented in Table 2-1.[36] Whenever an anomaly is found in the vaginal area, a search of the upper reproductive organs may yield other anomalies. Abnormal sex development and chromosomal abnormalities may also lead to malformations in the vagina.

TABLE 2-1 Summary of Adverse Effects of in Utero Exposure to Diethylstilbestrol (DES)[36]

EFFECTS OF IN UTERO EXPOSURE TO DES ON FEMALE PROGENY
Anatomic abnormalities
Lower müllerian tract
Adenosis and clear cell adenocarcinoma
Cervicovaginal structural abnormalities
Collars, hoods, septa, and cockscombs
Cervical mucus effects
Cervical stenosis (after "therapy")
Cervical incompetence
Upper müllerian tract
Uterine structural abnormalities
Fallopian tube structural abnormalities
Reproductive abnormalities
Menstrual dysfunction
Reproductive dysfunction
Infertility
Adverse pregnancy outcome
Spontaneous abortion
Ectopic pregnancy
Premature delivery
Perinatal death
Term delivery
Overall adverse pregnancy outcome
EFFECTS OF IN UTERO EXPOSURE TO DES ON MALE PROGENY
Anatomic abnormalities
Reproductive dysfunction
Altered semen analysis
Altered fertility potential

From Stilman RJ: *Am J Obstet Gynecol* 142:905-921, 1982, with permission.

Inflammatory and infectious diseases are among the most common disorders of the vagina. Polypoid areas of granulation tissue may be seen in the vaginal cuff (Figure 2-4) as the result of healing from a previous hysterectomy. Candidiasis is a common infection involving the vagina and is often seen in patients who are pregnant or on antibiotic therapy. Nonspecific vaginitis may be related to the organism *Gardnerella vaginalis.* Papanicolaou (Pap) smears may contain epithelial cells with adherent bacteria (clue cells) with this infection. *Trichomonas vaginalis, Neisseria gonorrhoeae,* and *Chlamydia trachomatis* infections are sexually transmitted diseases that may cause vaginitis. The human papillomavirus (HPV) causes condyloma acuminatum and is also implicated in the development of vaginal intraepithelial neoplasia (VAIN). Occasionally chronic infections, especially those caused by gram-negative rods such as *Escherichia coli,* may lead to a condition known as malakoplakia. Malakoplakia (Figure 2-5) shows a mixture of chronic inflammatory cells with lymphocytes, plasma cells, and numerous histiocytes containing eosinophilic cytoplasm. Characteristic basophilic spherials (Michaelis-Gutmann bodies) are seen in this condition. Emphysematous vaginitis[22] is an unusual response of the vagina to a variety of organisms. The infection gives rise to numerous gas-filled pockets (Figure 2-6) similar to emphysematous blebs in the lung.

Occasionally a prolapsed fallopian tube may occur in the upper vagina and present as granulation tissue or a polypoid mass (Figure 2-7). The epithelium is usually edematous with chronic inflammation. Endometriosis also presents in the vagina as isolated foci of blue domed cysts (Figure 2-8). A variety of cysts may arise in the vagina.[32] Epidermal inclusion cysts (Figure 2-9) are usually the result of invaginated squamous epithelium, often as a result of a laceration. The cysts are lined by reactive squamous epithelium and are filled with degenerating squamous cells, inflammation, and keratinous debris. One of the more common cysts of the vagina is Gartner's duct cyst (Figure 2-10), which is a cystic dilatation of residual mesonephric duct epithelium. The cyst is usually smooth walled and contains clear fluid. The epithelium is flattened and cuboidal.

Fibroepithelial polyps of the vagina[11,16,27,29,30,31] are polypoid lesions lined with benign squamous epithelium (Figure 2-11). The stroma contains a loose edematous proliferation of fibroblasts that may have a pseudosarcomatous pattern (Figure 2-12). When squamous VAIN occurs,[23] it presents colposcopically findings similar to those seen in the cervix. Low-grade squamous intraepithelial lesions (Figure 2-13) are often a combination of mild dysplasia and HPV (VAIN I). High-grade lesions (VAIN II and III) contain a larger population of neoplastic cells replacing more of the squamous epithelium (Figure 2-14). A careful examination of the vulva and vagina is required when there is a persistent unexplained abnormal Pap smear. Squamous cell carcinoma (Figures 2-15 and 2-16) is the most common malignant tumor of the vagina.[25] Most of these are of the large cell type, but several variants may occur (see box on 36). Clear cell adenocarcinoma is rare, with a higher incidence in DES-exposed offspring.[26,34,40] Clear cell adenocarcinoma may present with a tubulocystic (Figure 2-17), papillary (Figure 2-18), or solid pattern (Figure 2-19). Other malignant epithelial tumors of the vagina less commonly seen are adenosquamous carcinoma, adenoid cystic carcinoma, carcinoid tumor, and small cell carcinoma (Figure 2-20).[14,21,28]

Mesenchymal tumors of the vagina are uncommon. Smooth muscle tumors[33,37] are occasionally seen as subepithelial nodules (Figure 2-21). Vaginal rhabdomyomas[13,18] occur as polypoid lesions lined with benign squamous epithelium showing a proliferation of bland rhabdomyoblasts (Figures 2-22 and 2-23). Embryonal rhabdomyosarcoma (sarcoma botryoides) (Figures 2-24 to 2-27) may be seen in the vagina or cervix.[17] Although this lesion is usually a very aggressive tumor that has been treated by radical surgery, the advances in chemotherapy have placed this form of childhood rhabdomyosarcoma in a more favorable prognostic category according to the National Cancer Institute classification scheme.[38,41]

Other malignant tumors seen in the vagina include lymphoma, malignant melanoma,[39] and germ cell tumors, especially endodermal sinus tumor.[10,24] Mixed epithelial and mesenchymal lesions may present as a benign mixed tumor (Figure 2-28)[12,15,35] adenosarcoma, or carcinosarcoma or malignant mixed tumors resembling synovial sarcomas.

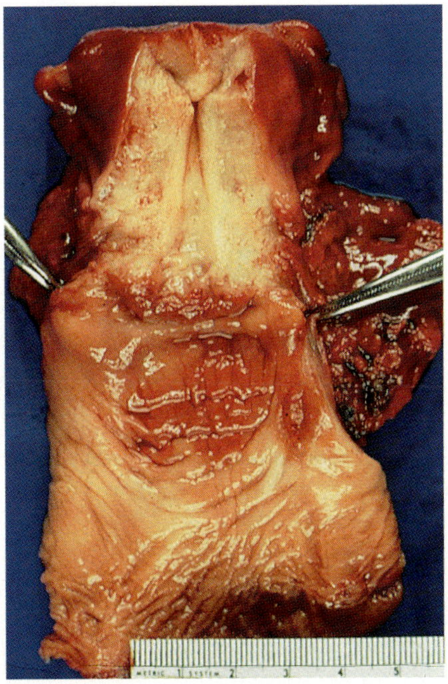

2.1 Gross photograph of a hysterectomy and radical upper vaginectomy from a diethylstilbestrol (DES)-exposed patient. In addition to clear cell adenocarcinoma, the patient has extensive adenosis involving the upper portion of the vagina, seen here by a red discoloration in the upper portion of the vagina. A fibrous rim (collar) also separates the ectocervix from the vagina. The cervix also contains an extensive ectropion.

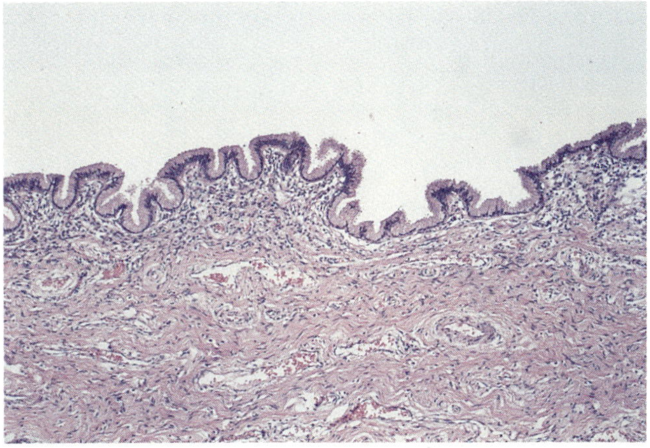

2.2 Photomicrograph of vaginal adenosis of endocervical type.

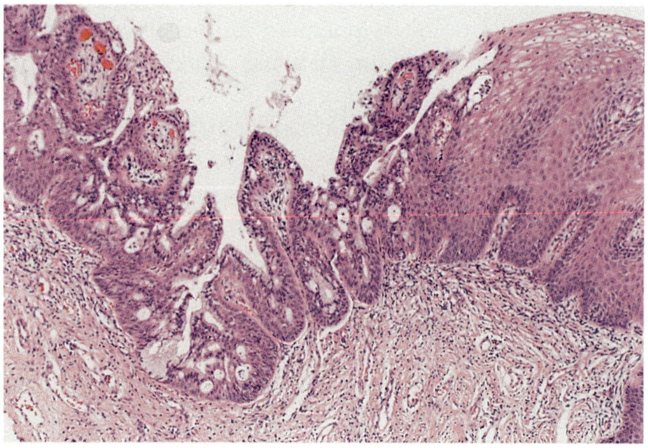

2.3 Example of vaginal adenosis undergoing squamous metaplasia. Although much of the epithelium is replaced by squamous metaplasia, residual mucinous glands are identified.

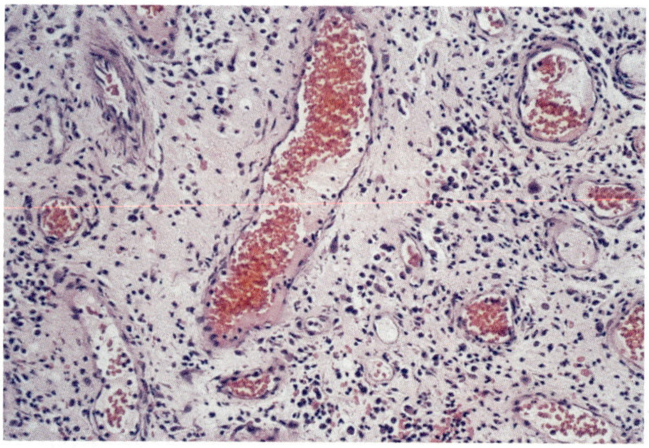

2.4 Granulation tissue of the vagina characterized by numerous dilated blood vessels surrounded by acute and chronic inflammatory cells

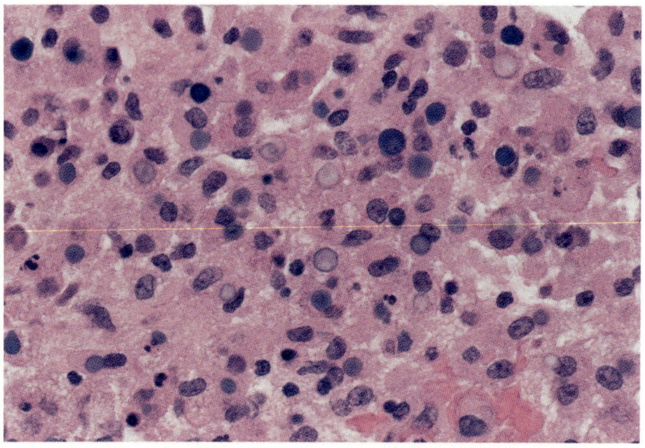

2.5 Malakoplakia of the vagina revealing a proliferation of histiocytes with eosinophilic cytoplasm and basophilic spherical calcification (Michaelis-Gutmann bodies).

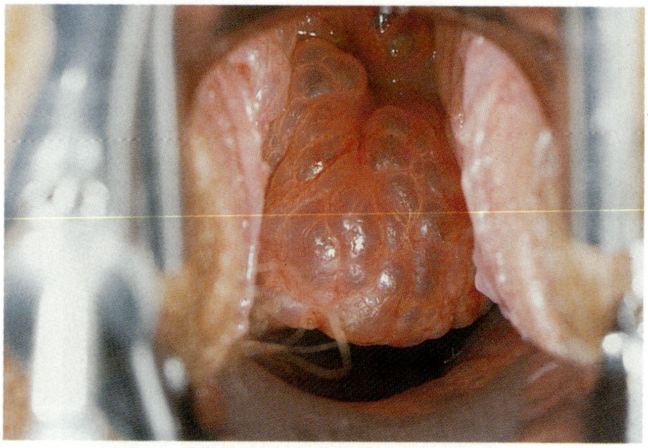

2.6 Clinical photograph of emphysematous vaginitis with multiple gas-filled cystic cavities in the vaginal mucosa and ectocervix. (Courtesy Dr. George Wendel.)

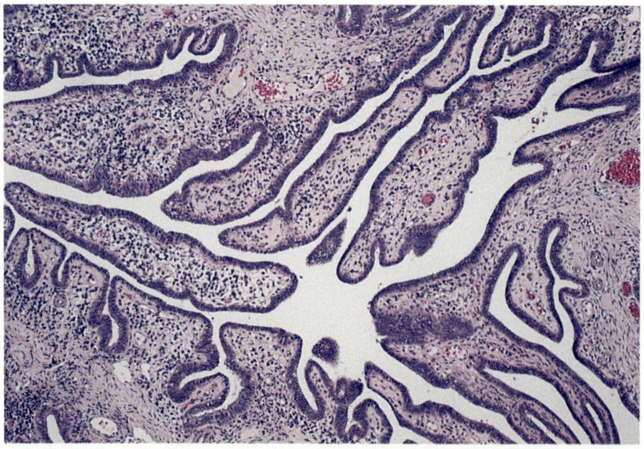

2.7 Prolapsed fallopian tube in the upper vagina after a hysterectomy. The tubal epithelium is edematous and contains chronic inflammation.

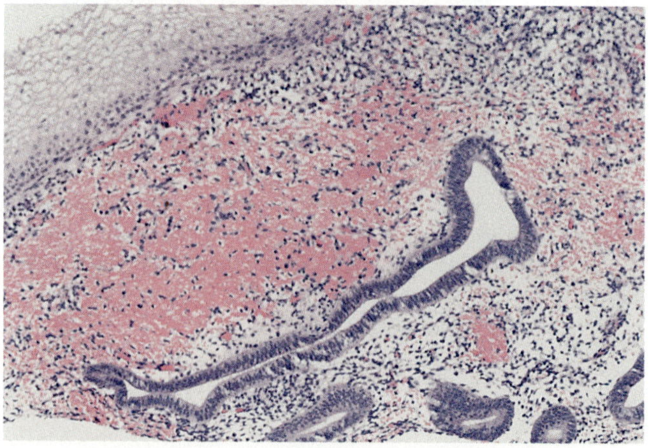

2.8 Endometriosis in the vagina demonstrating endometrial glands surrounded by endometrial stroma with hemorrhage.

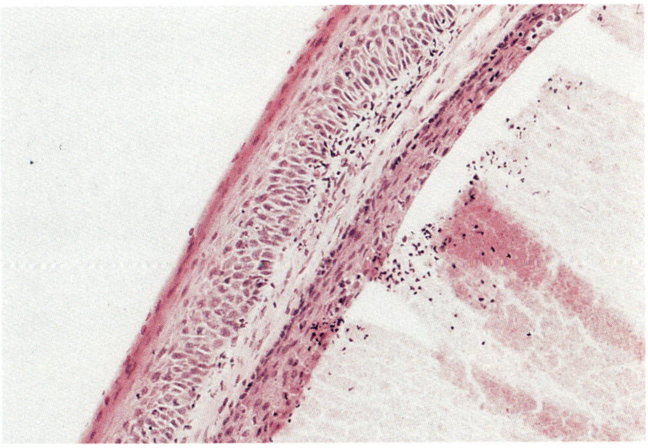

2.9 Epidermal inclusion cyst lined by reactive squamous epithelium and containing keratinous debris.

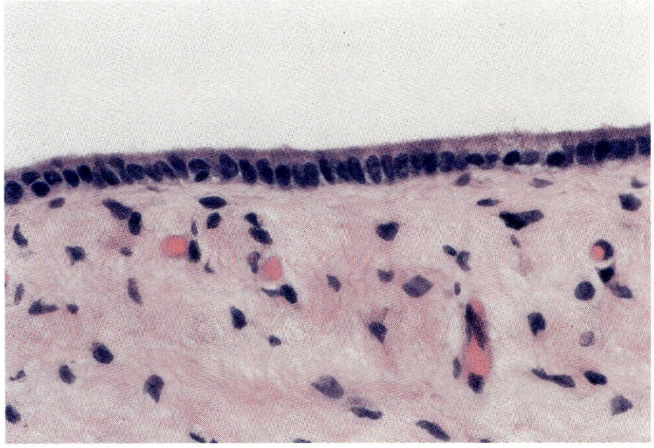

2.10 Gartner's duct cyst lined with flattened cuboidal epithelium.

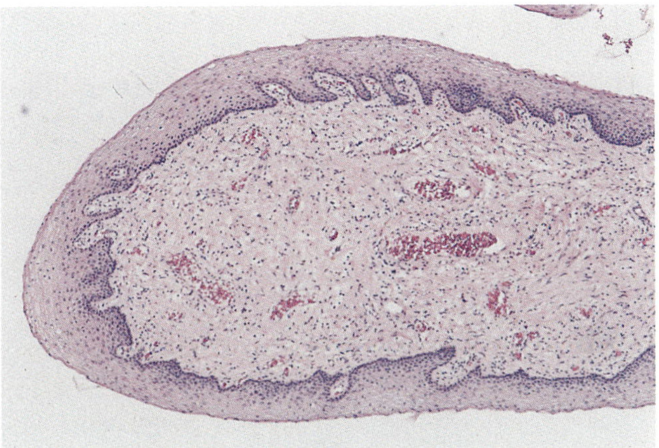

2.11 Fibroepithelial polyp of the vagina lined by squamous epithelium. The stroma shows a loose edematous fibrovascular proliferation.

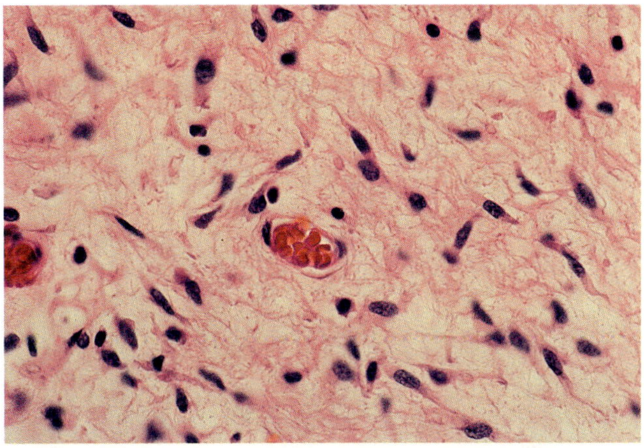

2.12 Higher-power view of a fibroepithelial polyp. The stromal cells have a stellate pattern that needs to be distinguished from a sarcoma.

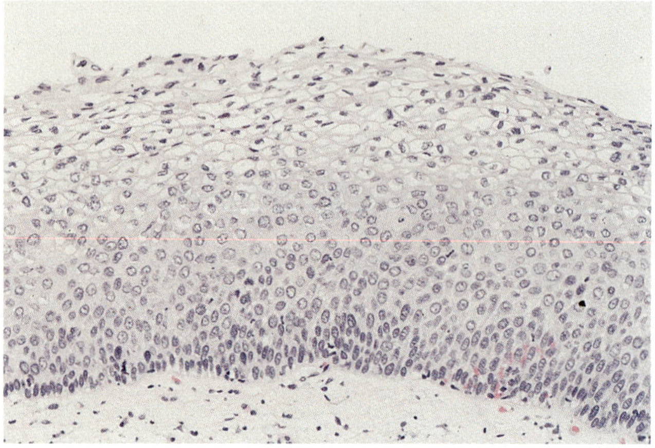

2.13 Low-grade squamous vaginal intraepithelial lesion (VAIN) (mild dysplasia, VAIN I) characterized by a proliferation of intraepithelial neoplastic squamous cells in the lower one third of the epithelium. The upper portion of the tissue reveals koilocytotic atypia consistent with human papillomavirus.

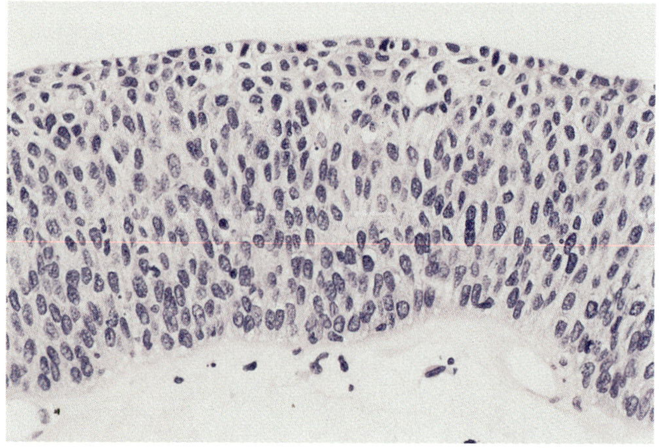

2.14 Example of a high-power squamous intraepithelial lesion (severe dysplasia, VAIN III). The neoplastic cells proliferate into the upper one third of the epithelium.

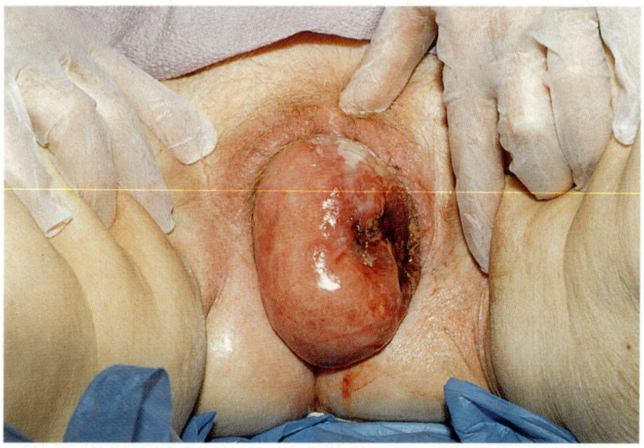

2.15 Clinical photograph of a prolapsed vagina containing ulcerated squamous cell carcinoma with surrounding hemorrhage. (Courtesy Dr. Steven Bernstein.)

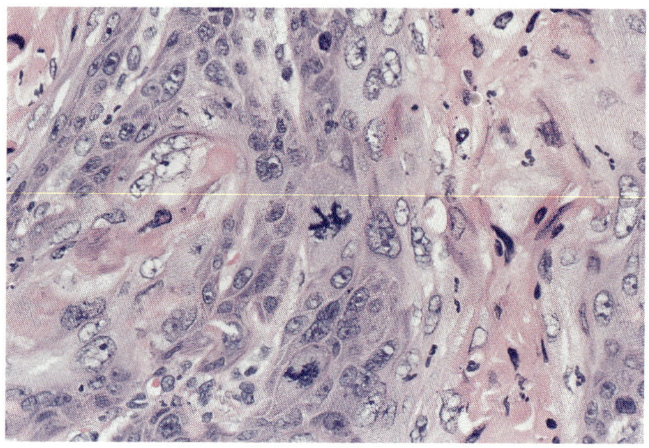

2.16 Invasive squamous cell carcinoma of the vagina demonstrating an abnormal mitotic figure. Most primary malignant vaginal tumors are squamous cell carcinomas.

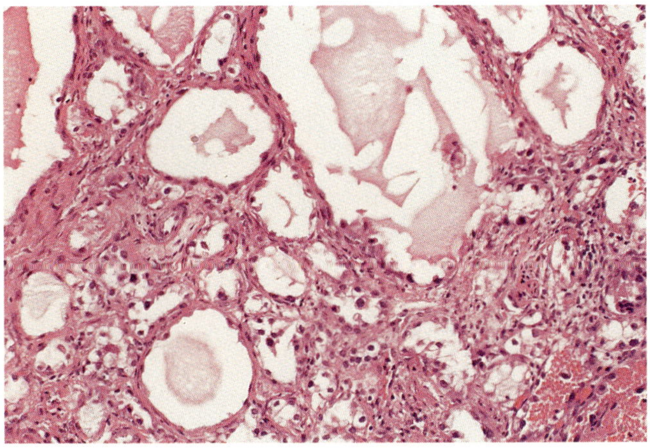

2.17 Tubulocystic variant of clear cell adenocarcinoma of the vagina. Numerous dilated cystic spaces are present, lined atypical cells showing hobnail features.

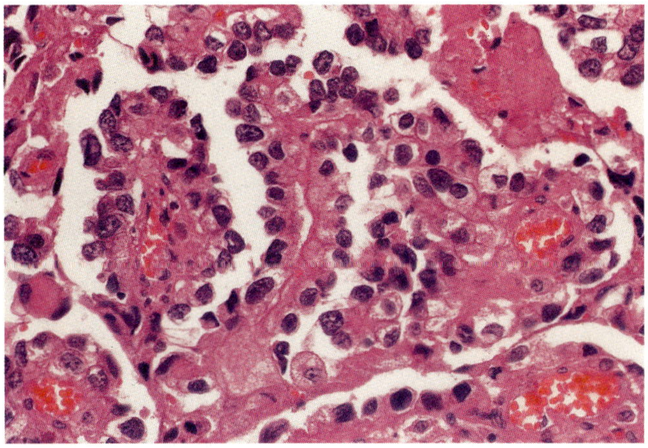

2.18 Papillary variant of clear cell adenocarcinoma of the vagina. The tumor contains papillary structures with a fibrovascular core lined with atypical, hobnail nuclei.

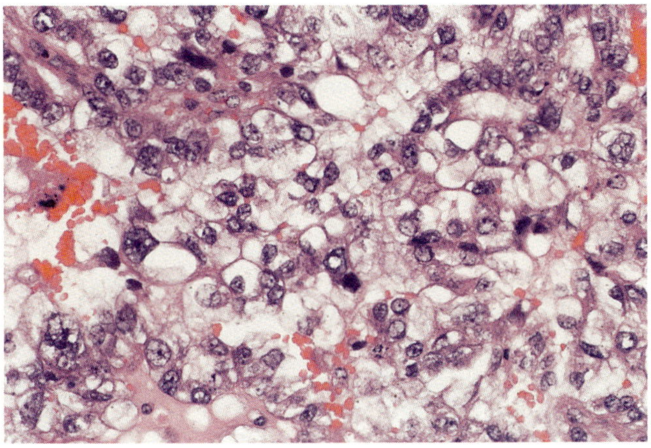

2.19 Solid variant of clear cell adenocarcinoma of the vagina. The cytoplasm is clear and there is nuclear atypia. This pattern is more common in the cervix.

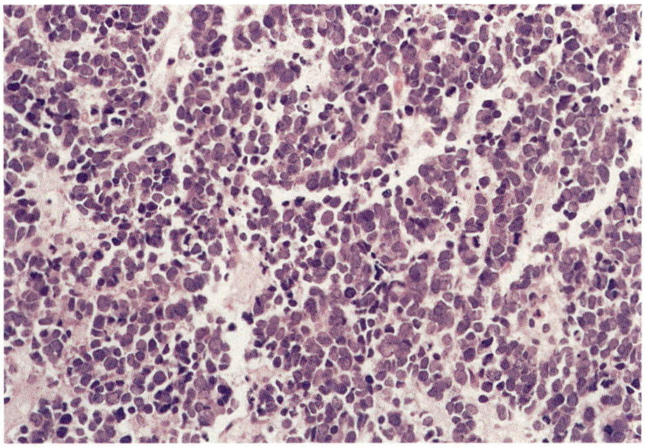

2.20 Small cell carcinoma of the vagina with neuroendocrine features.

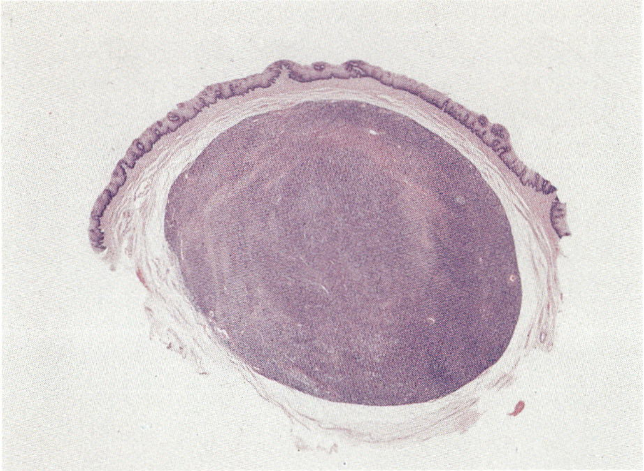

2.21 Well-circumscribed leiomyoma of the vagina lined with unremarkable squamous epithelium.

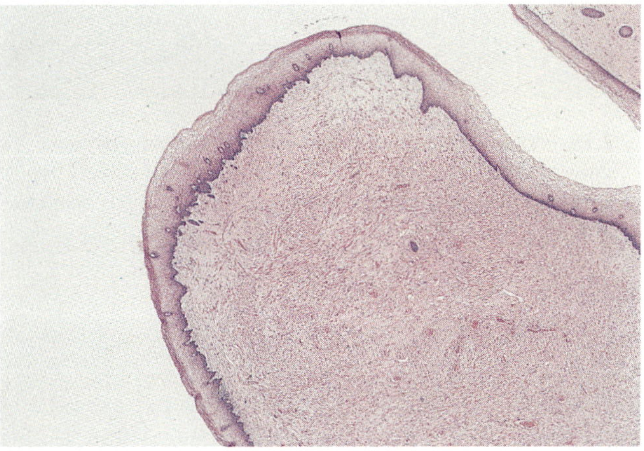

2.22 Polypoid rhabdomyoma of the vagina lined with unremarkable squamous epithelium.

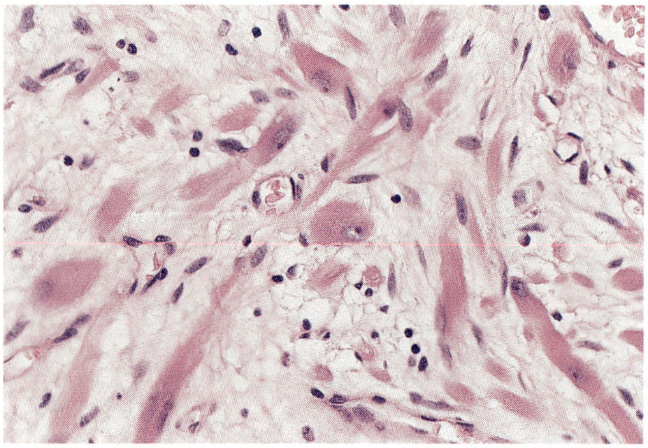

2.23 Higher-power view of vaginal rhabdomyoma showing numerous rhabdomyoblasts without significant nuclear atypia.

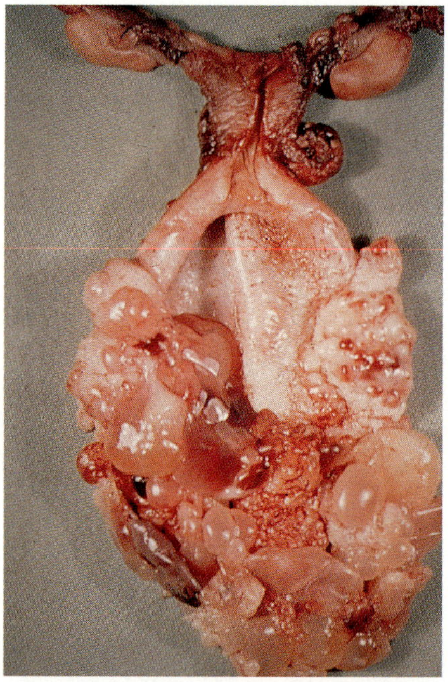

2.24 Gross view of vaginal embryonal rhabdomyosarcoma (sarcoma botryoides). Note the grapelike polypoid tumor replacing much of the vagina. (This photograph was also used in the CREOG set as slide C-111, reproduced with permission from and courtesy of Dr. Frank Vellios.)

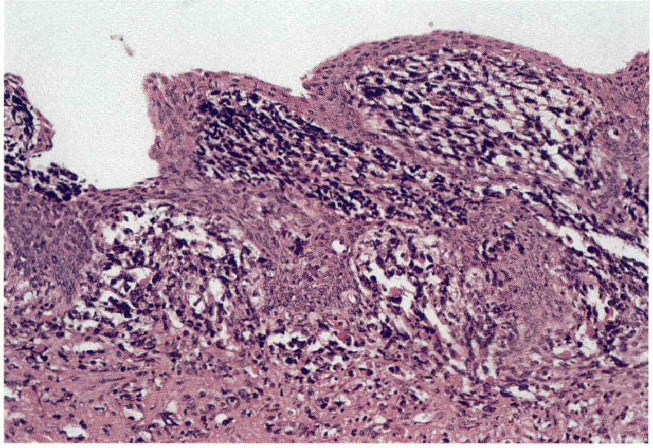

2.25 Photomicrograph of an embryonal rhabdomyosarcoma showing the characteristic cambium layer. This is a densely populated area of undifferentiated cells beneath the squamous epithelium.

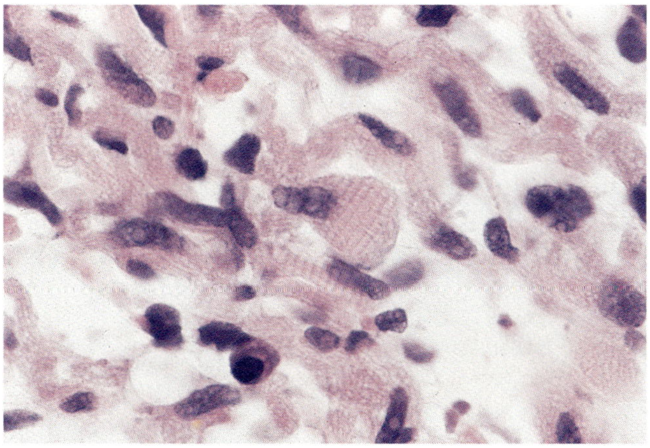

2.26 Embryonal rhabdomyosarcoma demonstrating cross-striations in rhabdomyoblastic cells.

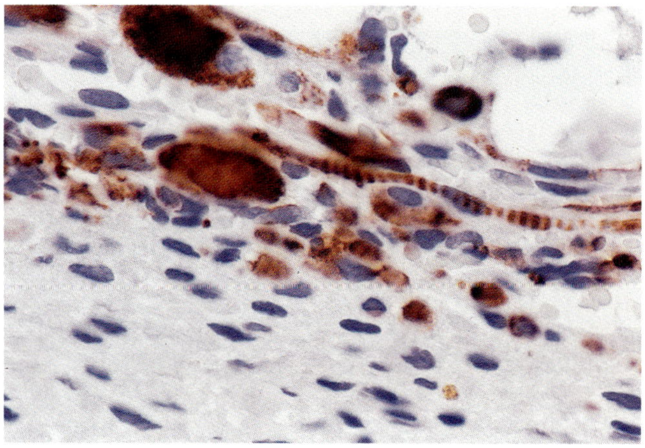

2.27 Positive immunoperoxidase stain for muscle-specific actin in an embryonal rhabdomyosarcoma. Cross-striations are also seen with this stain.

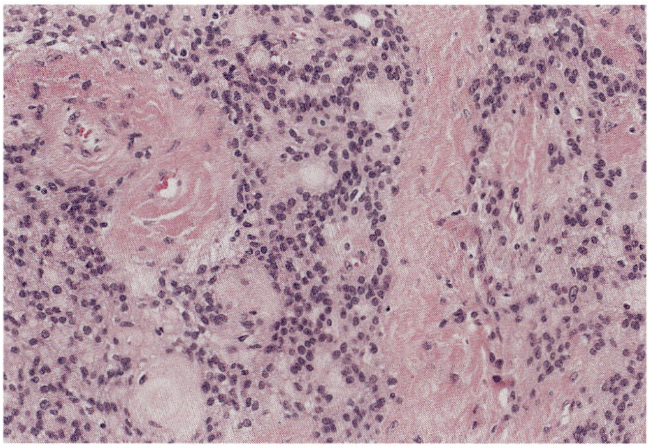

2.28 Benign mixed tumor of the vagina demonstrating a biphasic population of epithelial and stromal cells.

World Health Organization (WHO) Histologic Classification of Tumors of the Vagina[6]

(with associated systematized nomenclature of medicine [SNOMED] codes)

	SNOMED
I. Epithelial Tumors and Related Lesions	**SNOMED**
A. Squamous lesions	
1. Squamous papilloma	80520
2. Condyloma acuminatum	76720
3. Transitional metaplasia	73260
4. Squamous atypia	69700
5. Squamous intraepithelial lesions (dysplasia–carcinoma in situ, vaginal intraepithelial neoplasia (VAIN))	
a. Mild dysplasia (VAIN I)	74006
b. Moderate dysplasia (VAIN II)	74007
c. Severe dysplasia (VAIN III)	74008
d. Carcinoma in situ (VAIN III)	80702
6. Squamous cell carcinoma	80703
a. Keratinizing	80713
b. Nonkeratinizing	80723
c. Verrucous	80513
d. Warty (condylomatous)	
B. Glandular lesions	
1. Müllerian papilloma	
2. Adenosis	74200
3. Atypical adenosis	
4. Adenocarcinoma	81403
a. Clear cell adenocarcinoma	83103
b. Endometrioid adenocarcinoma	83803
c. Mucinous adenocarcinoma	84803
(1) Endocervical type	
(2) Intestinal type	81443
d. Mesonephric adenocarcinoma	91103
C. Other epithelial tumors	
1. Adenosquamous carcinoma	85603
2. Adenoid cystic carcinoma	82003
3. Adenoid basal carcinoma	80923
4. Carcinoid tumor	82403
5. Small cell carcinoma	80413
6. Undifferentiated carcinoma	80203
II. Mesenchymal Tumors	
A. Leiomyoma	88900
B. Rhabdomyoma	89000
C. Leiomyosarcoma	88903
D. Sarcoma botryoides (embryonal rhabdomyosarcoma)	89103
E. Endometrioid stromal sarcoma	89303
F. Others	
III. Mixed Epithelial and Mesenchymal Tumors	
A. Mixed tumor	89400
B. Adenosarcoma	89333
C. Malignant mesodermal mixed tumor (malignant müllerian mixed tumor, carcinosarcoma)	89513
D. Mixed tumor resembling synovial sarcoma	
IV. Miscellaneous Tumors	
A. Melanocytic nevus	87200
B. Blue nevus	87800
C. Malignant melanoma	87203
D. Tumors, germ cell type	
1. Yolk sac tumor (endodermal sinus tumor)	90713
2. Dermoid cyst (mature cystic teratoma)	90840
E. Adenomatoid tumor	90540
F. Villous adenoma	92610
G. Lymphoma and leukemia	95903
V. Secondary Tumors	
VI. Tumor-Like Lesions	
A. Stromal polyp (pseudosarcoma botryoides)	76800
B. Postoperative spindle cell nodule	
C. Vault granulation tissue	45020
D. Prolapse of fallopian tube	31050
E. Endometriosis	76500
F. Ectopic decidua	79510
G. Cysts	
1. Epidermal	33410
2. Müllerian	
3. Mesonephric	26370
H. Microglandular hyperplasia	72480
I. Lymphoma-like lesion	72290

TNM Staging Classification of Vaginal Carcinoma

International Union Against Cancer (UICC)

Primary Tumor (T)

- TX Primary tumor cannot be assessed
- T0 No evidence of primary tumor
- Tis Carcinoma in situ (preinvasive carcinoma)
- T1 Tumor confined to the vagina
- T2 Tumor invades paravaginal tissues but not to the pelvic wall
- T3 Tumor extends to the pelvic wall
- T4 Tumor invades the mucosa of the bladder or rectum and/or extends beyond the true pelvis

Regional Lymph Nodes (N)

- NX Regional lymph nodes cannot be assessed
- N0 No regional lymph node metastasis

Upper Two Thirds of the Vagina:

- N1 Pelvic lymph node metastasis

Lower One Third of the Vagina:

- N1 Unilateral regional lymph node metastasis
- N2 Bilateral regional lymph node metastasis

Distant Metastases (M)

- MX Presence of distant metastasis cannot be assessed
- M0 No distant metastases
- M1 Distant metastasis

Grading (G)

- GX Grade cannot be assessed
- G1 Well differentiated
- G2 Moderately differentiated
- G3 Poorly differentiated
- G4 Undifferentiated

Stage Grouping of Vaginal Carcinoma

The International Federation of Gynecology and Obstetrics (FIGO)
International Union Against Cancer (UICC)
American Joint Committee on Cancer (AJCC)

STAGE	TNM	
Stage 0	Tis	Carcinoma in situ, intraepithelial carcinoma
Stage I	T1 N0 M0	Tumor confined to the vagina
Stage II	T2 N0 M0	Tumor invades paravaginal tissues but does not extend to the pelvic wall
Stage III	T1 N1 M0 T2 N1 M0 T3 N0 M0	Tumor extends to the pelvic wall
Stage IVA	T1 N2 M0 T2 N2 M0 T3 N2 M0 T4 any N M0	Tumor invades the mucosa of the bladder or rectum and/or extends beyond the true pelvis
Stage IVB	Any T any N M1	Distant metastasis

The presence of a bullous edema or a growth building into the bladder or the rectum does not permit consignment of a case to Stage IV, unless the invasion of the bladder is proved by biopsy. Ridges and furrows into the bladder should be interpreted as signs of involvement only if they remain fixed to the growth on examination, thus confirming that the carcinoma has invaded the submucosa of the bladder.

BIBLIOGRAPHY

General Reading

1. Frierson HF, Mills SE: *The vulva and vagina.* In Sternberg SS, editor: *Diagnostic surgical pathology,* ed 2, New York, 1994, Raven Press.
2. Fu Y, Reagan J: *Pathology of the uterine cervix, vagina, and vulva,* Philadelphia, 1989, WB Saunders.
3. Kaufman RH, Faro S: *Benign diseases of the vulva and vagina,* ed 4, St. Louis, 1994, Mosby-Year Book.
4. Kurman RJ, Norris HJ, Wilkinson EJ: *Tumors of the cervix, vagina, and vulva. Atlas of tumor pathology,* 3rd series, fascicle 4, Washington, DC, 1992, Armed Forces Institute of Pathology.
5. Robboy SJ, Welch WR: Selected topics in the pathology of the vagina, *Hum Pathol* 22:868-876, 1991.
6. Scully RE, Bonfiglio TA, Kurman RJ, Silverberg SG, Wilkinson EJ: *World Health Organization. Histological classification of tumors of the female genital tract,* New York, 1994, Springer-Verlag.
7. Wilkinson EJ, editor: *Pathology of the vulva and vagina,* New York, 1987, Churchill Livingstone.
8. Woodruff JD, Angtuaco TL, Parmley TH: *Atlas of gynecologic pathology,* ed 2, New York, 1993, Raven Press.
9. Zanio RJ, Robboy SJ, Bentley R, Kurman RJ: *Diseases of the vagina.* In Kurman RJ, editor: *Blaustein's pathology of the female genital tract,* ed 4, New York, 1994, Springer-Verlag.

References

10. Aartsen EJ, Delemarre JFM, Gerretsen G: Endodermal sinus tumor of the vagina: radiation therapy and progeny, *Obstet Gynecol* 81:893-895, 1993.
11. Al-Nafussi AI, Rebello G, Hughes D, Blessing K: Benign vaginal polyp: a histological, histochemical and immunohistochemical study of 20 polyps with comparison to normal vaginal subepithelial layer, *Histopathology* 20:145-150, 1992.
12. Branton PA, Tavassoli FA: Spindle cell epithelioma, the so-called mixed tumor of the vagina: a clinicopathologic, immunohistochemical, and ultrastructural analysis of 28 cases, *Am J Surg Pathol* 17:509-515, 1993.
13. Chabrel CM, Beilby JOW: Vaginal rhabdomyoma, *Histopathology* 4:645-651, 1980.
14. Chafe W: Neuroepithelial small cell carcinoma of the vagina, *Cancer* 64:1948-1951, 1989.
15. Chen KTK: Benign mixed tumor of the vagina, *Obstet Gynecol* 57:89S, 1981.
16. Chirayil SJ, Tobon HJ: Polyps of the vagina: a clinicopathologic study of 18 cases, *Cancer* 47:2904-2907, 1981.
17. Copeland LH, Gershenson DM, Saul PB, Sncige N, Stringer CA, Edwards CL: Sarcoma botryoides of the female genital tract, *Obstet Gynecol* 66:262-266, 1985.
18. Gold JH, Bossen EH: Benign vaginal rhabdomyoma. A light and electron microscopic study, *Cancer* 37:2283-2294, 1976.
19. Herbst AL, editor: *Intrauterine exposure to diethylstilbestrol in the human,* Chicago, 1978, American College of Obstetricians and Gynecologists.
20. Herbst AL, Bern HA, editors: *Developmental effects of diethylstilbestrol (DES) in pregnancy,* New York, 1981, Thieme-Stratton.
21. Joseph RE, Enghardt MH, Doering DL, Brown BF, Shaffer DW, Raval HB: Small cell neuroendocrine carcinoma of the vagina, *Cancer* 70:784-789, 1992.
22. Kramer K, Tobon H: Vaginitis emphysematosa, *Arch Pathol Lab Med* 111:746-749, 1987.
23. Lenehan PM, Meffe F, Lickrish GM: Vaginal intraepithelial neoplasia: biologic aspects and management, *Obstet Gynecol* 68:333-337, 1986.
24. Liebhart M: Histopathological diagnosis of vaginal endodermal sinus tumors in infants, *Int J Gynecol Pathol* 5:217-222, 1986.
25. Manetta A, Pinto JL, Larson JE, Stevens CW, Pinto JS, Podczaski ES: Primary invasive carcinoma of the vagina, *Obstet Gynecol* 72:77-81, 1988.
26. Melnick S, Cole P, Anderson D, Herbst A: Rates and risks of diethylstilbestrol-related clear-cell adenocarcinoma of the vagina and cervix: an update, *N Engl J Med* 316:514-516, 1987.
27. Miettinen M, Wahlström T, Vesterinen E, Saksela E: Vaginal polyps with pseudosarcomatous features: a clinicopathologic study of seven cases, *Cancer* 51:1148-1151, 1983.
28. Miliauskas JR, Leong ASY: Small cell (neuroendocrine) carcinoma of the vagina, *Histopathology* 21:371-374, 1992.
29. Mucitelli DR, Charles EZ, Kraus FT: Vulvovaginal polyps: histologic appearance, ultrastructure, immunocytochemical characteristics, and clinicopathologic correlations, *Int J Gynecol Pathol* 9:20-40, 1990.
30. Norris HJ, Taylor HB: Polyps of the vagina: a benign lesion resembling sarcoma botryoides, *Cancer* 19:227-232, 1966.
31. Östör AG, Fortune DW, Riley CB: Fibroepithelial polyps with atypical stromal cells (pseudosarcoma botryoides) of vulva and vagina: a report of 13 cases, *Int J Gynecol Pathol* 7:351-360, 1988.

32. Pradhan S, Tobon H: Vaginal cysts. A clinicopathological study of 41 cases, *Int J Gynecol Pathol* 5:35-46, 1986.
33. Rastogi BL, Bergman B, Angervall L: Primary leiomyosarcoma of the vagina: a study of five cases, *Gynecol Oncol* 18:77-86, 1984.
34. Sharp GB, Cole P, Anderson D, Herbst AL: Clear cell adenocarcinoma of the lower genital tract: correlation of mother's recall of diethylstilbestrol history with obstetrical records, *Cancer* 66:2215-2220, 1990.
35. Sirota RL, Dickersin GR, Scully RE: Mixed tumors of the vagina: a clinicopathological analysis of eight cases, *Am J Surg Pathol* 5:413-422, 1981.
36. Stilman RJ: In utero exposure to diethylstilbestrol: adverse effects on the reproductive tract and reproductive performance in male and female offspring, *Am J Obstet Gynecol* 142:905-921, 1982.
37. Tavassoli FA, Norris HJ: Smooth muscle tumors of the vagina, *Obstet Gynecol* 53:689-693, 1979.
38. Tsokos M: The diagnosis and classification of childhood rhabdomyosarcoma, *Semin Diagn Pathol* 11:26-38, 1994.
39. Van Nostrand KM, Lucci JA, Schell M, Berman ML, Manetta A, DiSaia PJ: Primary vaginal melanoma: improved survival with radical pelvic surgery, *Gynecol Oncol* 55:234-237, 1994.
40. Waggoner SE, Mittendorf R, Biney N, Anderson D, Herbst AL: Influence of in utero diethylstilbestrol exposure on the prognosis and biologic behavior of vaginal clear cell adenocarcinoma, *Gynecol Oncol* 55:238-244, 1994.
41. Wijnaendts LCD, van der Linder JC, van Unnik AJM, Delemarre JFM, Voute PA, Meijer CJLM: Histopathological classification of childhood rhabdomyosarcomas: relationship with clinical parameters and prognosis, *Hum Pathol* 25:900-907, 1994.

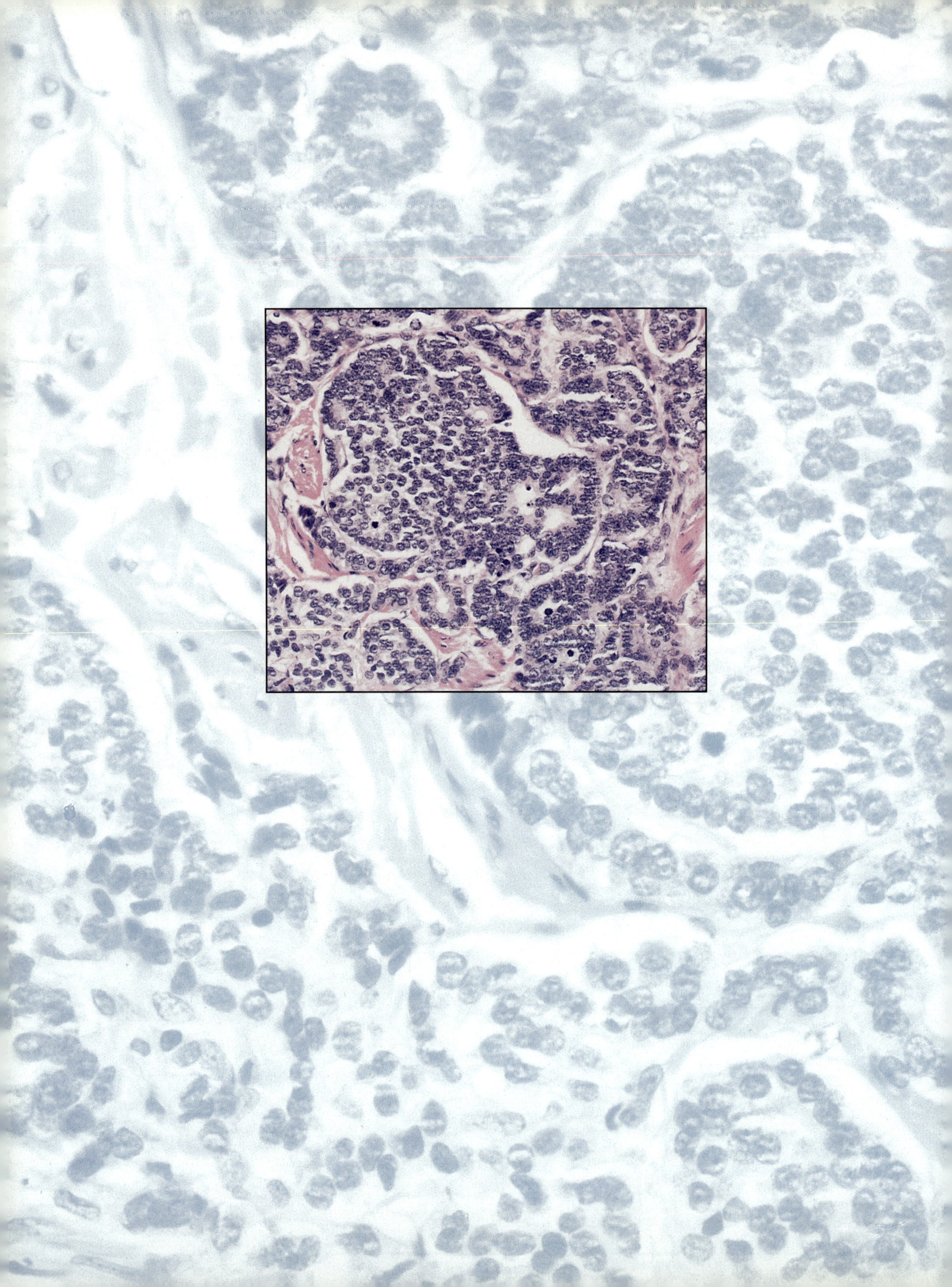

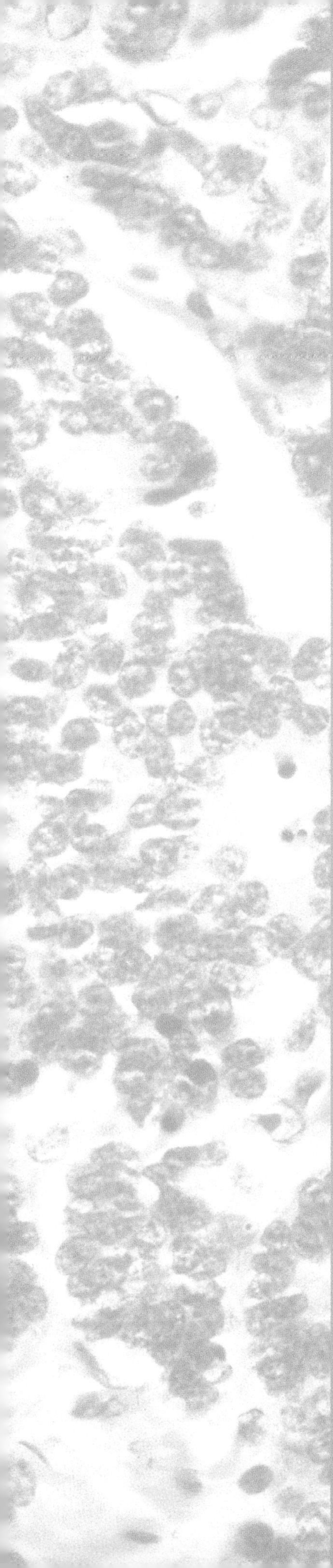

Chapter 3

Pathology of the Uterine Cervix

EPITHELIAL TUMORS AND RELATED LESIONS

Inflammation

Acute cervicitis may occur from a primary infection or as a secondary reaction from chemical or foreign body injuries. Among the more common infections are *Neisseria gonorrhoeae, Trichomonas vaginalis, Chlamydia trachomatis* (Figure 3-1), and *Candida albicans* (Figure 3-2). Acute cervicitis is usually characterized by a purulent discharge and marked erythema. Cervical tenderness may or may not be present. The histologic appearance is of marked stromal edema and an infiltration of neutrophils. Focal superficial erosion and/or ulceration may also be present. Bacteriologic cultures and wet mounts are useful in the diagnosis of these disorders.

Chronic cervicitis has often been erroneously used, as has erosion, to refer to the presence of endocervical glandular tissue on the ectocervix. The term chronic cervicitis should be reserved for the condition in which there is an infiltration of lymphocytes and plasma cells in the submucosa of the cervix. This condition often causes a persistent discharge, which may or may not reveal organisms. The discharge may be a reflection of the chronically irritated condition of the cervix with enhanced mucin production. Persistent infection with *T. vaginalis* often leads to chronic cervicitis that may extend into follicular cervicitis. Follicular cervicitis refers to the condition in which lymphoid follicles are present. The word "follicular" can often be misleading and is dependent on the site being described. For example, follicular salpingitis refers to the condition of the fallopian tube in which destruction of the villi with anastomosis and adhesions gives a pattern that resembles thyroid follicles (see Chapter 5). *Gardnerella vaginalis* (formerly *Haemophilus vaginalis*) can also cause chronic cervicitis. Chronic cervicitis may give rise to abnormal cytologic smears. The marked inflammatory component often causes reactive and reparative changes that may be difficult to distinguish from dysplasia (Figure 3-3).

Herpesvirus infection of the cervix is usually asymptomatic, although it often accompanies vulvar or vaginal herpes, which is markedly painful. The early lesion on the cervix is a vesicle that rapidly transforms into a well-circumscribed shallow ulcer. These ulcers can become secondarily infected. A biopsy or cytologic smear for herpetic lesions usually reveals the characteristic intranuclear inclusions of the herpesvirus.

Syphilitic cervicitis initially presents with a single ulcerated chancre that is painless and asymptomatic. It is for this reason that many primary syphilitic lesions of the cervix are not observed clinically. Although syphilitic cervicitis has been considered a rare presentation, it is probably much more common than has been observed. Secondary syphilis of the cervix can present with a chronic granulomatous inflammation containing multinucleated giant cells and spirochetal organisms (Figures 3-4 to 3-6). Occasionally, secondary and tertiary syphilis of the cervix presents with such marked irregularity and firmness of the cervix that it clinically mimics invasive carcinoma of the cervix.

Tuberculous cervicitis is rare and is usually the result of secondary infection from the fallopian tube and peritoneum. Typical caseating granulomas are identified, and acid-fast stains reveal the mycobacterium. Other unusual infections of the cervix include parasitic infections such as echinococcosis, amebiasis, and schistosomiasis. Actinomycosis has also been observed in the cervix. Another unusual presentation of cervical inflammation is cervical vaginitis emphysematosa. This condition is caused by gas-forming bacteria and leads to characteristic multiple blue-gray, subepithelial, air-containing cysts of the portio vaginalis and ectocervix. This condition is possibly related to *T. vaginalis*.

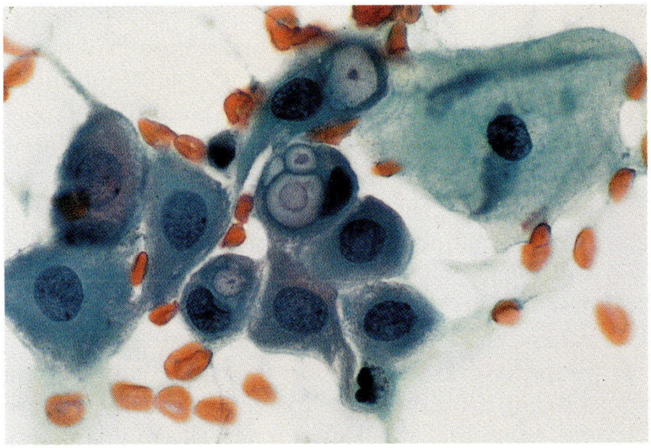

3.1 Cytologic smear from a patient with *Chlamydia* infection demonstrating the characteristic cytoplasmic inclusions.

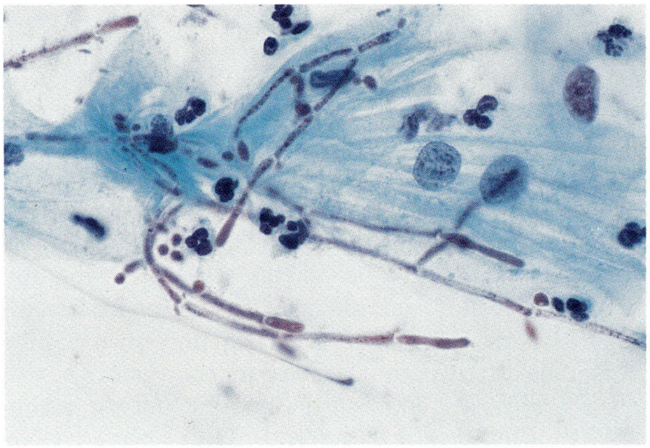

3.2 Cytologic smear from a patient with *Candida albicans* infection demonstrating the characteristic fungal hyphae.

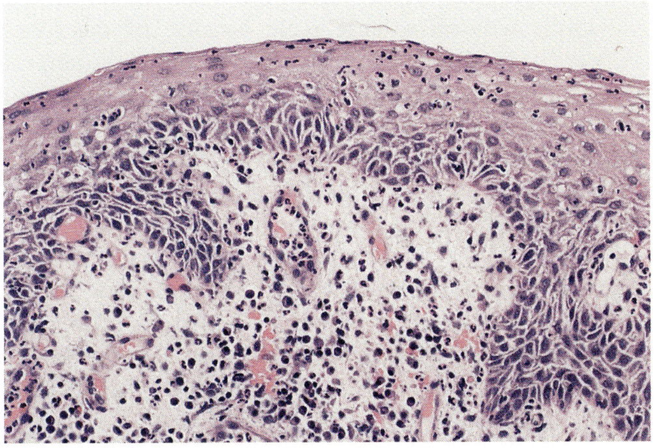

3.3 Biopsy from a patient with acute and chronic cervicitis. Squamous atypia is present at the base of the epithelium as a response to the inflammatory stimulus.

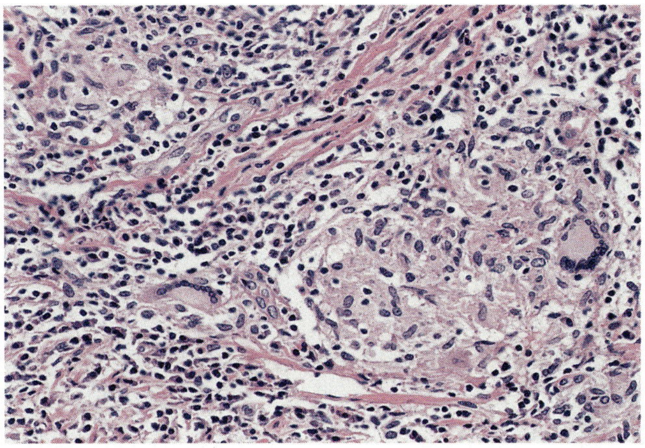

3.4 Cervical biopsy from a patient with syphilis demonstrating a marked inflammatory infiltrate with granulomatous inflammation containing multinucleated giant cells.

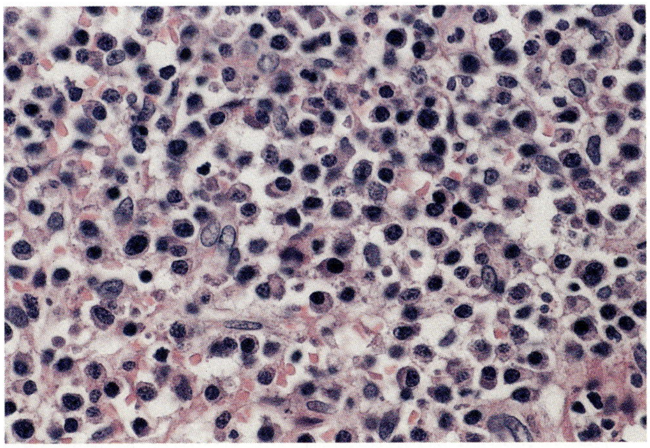

3.5 Syphilis of the cervix with an inflammatory infiltrate containing increased numbers of plasma cells.

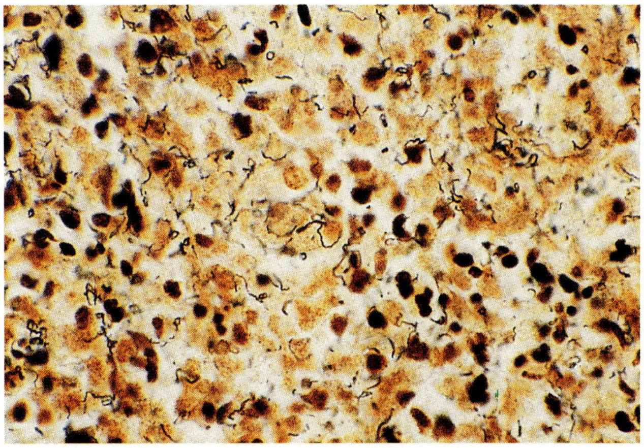

3.6 Warthin-Starry stain demonstrating numerous spirochetes in cervical syphilis.

Human Papillomavirus

The human papillomavirus (HPV), a subgroup of the papovavirus family, consists of a heterogeneous group of viruses that are responsible for various lesions ranging from common cutaneous warts to condylomatous lesions of mucous membranes.[14] The different types of HPVs are distinguished by molecular hybridization techniques. The type of HPV determines the appearance, location, and biologic behavior of the lesion.

Condyloma acuminatum has been known as a disease of the external genitalia and perianal region. The diagnosis is usually established clinically, and the lesion has characteristic papillary fronds. Occasional condylomata acuminata appear on the vagina and cervix, but this is unusual. Cellular manifestations of HPV infection (Figure 3-7) of the cervix were first observed in 1949 by Ayre.[11] In 1960[12] the same author indicated a viral etiology as the mechanism producing the cellular abnormalities, but the true significance of these findings were not recognized until later. The term "koilocytotic atypia" for these abnormal cellular changes was coined by Koss.[36] Meisels and co-workers documented the HPV etiology of the koilocytotic changes.[35,36] They found that when these lesions were on the cervix or vagina, they were usually flat and noncondylomatous. These lesions were referred to as "flat" condylomata. A review of the cervical biopsies obtained during the year 1972 was compared with the results from 1982 at Parkland Memorial Hospital.[15] Approximately 48% of the biopsies from both years revealed evidence of HPV infection.

The following criteria are used to identify HPV infection in histologic preparations: koilocytosis, dyskeratosis, parakeratosis, multinucleation, and a spiked surface (Figures 3-8 and 3-9). Histologic criteria for diagnosing cervical intraepithelial neoplasia (CIN) include loss of the basal/parabasal interface, upward polarity of nuclei, loss of maturation, mitotic activity, and abnormal mitoses. The presence of abnormal mitotic figures appears to be one of the best histologic correlates for CIN.[17,47]

HPV infection of the cervix continues to be incriminated by circumstantial evidence in the genesis of intraepithelial and invasive squamous neoplasms of the entire female genital tract.* The clinical appearance of some condylomatous lesions of the female genital tract can be very similar to that of intraepithelial neoplasia. Many investigators are now postulating that the entire CIN dysplasia continuum may begin at the lower levels with an HPV infection. As a higher-grade dysplasia or CIN develops, the viral nature of the lesion is not expressed by typical morphologic findings and can be demonstrated only by DNA molecular hybridization techniques. Molecular hybridization studies have revealed that numerous subtypes of HPV infection contribute to cervical lesions. Types 6 and 11 are thought to represent a reversible type of viral infection that produces the typical flat condyloma. Types 16, 18, 31, 33, and 35 are seen in higher-grade CIN lesions.

The treatment of genital condylomatous lesions is still a major challenge for both patient and physician. A definitive treatment has yet to be established and a wide variety of therapies have been used. Physicians who routinely deal with the disease know that recurrence is a major problem. The virus is not usually confined to one portion of the genital tract. The vagina is thought to be a major reservoir. The development of systemic therapy appears to be the only approach that will eradicate the virus throughout the entire genital tract. Autogenous vaccines have been used but are difficult to implement on a large scale because of the time and work involved in preparation and administration. Another theoretical disadvantage is the systemic administration of a possible carcinogenic agent. Local destruction techniques have been used with marginal results, producing eradication in 20% to 80% of cases. Condylomata acuminata have been treated by interferon.[39] Enhanced immunologic functions and interference with viral replication are the suspected mechanisms of action. Other investigators have used a topically applied interferon gel preparation with some success. Topical 5-fluorouracil (5-FU) cream has been recommended for the treatment of vaginal condylomata. Its effect is to create a thymidine deficiency and thus interfere with DNA and RNA synthesis.

The incidence of HPV infections of the genital tract is rising. The clinical management of these lesions has assumed great importance because of the potential neoplastic transformation. The transmission of this infection is becoming an important social problem because of inadequate therapy for eradication. Although the genomes of many of the papillomaviruses have been molecularly cloned and maps of the viral DNA have been constructed, the major impediment to analysis of this virus is the lack of a culture system that will allow replication. The rejection of papilloma is associated with the cell-mediated phenomenon. The transformation of papillomas to carcinomas appears to involve not only the virus but probably other intrinsic factors such as genetic background and environment. Further scientific investigation of the complex biology of these lesions is needed to provide a rational basis of treatment.

*References 13, 18, 29, 46, 48, 54, 65, 66.

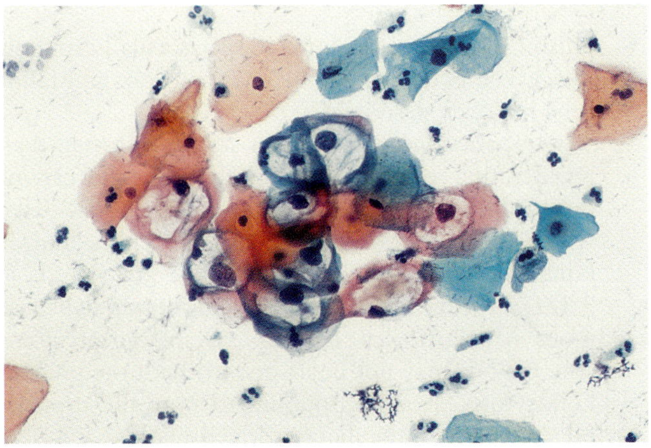

3.7 Cervical smear from a patient with human papillomavirus (HPV) infection. The squamous cells reveal characteristic koilocytotic atypia.

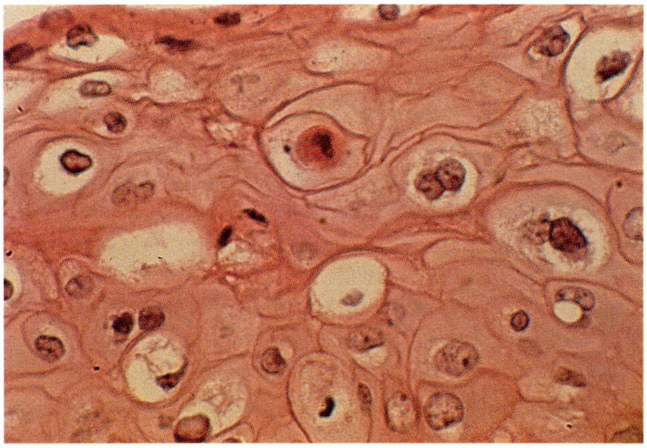

3.8 Cervical biopsy from a patient with HPV infection. The upper half of the epithelium is demonstrated and shows koilocytosis, dyskeratosis, and double nuclei.

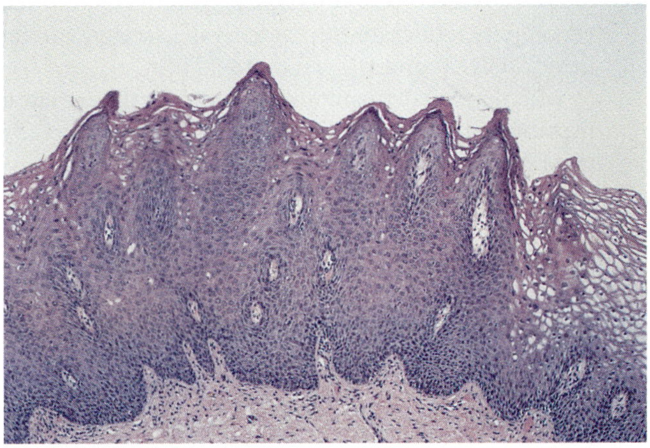

3.9 Cervical biopsy from a patient with HPV infection demonstrating the mild papillomatosis also referred to as a "spiked" surface.

Squamous Lesions

Squamous metaplasia begins as reserve cell hyperplasia beneath the columnar cells of the endocervical epithelium. These pluripotential cells, which are presumed to replenish the columnar epithelium, are now beginning their earliest commitment to squamous cells. Reserve cells are relatively small with bland nuclei, but they contain a high nuclear-to-cytoplasmic (NC) ratio that may cause confusion with dysplasia and carcinoma in situ. The high degree of nuclear density is also responsible for the whiteness of the epithelium after the application of acetic acid during colposcopic examination. Immature squamous metaplasia (Figure 3-10) is the next stage of the transformation in which the reserve cells begin to differentiate, showing cytoplasmic features of squamous cells. Again, the high NC ratio may lead to an erroneous diagnosis of dysplasia. Mature squamous metaplasia is the end product of the transformational process. The maturation usually does not reach the degree of organization of original squamous epithelium and may contain less glycogen.

Squamous atypia refers to reactive squamous epithelial changes due to a variety of causes, including inflammatory reactive/reparative reactions and alterations resulting from irradiation. Included in this group are those epithelial changes characterized by minor nuclear abnormalities and nonspecific perinuclear halos. Some of these lesions may or may not be related to HPV, but they cannot be definitively classified as such.[43] Diagnostic and therapeutic procedures may also cause artifacts and atypia in the squamous epithelium.[57]

Dysplasia literally means "bad molding" and is a term used (and misused) with widely varying definitions. Dysplastic kidneys are developmental abnormalities. Mammary dysplasia is used synonymously with fibrocystic disease, and cervical dysplasia is a neoplastic process. In cervical dysplasia the uniform neoplastic cells proliferate within the epithelium to various levels (mild, moderate, or severe) before differentiation occurs. The junction of the uniform neoplastic cells and the differentiated cells is the cut-off point for grading the dysplasia. Although maturation occurs, it is usually abnormal since the cells are derived from the underlying neoplasia. The degree of atypia in the superficial layers (the region sampled by a cytologic smear) is a function of the time allowed for maturation. Therefore, mild dysplasia will have greater maturation and less atypia on a cytologic smear even though the dysplastic cells at the base have the same malignant criteria as severe dysplasia.

Carcinoma in situ is the situation in which the entire thickness of the epithelium is replaced by neoplastic cells with no evidence of maturation. It may have several morphologic forms with variations in the size of the cells composing the lesion and in the degree of cell pleomorphism. Although carcinoma in situ is usually confined to the cervix, extension to the endometrium and fallopian tube has been described.[60]

CIN is a concept based on studies showing that the proliferating cells in all levels of dysplasia and carcinoma in situ show the same malignant criteria.[50] The extent to which the neoplastic cells replace the epithelium determines the grade (CIN I, II, or III) (Figures 3-11, 3-12, 3-13, 3-14, 3-15, and 3-16). The intraepithelial squamous neoplastic lesions, CIN, dysplasia/carcinoma in situ, may or may not be associated with the presence of koilocytosis. It is appropriate to note the presence of HPV changes in the diagnostic terminology, e.g., "moderate dysplasia with HPV changes." Squamous intraepithelial lesion (SIL) is a term introduced by the Bethesda System for cervical-vaginal cytology reporting (see box on p. 65). Low-grade lesions (LSIL) encompass HPV and mild dysplasia (CIN I). High-grade lesions (HSIL) encompass moderate to severe dysplasia and carcinoma in situ (CIN II and III) (Figure 3-17).

Microinvasive squamous carcinoma is the earliest manifestation of stromal invasion (Figure 3-18). Currently the most commonly used definition is of a lesion that invades to a depth of no greater than 3 mm when measured from the basement membrane of its point of origin and which does not demonstrate vascular space invasion (Figure 3-19). This definition is endorsed by the Society of Gynecologic Oncologists. The most recent FIGO staging of cervical tumors (see box on p. 64) classifies tumors with a depth of less than 5 mm and a horizontal growth less than 7 mm as Stage Ia2.

Squamous cell carcinoma of the cervix[34] is often exophytic (Figure 3-20) and expands locally (Figure 3-21). Cytologically the tumor demonstrates pleomorphic epithelial cells with nucleoli (Figure 3-22). Nonkeratinizing carcinoma (Figure 3-23) is the most frequent subtype and is composed of cells with a moderate amount of cytoplasm, occasionally containing individually keratinized cells, but no keratin pearls. Keratinizing carcinoma (Figure 3-24) is characterized by the presence of relatively large cells with abundant cytoplasm and with keratin pearls. This category includes those small cell carcinomas that show some squamous differentiation but does not include those tumors that resemble small cell carcinoma of the lung with neuroendocrine differentiation. Keratinizing carcinomas with a prominent HPV appearance are referred to as warty carcinomas (Figure 3-25). A well-differentiated variant of keratinizing carcinoma of the cervix is verrucous carcinoma. The papillary variant of squamous carcinoma (Figure 3-26) may present problems in assessing invasion.[45] A lymphoepithelioma-like pattern (Figures 3-27 and 3-28) may also be seen in the cervix.[27,28,32,37]

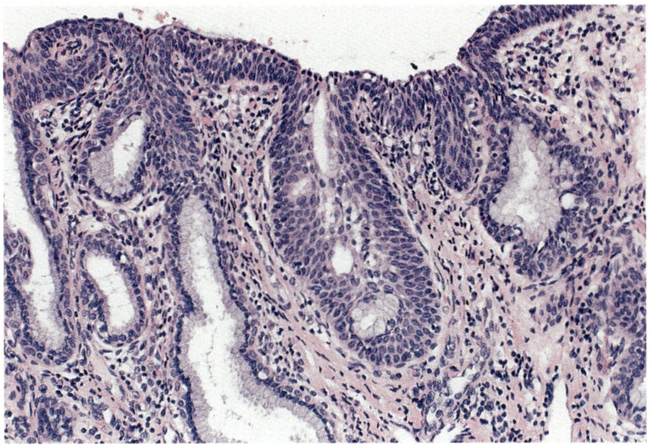

3.10 Cervical biopsy demonstrating immature squamous metaplasia. There is an increased nuclear-cytoplasmic (NC) ratio that may be confused with cervical intraepithelial neoplasia.

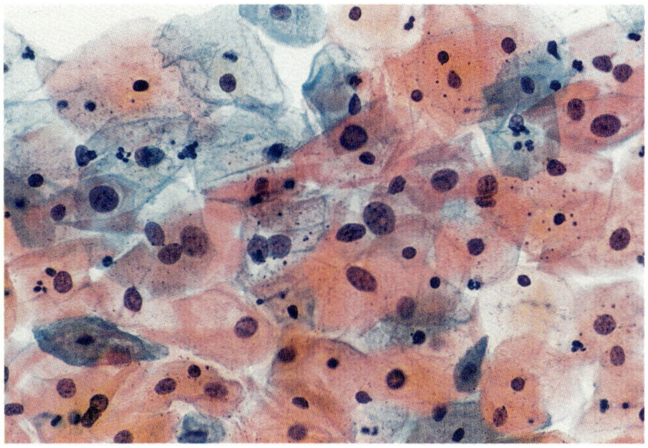

3.11 Cytologic smear demonstrating a low-grade squamous intraepithelial lesion encompassing mild dysplasia (CIN I) and HPV changes.

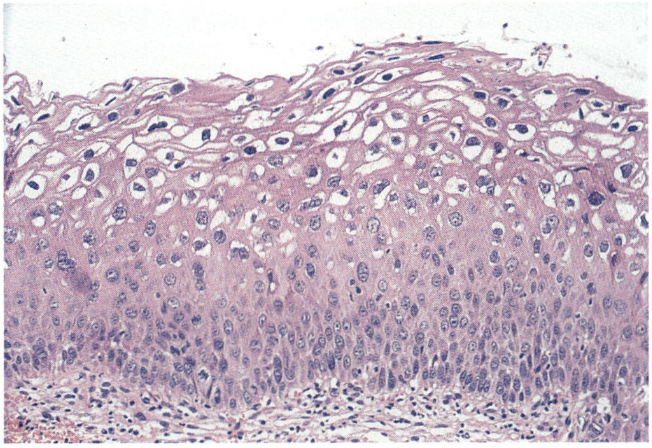

3.12 Cervical biopsy from a patient with mild dysplasia (CIN I) and HPV changes. The koilocytotic changes are in the upper half of the epithelium.

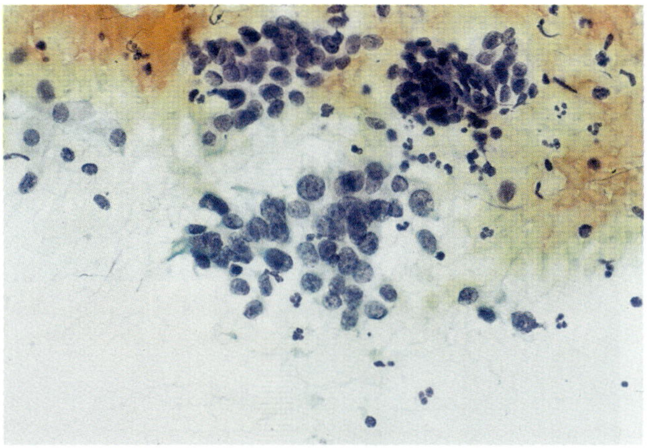

3.13 Cytologic smear from a patient with a high-grade squamous intraepithelial lesion. The abnormal cells reveal a high nuclear-to-cytoplasmic (NC) ratio that correlated with severe dysplasia (CIN III).

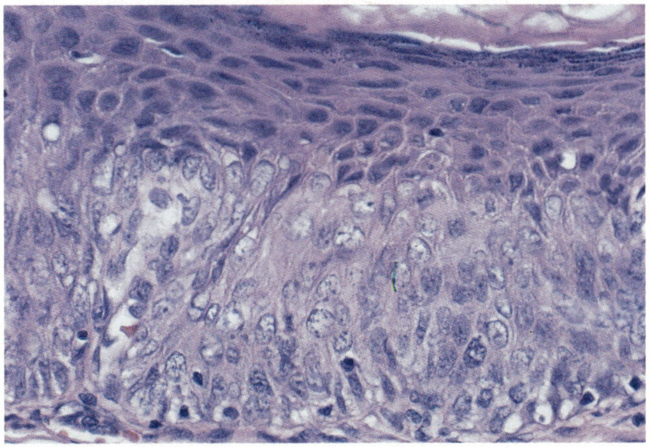

3.14 Cervical biopsy from a patient with CIN II demonstrating the intraepithelial neoplastic cells extending into the middle one third of the epithelium

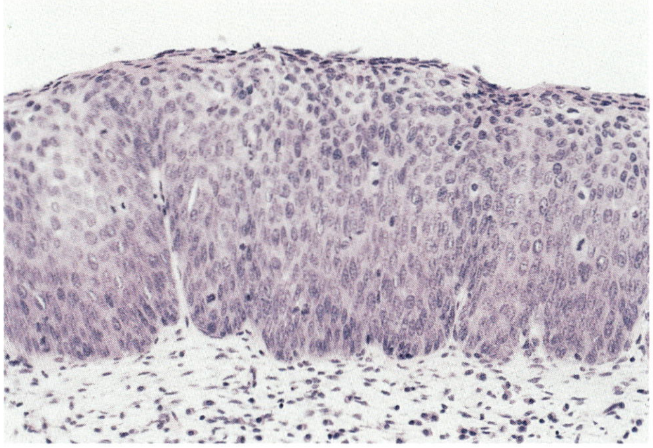

3.15 Cervical biopsy from a patient with CIN III demonstrating intraepithelial proliferation in the upper one third of the epithelium.

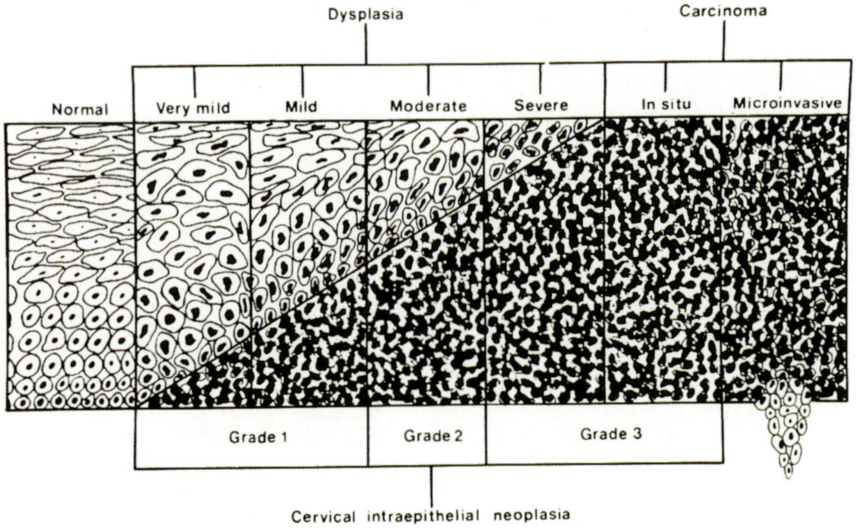

3.16 Diagram representing the correlation of dysplasia and cervical intraepithelial neoplasia. (Modified from Ferenczy A, Winkler B: *Cervical intraepithelial neoplasia and condyloma.* In Kurman RL, editor: *Blaustein's pathology of the female genital tract,* ed 3, New York, 1987, Springer-Verlag, pp 156-177.)

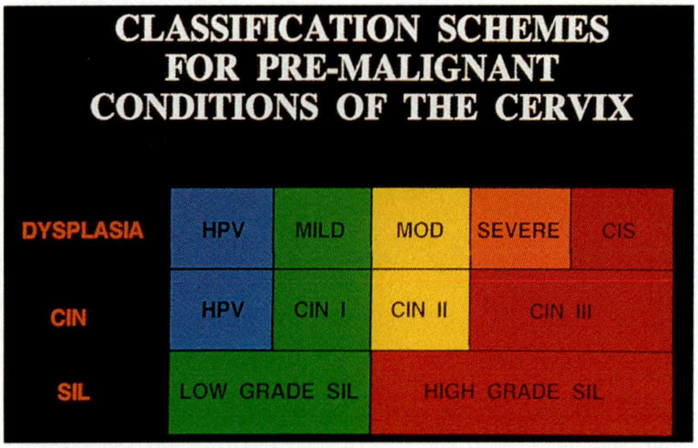

3.17 Diagram representing classification schemes for premalignant cervical lesions.

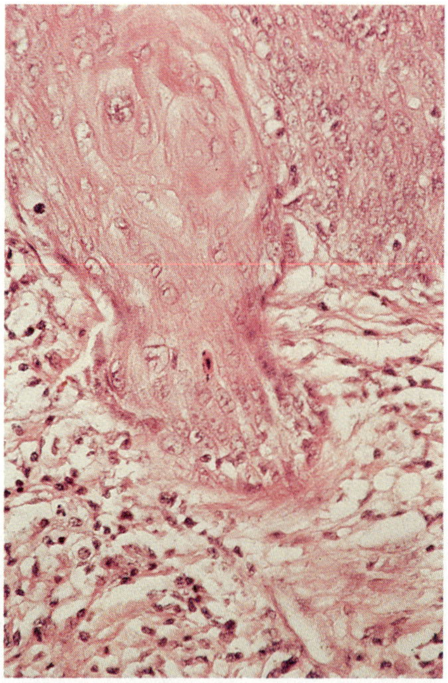

3.18 Cervical biopsy demonstrating minimal superficial invasion corresponding with a FIGO Stage Ia1. The invasive tumor brakes through the basement membrane and has an increased amount of cytoplasm with eosinophilia.

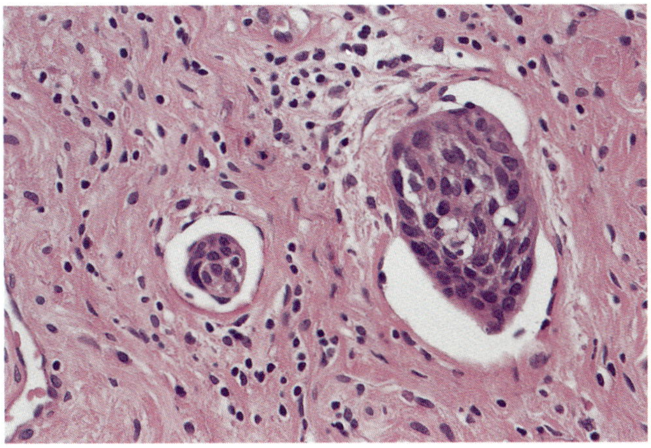

3.19 Vascular space involvement in squamous carcinoma of the cervix. The larger tumor fragment on the right is adherent to the vascular wall.

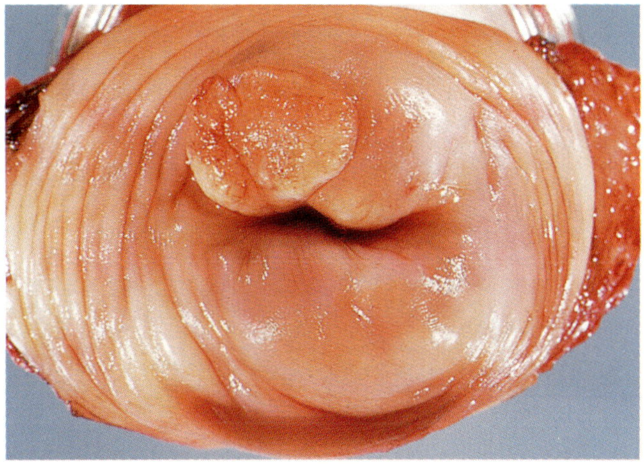

3.20 Gross view demonstrating exophytic invasive squamous cell carcinoma of the cervix.

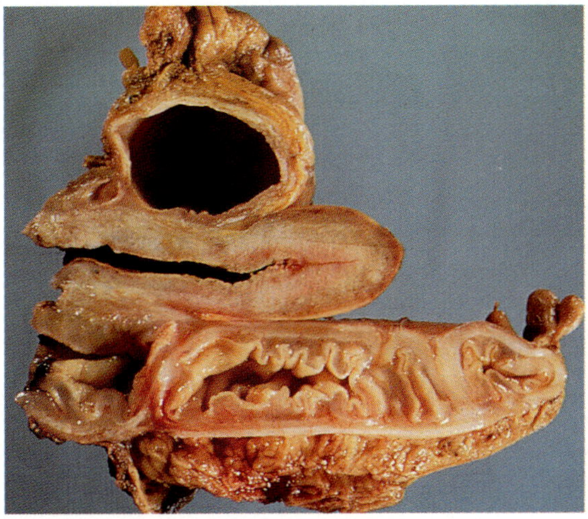

3.21 Sagittal cross-section of pelvic exenteration for recurrent cervical carcinoma. The tumor infiltrated the anterior wall of the cervix into the bladder.

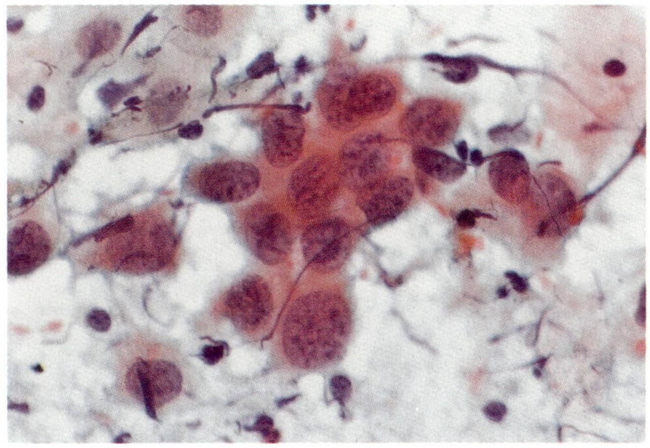

3.22 Cervical smear from a patient with invasive squamous cell carcinoma. The nuclei are hyperchromatic and irregular with markedly increased nuclear size.

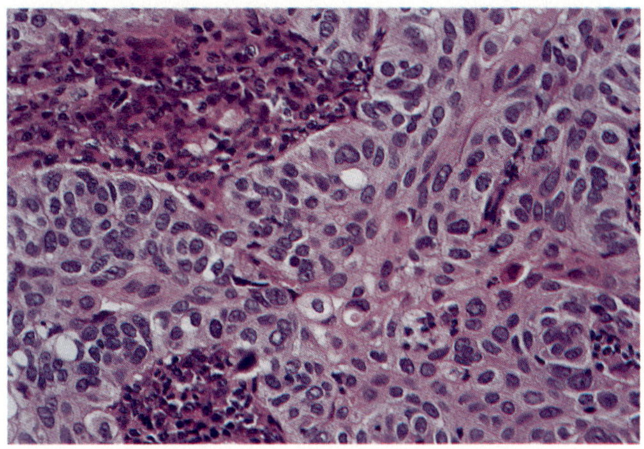

3.23 Large cell nonkeratinizing squamous carcinoma of the cervix.

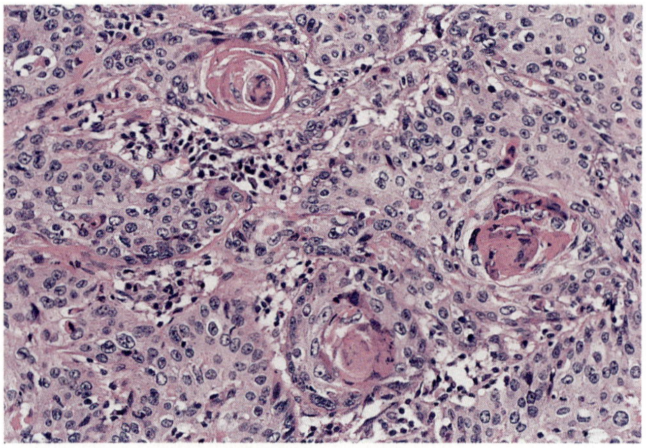

3.24 Keratinizing squamous cell carcinoma of the cervix demonstrating keratin pearl formation.

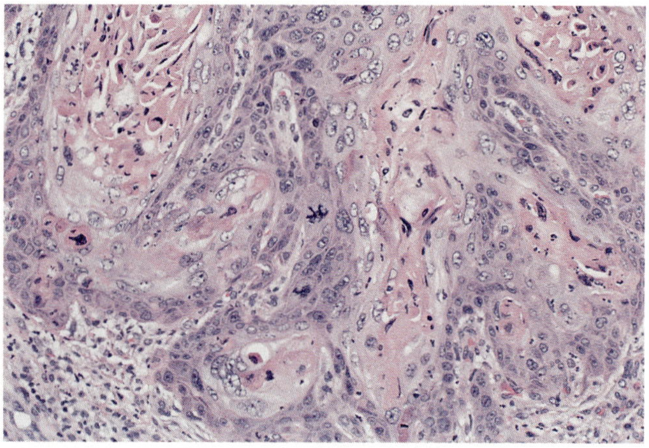

3.25 Warty squamous cell carcinoma of the cervix exhibiting HPV changes.

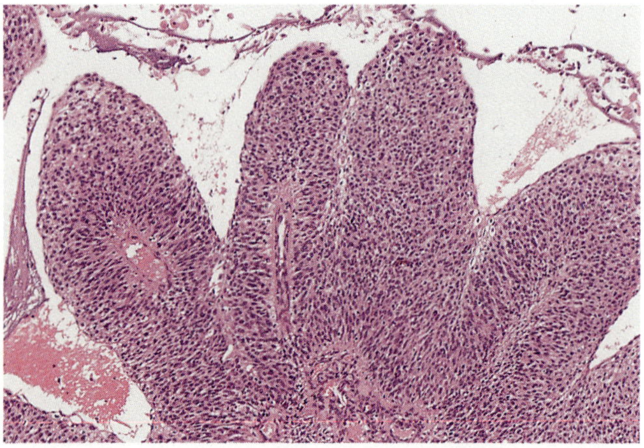

3.26 Papillary squamous carcinoma of the cervix demonstrating finger-like projections with a fibrovascular core.

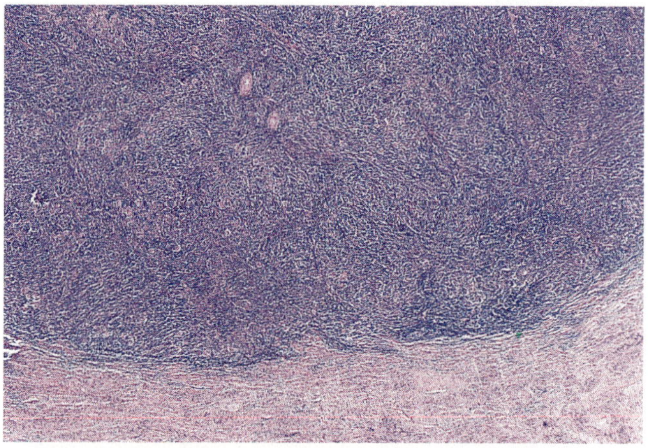

3.27 Lymphoepithelioma-like squamous carcinoma of the cervix showing a well-demarcated border.

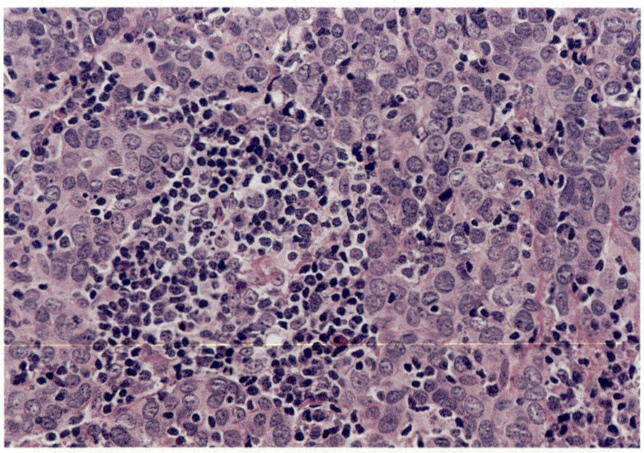

3.28 Higher-power view of lymphoepithelioma-like carcinoma of the cervix. There is a poorly differentiated epithelial tumor infiltrated with lymphocytes.

Glandular Lesions

The endocervical mucosa is composed of mucinous epithelium of the müllerian type. Clusters of these cells or metaplastic cells are required for a satisfactory cervical smear (Figure 3-29). The endocervical crypts may become obstructed by metaplastic epithelium, forming nabothian cysts (Figure 3-30). Endocervical tunnel clusters may extend into the fibromuscular stroma (Figure 3-31) and need to be distinguished from minimum deviation adenocarcinoma.[20,51]

Microglandular hyperplasia[64,68] is usually associated with pregnancy or the use of oral contraceptives, although this concept has recently been challenged.[26] It is a benign proliferation with a characteristic pattern (Figure 3-32). This may also occur in areas of adenosis and may be confused with adenocarcinoma.[70]

Mesonephric duct remnants[23] are found deep in the fibromuscular stroma of the cervix (Figures 3-33 and 3-34). They can be confused with adenosis and adenocarcinoma. In some cases of mesonephric duct hyperplasia a moderate degree of nuclear atypia may be noted. Tubal (Figure 3-35) and epidermoid (Figure 3-36) metaplasia are often seen in the cervix.[41] Endometriosis can occur on the cervix (Figure 3-37) and presents in the same fashion as in other sites. Blue-domed cysts containing old hemorrhagic fluid can be seen clinically. Mucosal endometriosis may occur after operative trauma such as a cone biopsy. Endocervical polyps are hyperplastic proliferations of the endocervical glands and stroma (Figures 3-38 and 39). They are a result of chronic inflammation, and the surface often undergoes squamous metaplasia. Müllerian papillomas of the cervix are polypoid lesions lined with flattened cuboidal epithelium (Figure 3-40).

Endocervical glandular atypia includes reactive epithelial changes that may be related to varied etiologies, including inflammatory and reparative alterations and epithelial alterations secondary to radiation. Also included in this category is the Arias-Stella change involving endocervical epithelium (Figure 3-41).[49] The term endocervical glandular dysplasia includes those glandular epithelial lesions characterized by nuclear atypia that is not as severe as that noted in adenocarcinoma in situ. These lesions have not been well studied and their biologic significance has not been established.

Adenocarcinoma in situ (Figure 3-42) often extends from normal endocervical glands and occurs at the same depth.[21,42,44,55] Adenocarcinoma of the endocervix (Figures 3-43 and 3-44) is being reported with increasing frequency.[38,61] Some studies suggest that this cell type is also related to HPV infection.[63] The most common type is mucinous adenocarcinoma. The mucinous differentiation can be of müllerian (Figure 3-45) or intestinal (Figure 3-46) type. An extremely well differentiated form of endocervical adenocarcinoma (Figure 3-47) has been referred to as "adenoma malignum" or "minimum deviation adenocarcinoma".[25,52,53] Endometrioid variants (Figures 3-48 and 3-49) have also been described.[71] Villoglandular adenocarcinoma cervix (Figures 3-50, 3-51 and 3-52) is a recently described pattern that appears to have a favorable prognosis.[30,68] The tumor is often superficial with little or no invasion. It resembles villous adenomas seen in the gastrointestinal tract.

Clear cell adenocarcinoma of the cervix (Figures 3-53 and 3-54) is a rare pattern found in some diethylstilbestrol (DES)-exposed offspring. The clear cell pattern is actually only one of three patterns, the others being papillary and tubulocystic. This tumor is associated with, but has not been conclusively shown to arise from, adenosis. It occurs more often with the tuboendometrial type of adenosis.

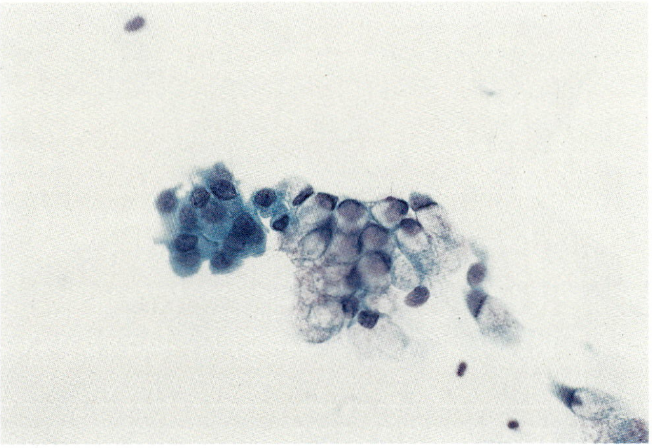

3.29 Cervical cytologic smear demonstrating endocervical cells (right side) and metaplastic cells (left side).

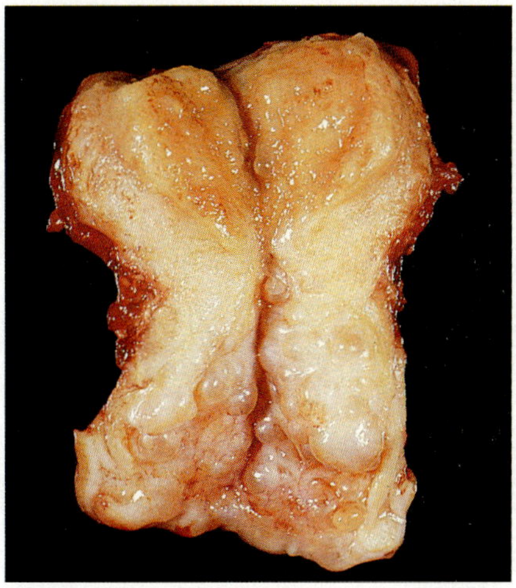

3.30 Hysterectomy specimen containing numerous nabothian cysts of the cervix.

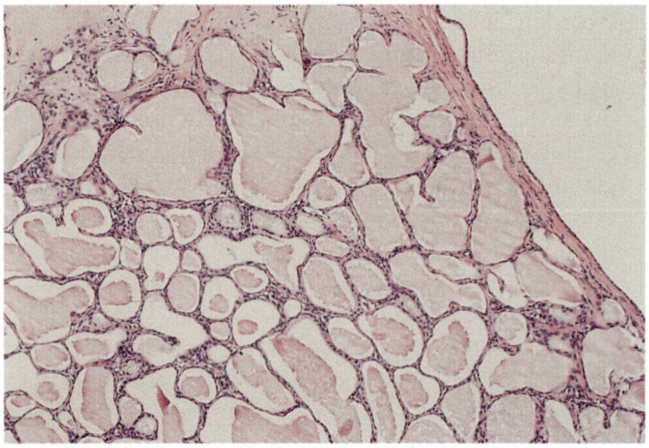

3.31 Endocervical tunnel clusters characterized by well-circumscribed aggregates of crowded glands with cystic dilatation and a flattened lining.

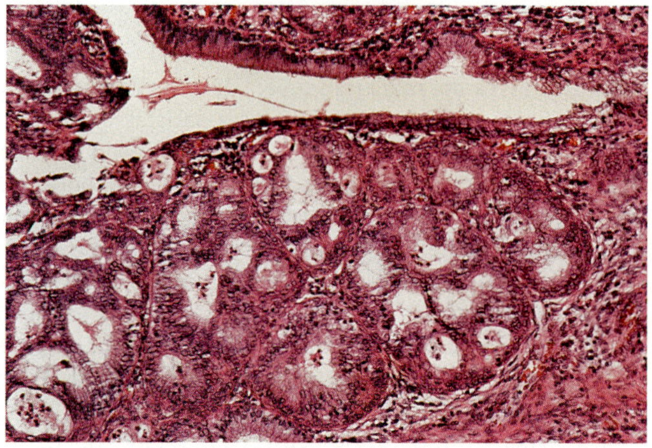

3.32 Microglandular hyperplasia characterized by small crowded glands with no significant nuclear atypia.

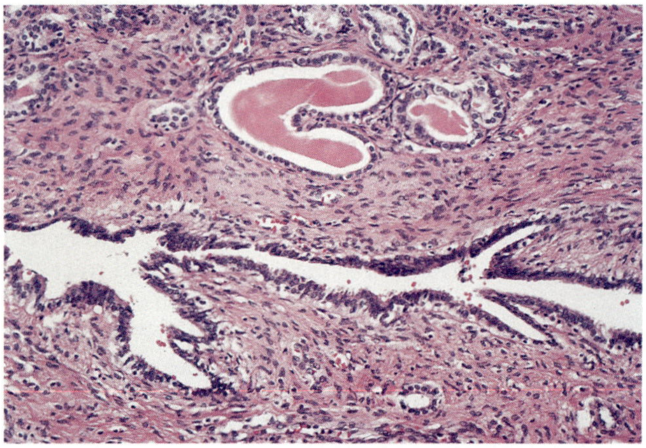

3.33 Mesonephric duct remnants showing tubular and ductal structures in the fibromuscular stroma of the cervix.

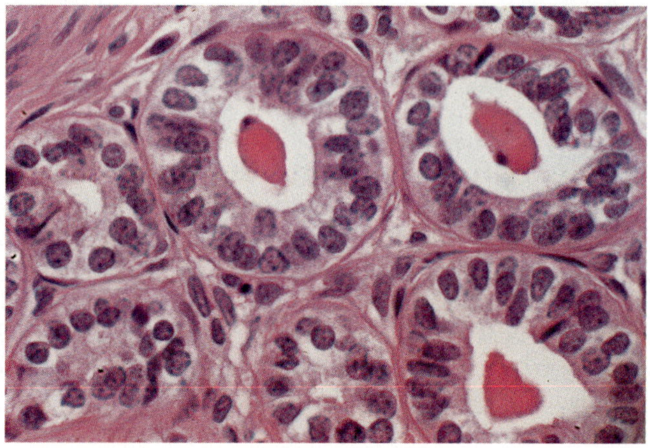

3.34 Higher-power view of mesonephric duct remnants showing the bland round nuclei and eosinophilic secretions in the lumen.

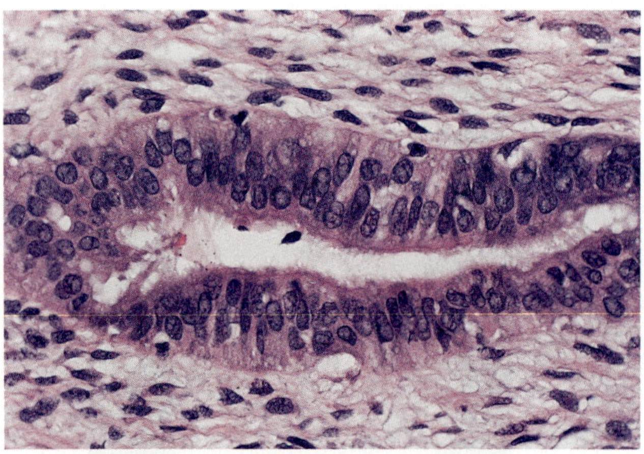

3.35 Tubal metaplasia of the cervix demonstrating ciliated epithelium with pseudostatified nuclei.

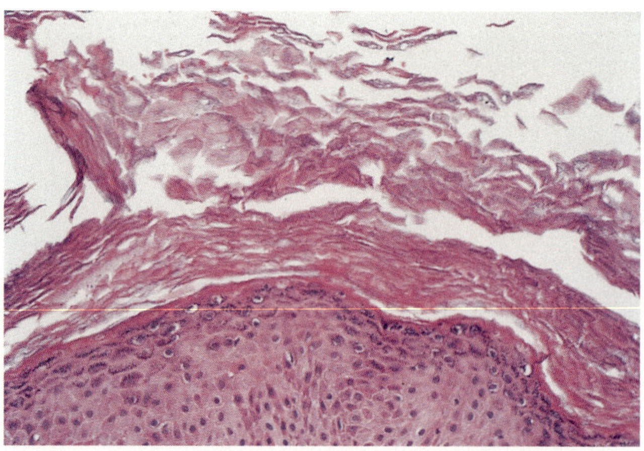

3.36 Epidermal metaplasia of the cervix characterized by a granular layer in the upper portion of the cervix with overlying hyperkeratosis.

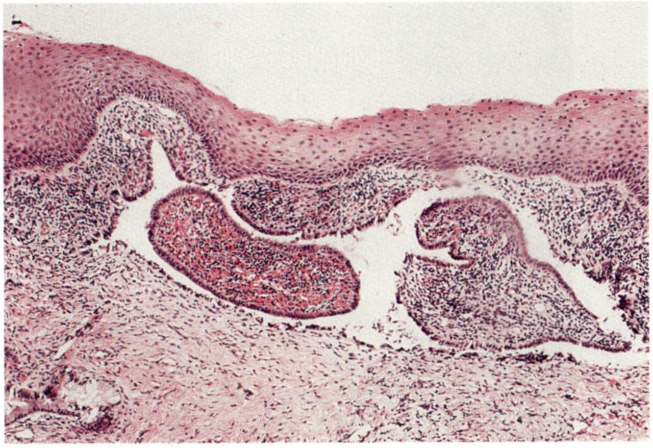

3.37 Endometriosis of the cervix with overlying squamous epithelium.

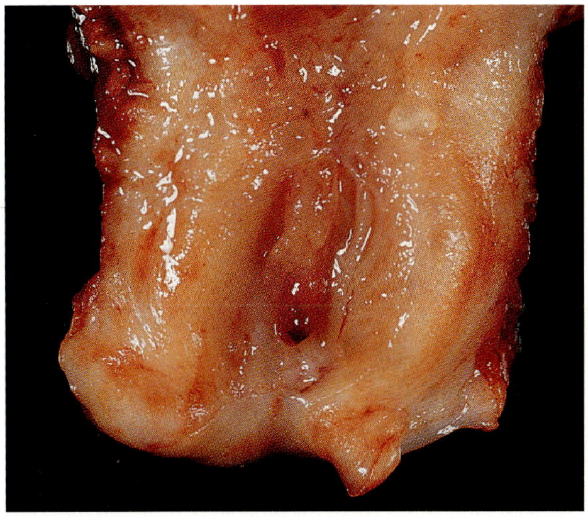

3.38 Gross view of an endocervical polyp.

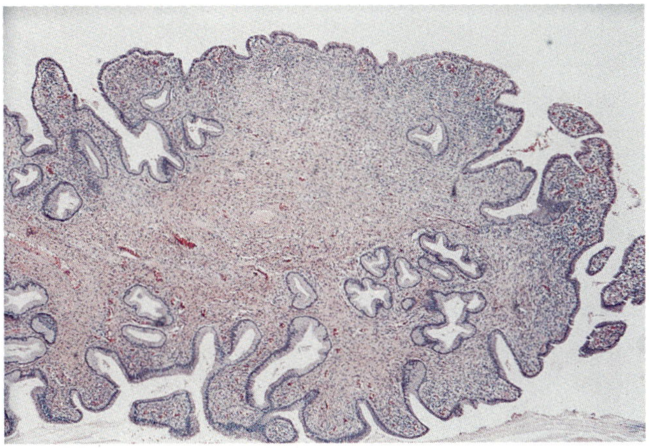

3.39 Endocervical polyp with cleftlike spaces and a chronic inflammatory infiltrate.

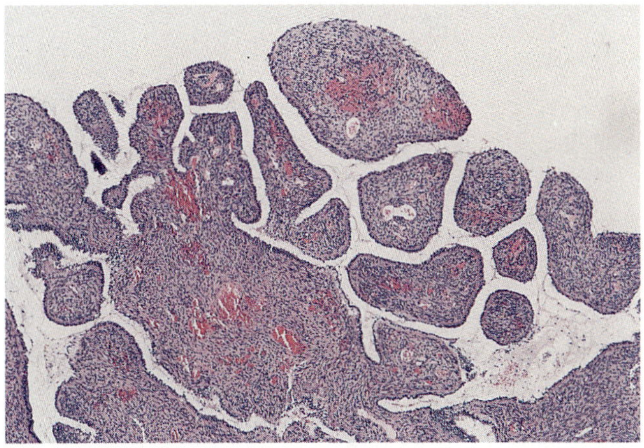

3.40 Müllerian papilloma of the cervix containing blunt papillary projections lined with bland müllerian epithelium and a fibrovascular stroma.

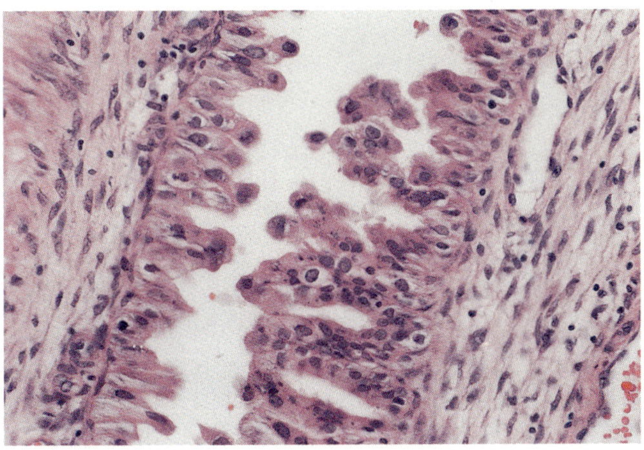

3.41 Arias-Stella reaction of the endocervix showing elongated glands with hobnail features.

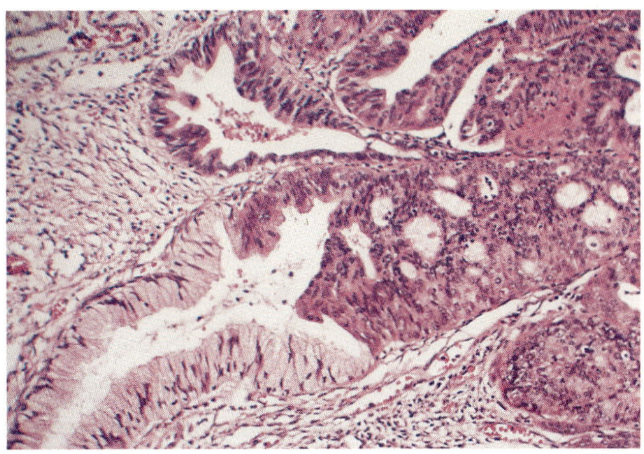

3.42 Adenocarcinoma in situ of the cervix partially involving an endocervical gland.

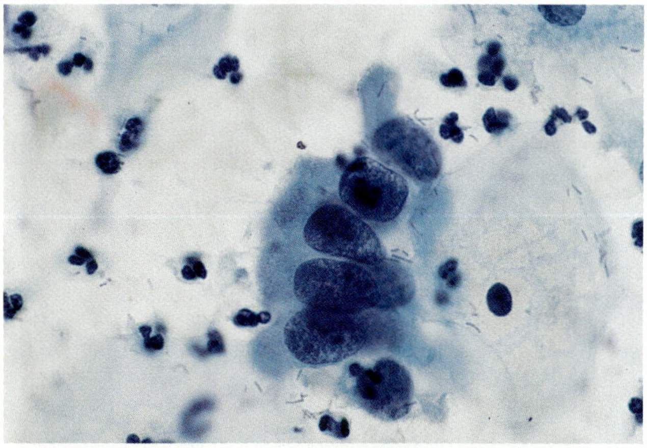

3.43 Cytologic smear of adenocarcinoma of the cervix. The cluster of malignant cells contains eccentric nuclei with hyperchromatism.

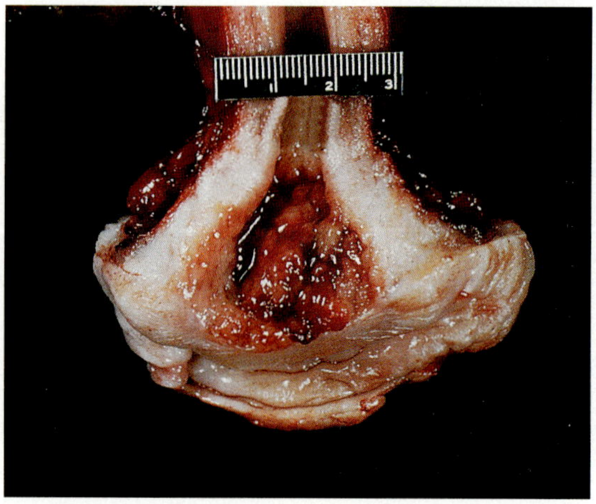

3.44 Gross view of invasive adenocarcinoma of the cervix demonstrating a polypoid tumor in the endocervical canal.

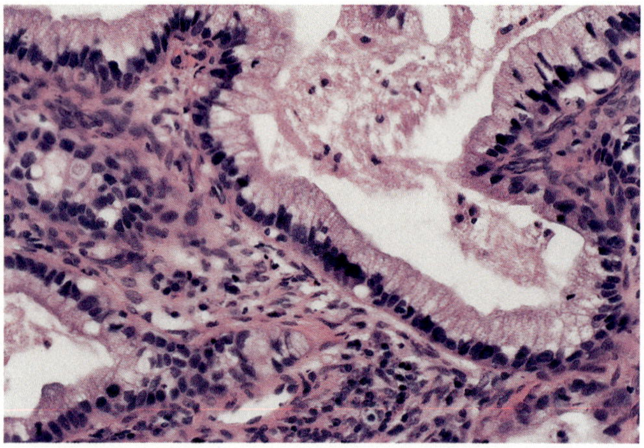

3.45 Adenocarcinoma of the cervix with an endocervical-type pattern. The epithelium contains basally oriented nuclei with mucinous epithelium.

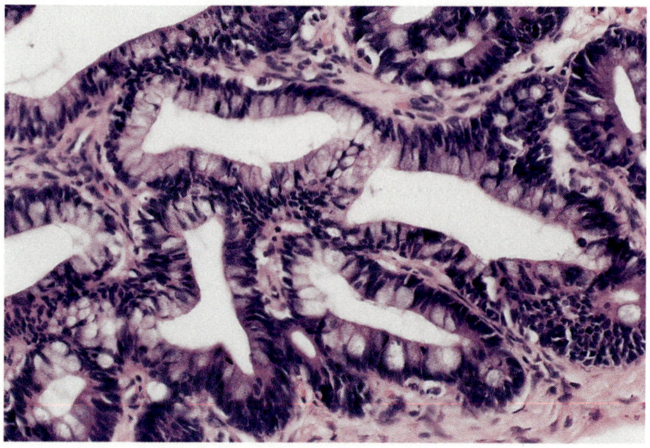

3.46 Adenocarcinoma of the endocervix with intestinal-type differentiation demonstrating numerous goblet cells.

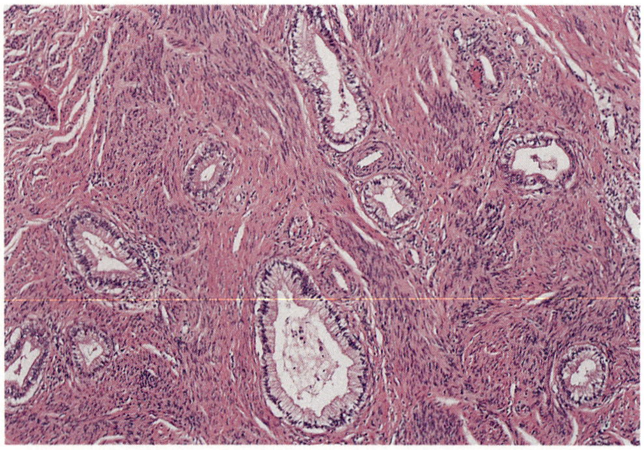

3.47 Minimum deviation adenocarcinoma of the cervix demonstrating well-differentiated mucinous adenocarcinoma infiltrating the cervical stroma with a minimal stromal response to the tumor.

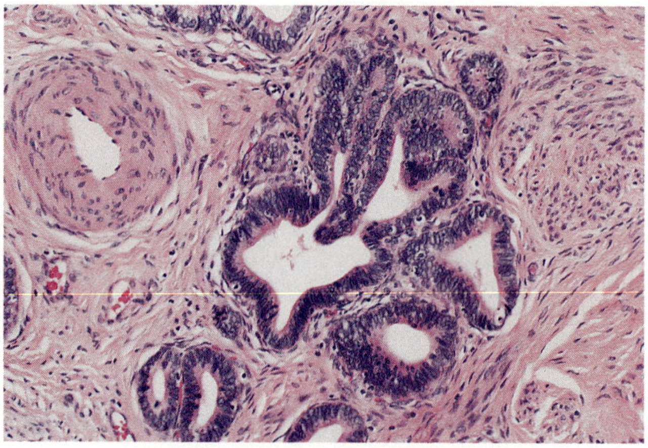

3.48 Minimum deviation adenocarcinoma of the cervix with endometrioid-type differentiation.

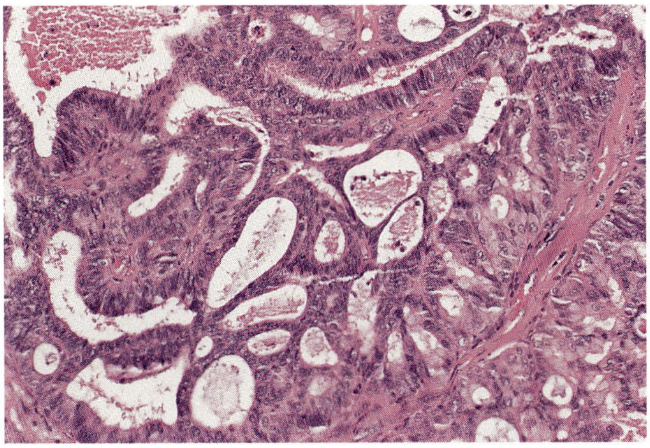

3.49 Adenocarcinoma of the cervix with endometrioid-type differentiation.

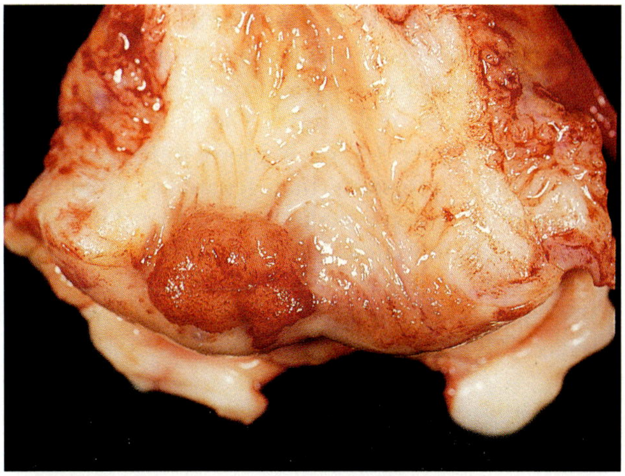

3.50 Gross view of villoglandular adenocarcinoma of the cervix demonstrating a polypoid, well-differentiated tumor.

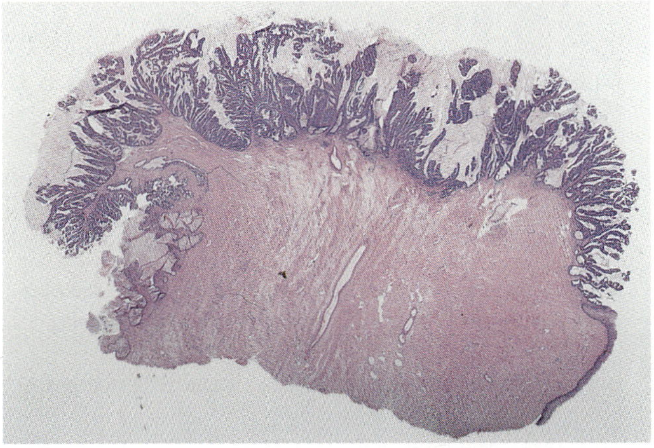

3.51 Low-power photomicrograph of villoglandular adenocarcinoma of the cervix.

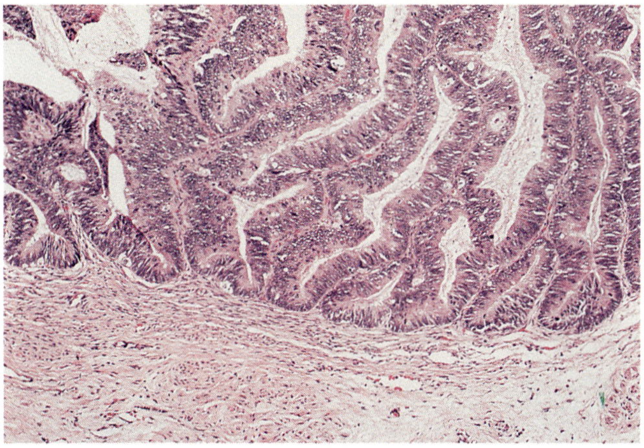

3.52 Villoglandular adenocarcinoma of the cervix showing a stromal interface with no destructive invasion.

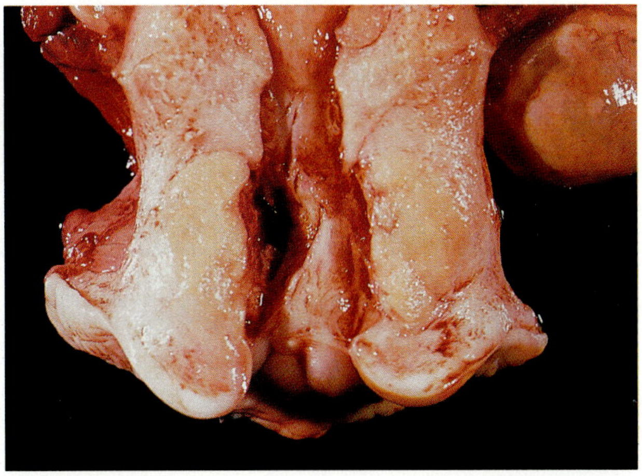

3.53 Gross view of clear cell carcinoma of the cervix showing deep cervical stromal involvement.

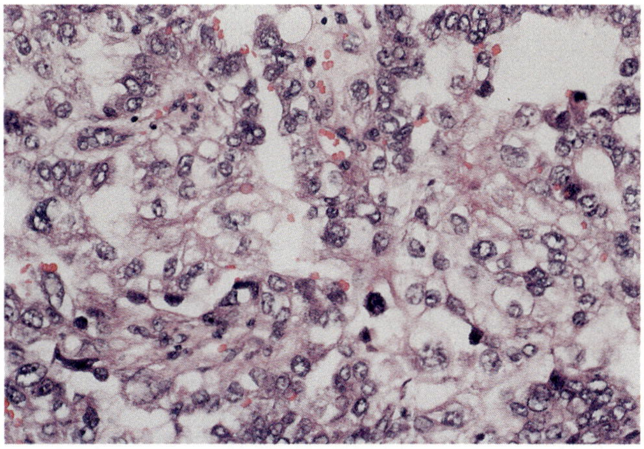

3.54 Clear cell adenocarcinoma of the cervix.

Other Epithelial Tumors

Serous papillary adenocarcinoma of the cervix (Figures 3-55 and 3-56) has a pattern similar to that of serous adenocarcinoma of the ovary. Glassy cell carcinoma of the cervix (Figure 3-57) is a poorly differentiated carcinoma with cytoplasm that resembles ground glass. Electron microscopic studies suggest that this lesion is a poorly differentiated adenosquamous carcinoma.[58] Adenoid cystic (Figure 3-58) and adenoid basal (Figures 3-59 and 3-60) carcinomas may also be seen in the cervix.[22]

Carcinoid tumors (Figure 3-61) and small cell carcinomas (Figure 3-62) of the cervix are recognized as including a heterologous group of tumors. Small cell carcinomas are examples of high-grade neuroendocrine carcinomas that resemble small cell carcinoma of the lung.[9,24,59] These tumors should be distinguished from small cell nonkeratinizing squamous cell carcinoma.

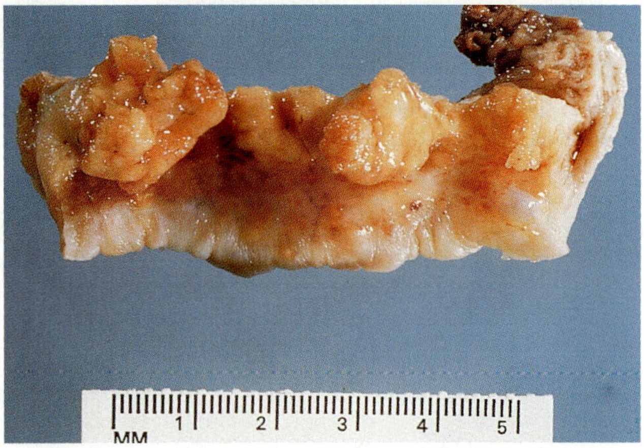

3.55 Gross view of serous papillary adenocarcinoma of the cervix.

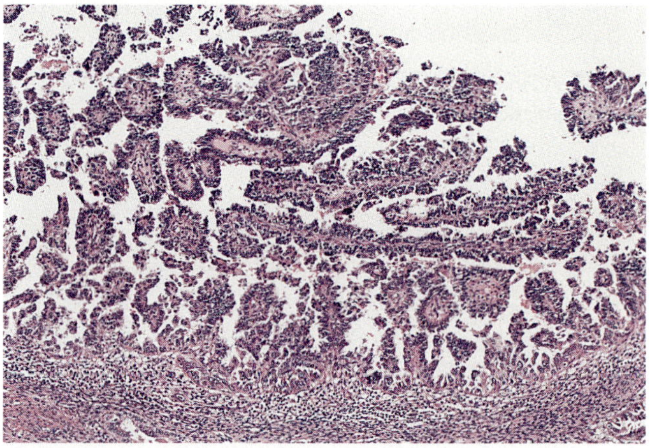

3.56 Serous papillary adenocarcinoma of the cervix showing fibrovascular cores lined with a papillary adenocarcinoma.

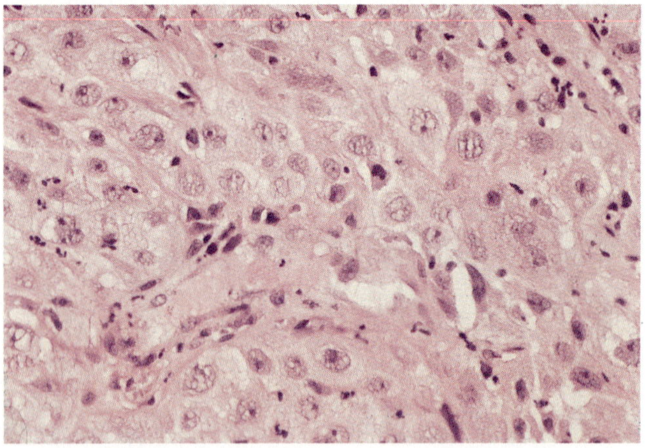

3.57 Glassy cell carcinoma of the cervix demonstrating pleomorphic nuclei with eosinophilic cytoplasm having a ground-glass appearance.

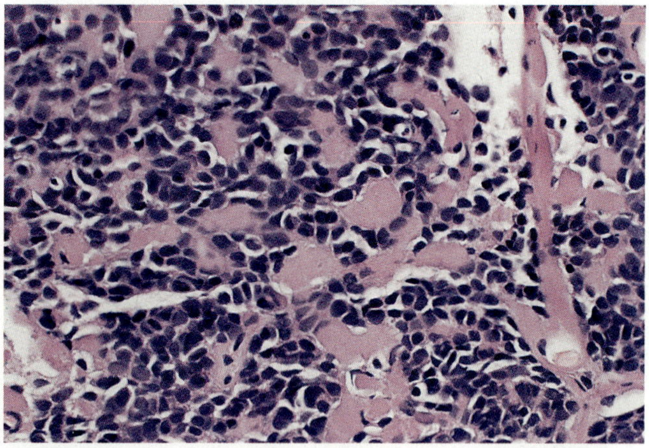

3.58 Adenoid cystic carcinoma of the cervix demonstrating a cribriform pattern with hyalinized stroma.

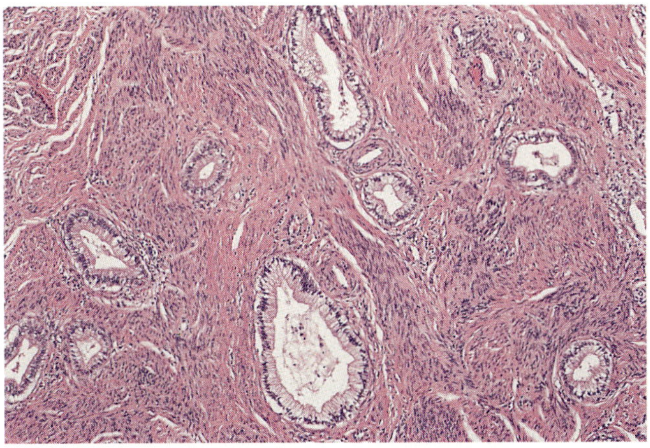

3.59 Adenoid basal carcinoma of the cervix showing a mixture of glandular and basaloid proliferation.

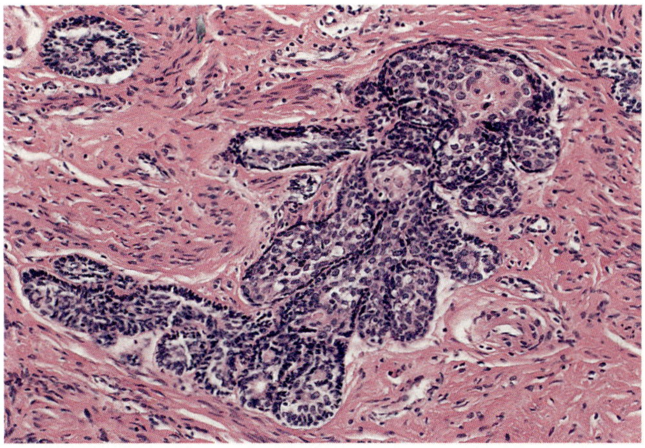

3.60 Adenoid basal cell carcinoma of the cervix showing basaloid cells with focal squamous differentiation.

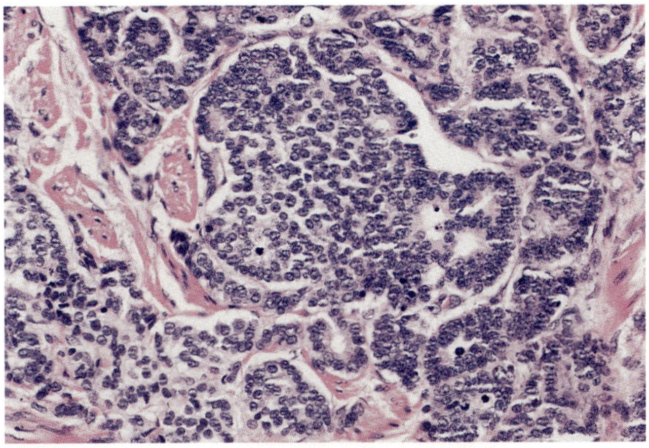

3.61 Carcinoid tumor of the cervix showing an insular pattern with focal glandular differentiation.

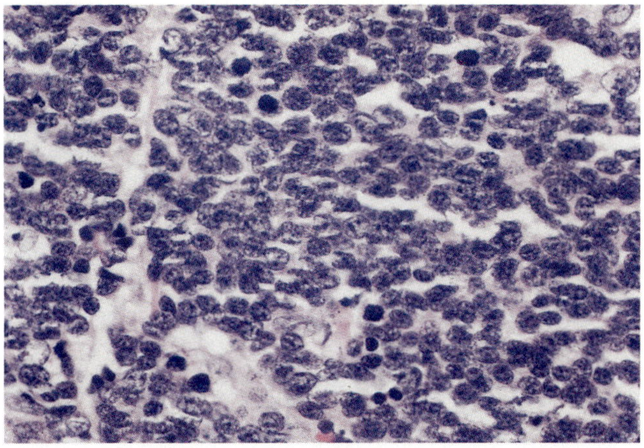

3.62 Small cell carcinoma of the cervix of the neuroendocrine type.

MESENCHYMAL TUMORS

Decidual changes are commonly seen in the cervix during pregnancy (Figure 3-63). A variety of benign soft tissue tumors, including hemangiomas (Figure 3-64), occur in the cervix. Smooth muscle neoplasms of the cervix can consist of benign leiomyomas, leiomyomas with unusual variants, smooth muscle neoplasms of indeterminate malignant potential, and leiomyosarcomas. Leiomyosarcomas (Figures 3-65 and 3-66) are rare in the cervix, but a smooth muscle neoplasm of the cervix is more likely to be malignant than a smooth muscle neoplasm of the uterus. Mitotic counts are necessary to determine the biologic behavior of these tumors. A complete discussion of this is presented in the section under mesenchymal tumors of the uterine corpus. Other sarcomas of the cervix include stromal sarcoma (Figure 3-67), embryonal rhabdomyosarcoma (sarcoma botryoides) (Figures 3-68 to 3-70), and alveolar soft-part sarcoma.[19,56,62]

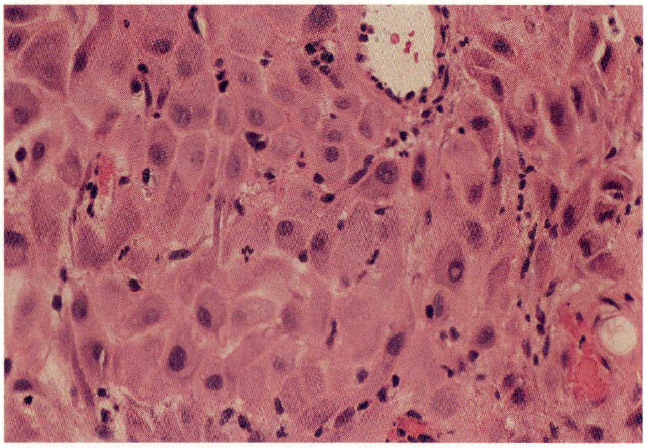

3.63 Decidual reaction of the cervix revealing abundant eosinophilic cytoplasm.

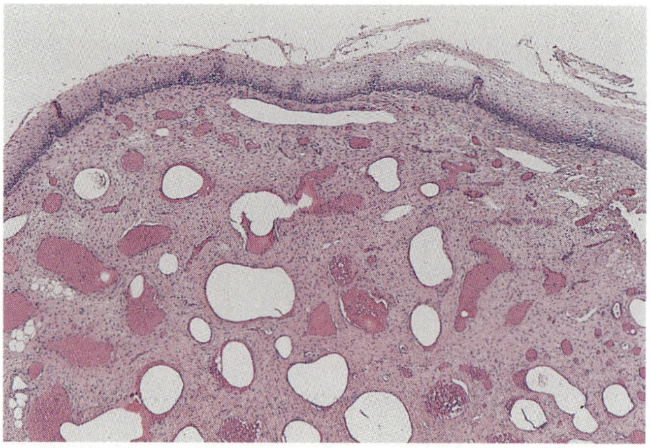

3.64 Hemangioma of the cervix with numerous dilated vascular spaces.

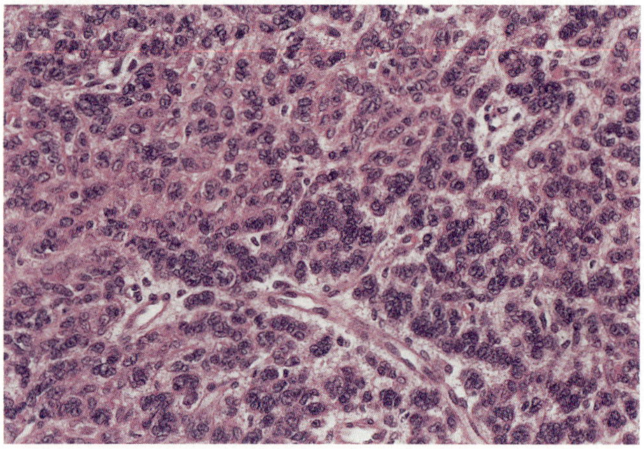

3.65 Epithelioid leiomyosarcoma of the cervix.

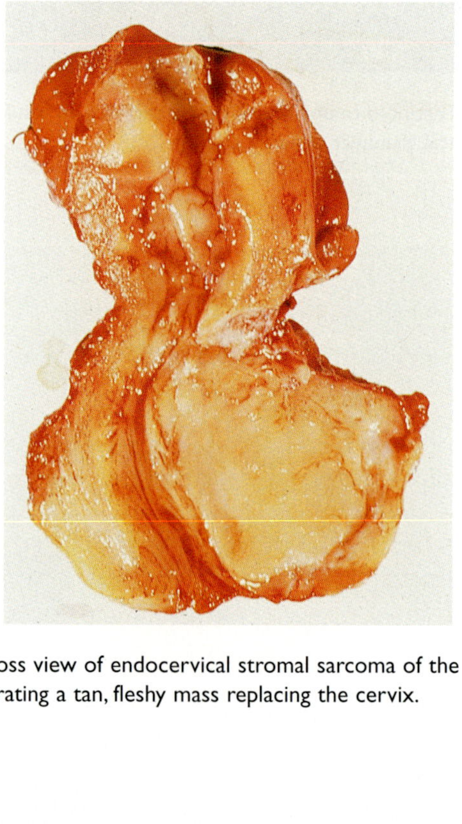

3.66 Gross view of endocervical stromal sarcoma of the cervix demonstrating a tan, fleshy mass replacing the cervix.

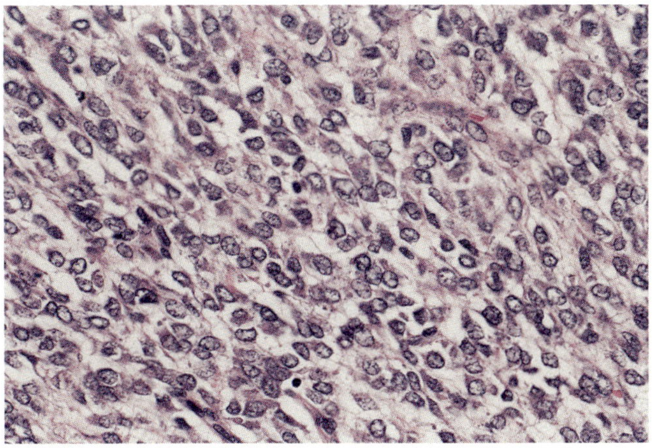

3.67 Endocervical stromal sarcoma characterized by spindle cell proliferation lacking specific differentiation.

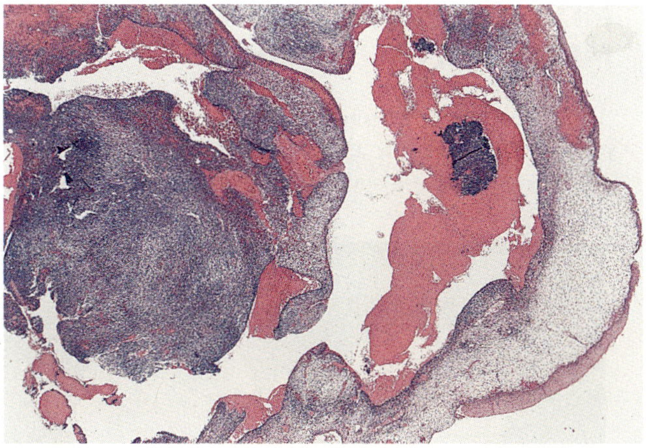

3.68 Low-power photomicrograph of sarcoma botryoides of the cervix.

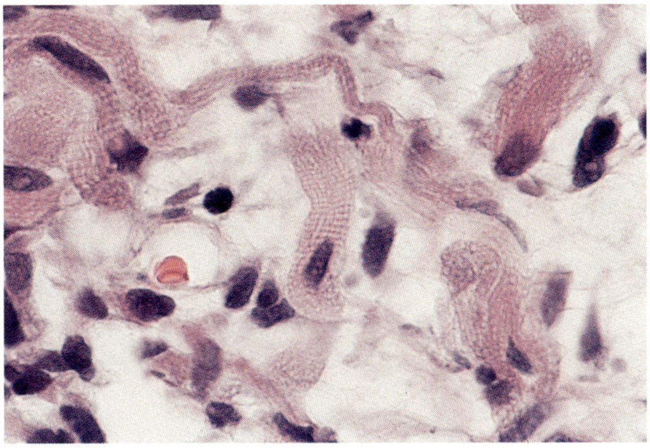

3.69 Sarcoma botryoides of the cervix with rhabdomyoblastic differentiation.

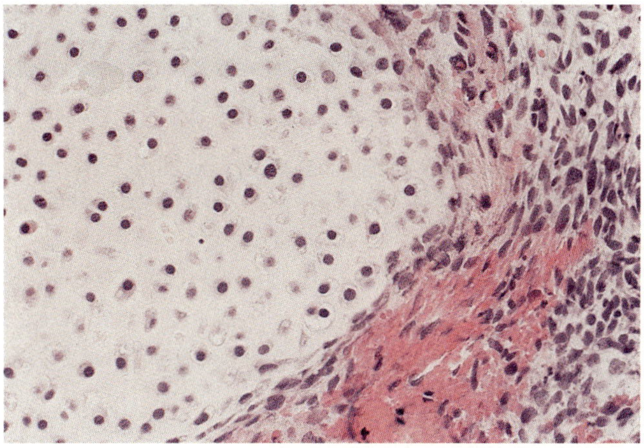

3.70 Sarcoma botryoides of the cervix showing focal cartilaginous differentiation.

MIXED EPITHELIAL AND MESODERMAL TUMORS

Adenofibroma is a benign tumor, usually papillary, composed of both glands and a fibrous stroma. It is seen in other areas of the female genital tract, but its malignant counterpart, adenosarcoma, is rarely seen in the cervix.[30] Malignant mesodermal mixed tumors (carcinosarcomas) (Figures 3-71 and 72) are tumors composed of malignant epithelium (usually adenocarcinoma) and a sarcoma that may be heterologous and/or homologous.

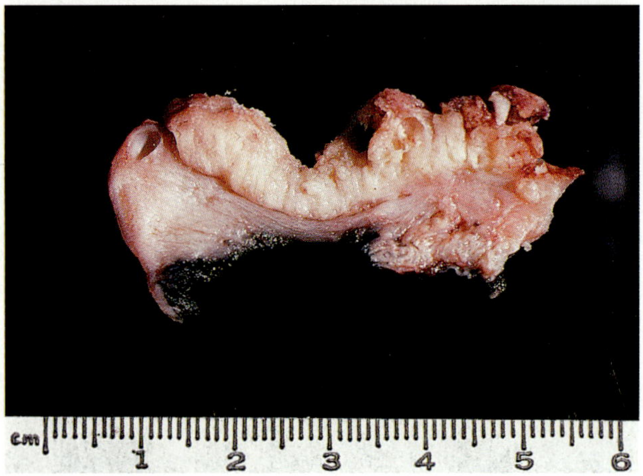

3.71 Gross view of a malignant mixed mesodermal tumor (carcinosarcoma) of the cervix. The tumor has a fleshy, polypoid appearance.

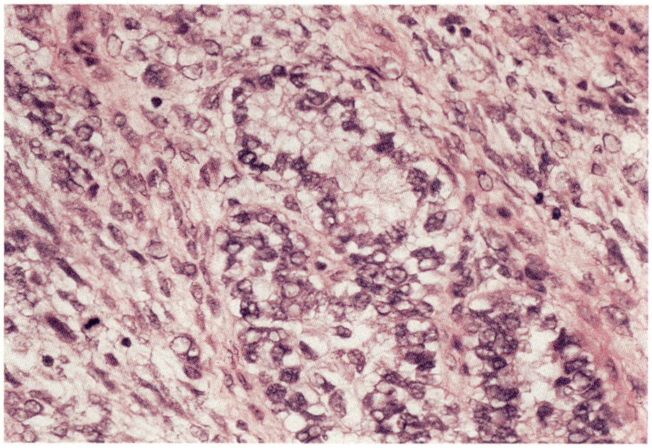

3.72 Malignant mixed müllerian tumor of the cervix showing a mixture of adenocarcinoma and undifferentiated sarcoma.

MISCELLANEOUS TUMORS

Malignant melanoma of the cervix (Figure 3-73) can also be a primary lesion.[40] On mucosal surfaces, such as the cervix and vagina, a definite Clark level cannot be ascertained, since there is a not a true papillary dermis. In these sites, depth of invasion is used as a prognostic factor. Lymphomas of the cervix (Figures 3-74 and 3-75) are usually the result of a metastatic presentation; however, primary lymphomas of the cervix have been described.[10,97]

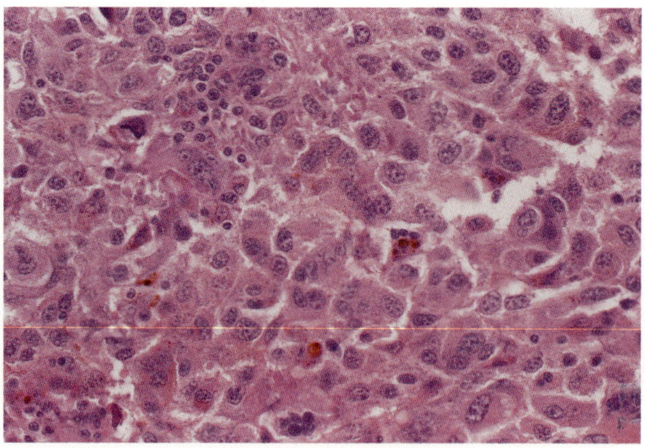

3.73 Malignant melanoma of the cervix with markedly pleomorphic cells containing scattered melanin pigment.

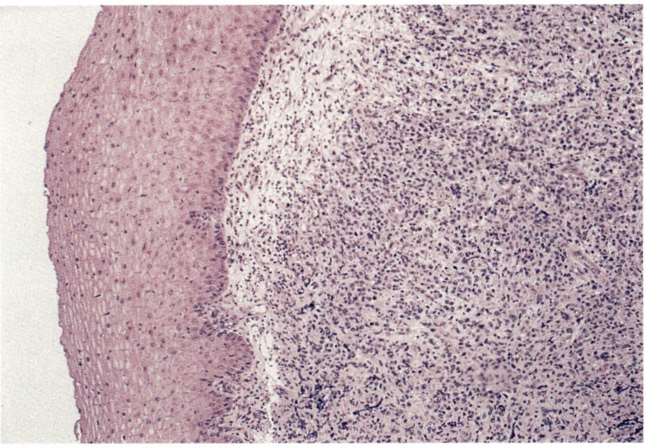

3.74 Primary lymphoma of the cervix showing a dense infiltration beneath the squamous epithelium.

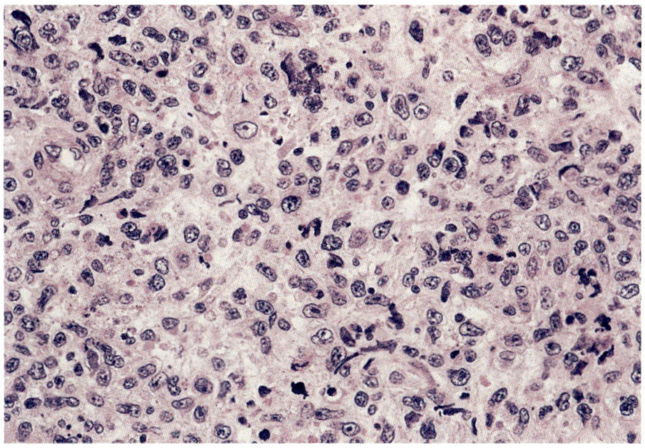

3.75 Large cell undifferentiated lymphoma of the cervix.

SECONDARY TUMORS

Metastatic carcinoma to the cervix[33] is most commonly that from either endometrium, fallopian tube, or ovary. Metastases from extragenital sites such as the breast (Figure 3-76), colon, and stomach have also been described.

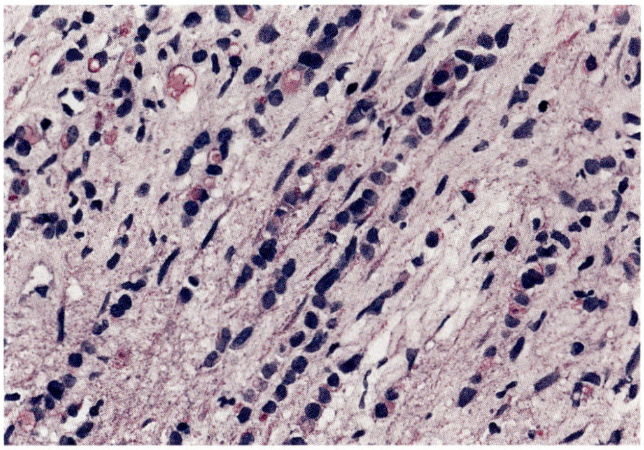

3.76 Metastatic lobular carcinoma of the breast showing the characteristic single file pattern with scattered signet-ring cells.

World Health Organization (WHO) Histologic Classification of Tumors of the Uterine Cervix[8]

(with associated systematized nomenclature of medicine [SNOMED] codes)

I. Epithelial Tumors and Related Lesions	**SNOMED**
A. Squamous lesions	
1. Squamous papilloma	80520
2. Condyloma acuminatum	76720
3. Squamous metaplasia	73220
4. Transitional metaplasia	73260
5. Squamous atypia	69700
6. Squamous intraepithelial lesions (dysplasia–carcinoma in situ, cervical intraepithelial neoplasia [CIN])	
a. Mild dysplasia (CIN I)	74002
b. Moderate dysplasia (CIN II)	74007
c. Severe dysplasia (CIN III)	74008
d. Carcinoma in situ (CIN III)	80702
7. Squamous cell carcinoma	80703
a. Keratinizing	80713
b. Nonkeratinizing	80723
c. Verrucous	80513
d. Warty (condylomatous)	
e. Papillary	80523
f. Lymphoepithelioma-like carcinoma	80823
B. Glandular lesions	
1. Endocervical polyp	76800
2. Müllerian papilloma	
3. Glandular atypia	
4. Glandular dysplasia	74000
5. Adenocarcinoma in situ	81402
6. Adenocarcinoma	81403
a. Mucinous adenocarcinoma	84803
(1) Endocervical type	
(2) Intestinal type	81443
b. Endometrioid adenocarcinoma	83803
c. Clear cell adenocarcinoma	83103
d. Serous adenocarcinoma	84413
e. Mesonephric adenocarcinoma	91103
C. Other epithelial tumors	
1. Adenosquamous carcinoma	85603
2. Glassy cell carcinoma	
3. Adenoid cystic carcinoma	82003
4. Adenoid basal carcinoma	80923
5. Carcinoid tumor	82403
6. Small cell carcinoma	80413
7. Undifferentiated carcinoma	80203

II. Mesenchymal Tumors	
A. Leiomyoma	88900
B. Leiomyosarcoma	88903
C. Endocervical stromal sarcoma	89303
D. Sarcoma botryoides (embryonal rhabdomyosarcoma)	89103
E. Endometrioid stromal sarcoma	89303
F. Alveolar soft-part sarcoma	95813
G. Others	
III. Mixed Epithelial and Mesenchymal Tumors	
A. Adenofibroma	90130
B. Adenomyoma	
1. Atypical polypoid adenomyoma (variant)	
C. Adenosarcoma	89333
D. Malignant mesodermal mixed tumor (malignant müllerian mixed tumor, carcinosarcoma)	89513
E. Wilms tumor	89603
IV. Miscellaneous Tumors	
A. Melanocytic nevus	87200
B. Blue nevus	87800
C. Malignant melanoma	87203
D. Lymphoma and leukemia	
E. Tumors of germ cell type	
1. Yolk sac tumor (endodermal sinus tumor)	90713
2. Dermoid cyst (mature cystic teratoma)	90840
V. Secondary Tumors	
VI. Tumor-Like Lesions	
A. Endocervical glandular hyperplasia	
B. Cysts	33400
C. Tunnel cluster	
D. Microglandular hyperplasia	72480
E. Arias-Stella change	79430
F. Mesonephric remnants	26370
G. Mesonephric hyperplasia	72580
H. Ciliated cell metaplasia	
I. Intestinal metaplasia	73320
J. Epidermal metaplasia	73220
K. Endometriosis	76500
L. Ectopic decidua	
M. Placental site nodule and plaque	
N. Stromal polyp (pseudosarcoma botryoides)	
O. Postoperative spindle cell nodule	
P. Traumatic (amputation) neuroma	49770
Q. Retention of fetal glial tissue	
R. Lymphoma-like lesions	72290

TNM Staging Classification for Cervical Carcinoma

International Union Against Cancer (UICC)

Primary Tumor (T)—see corresponding FIGO stages

TX	Primary tumor cannot be assessed
T0	No evidence of primary tumor
Tis	Carcinoma in situ (Stage 0)
T1a, 1b	
T2a, 2b	
T3a, 3b	
T4a, 4b	

Nodal Involvement (N)

NX	Minimum requirements to assess the regional nodes cannot be met	
N0	No involvement of regional nodes	
N1	Evidence of regional node involvement	
	N1a	Metastasis in one or two regional lymph nodes below the common iliac artery
	N1b	Metastasis in three or more regional lymph nodes below the common iliac artery
	N1c	Metastasis in any lymph node along the common iliac artery
N2	Involvement of lumboaortic nodes	

Distant Metastasis (M)

MX	Minimum requirements to assess the presence of distant metastasis cannot be met	
M0	No (known) distant metastasis	
M1	Distant metastasis present	
	M1a	Distant metastasis in para-aortic lymph nodes below the diaphragm only
	M1b	Distant metastasis in other sites (specify)

Residual Tumor (R)—postsurgical treatment

R0	No residual tumor
R1	Microscopic residual tumor
R2	Macroscopic residual tumor (specify site)

Stage Grouping of Cervical Carcinoma

The International Federation of Gynecology and Obstetrics (FIGO)
International Union Against Cancer (UICC)
American Joint Committee on Cancer (AJCC)

STAGE	TNM		
Stage 0	Tis	N0	M0
Stage IA	T1a	N0	M0
Stage IB	T1b	N0	M0
Stage IIA	T2a	N0	M0
Stage IIB	T2b	N0	M0
Stage IIIA	T3a	N0	M0
Stage IIIB	T1	N1	M0
	T2	N1	M0
	T3a	N1	M0
	T3b	Any N	M0
Stage IVA	T4	Any N	M0
Stage IVB	Any T	Any N	M1

FIGO Staging Classification for Cervical Carcinoma

The International Federation of Gynecology and Obstetrics (FIGO)

Stage 0 Carcinoma in situ, intraepithelial carcinoma

Stage I The carcinoma is strictly confined to the cervix (extension to the corpus should be disregarded)

- Stage Ia Preclinical carcinomas of the cervix, those diagnosed microscopically
  - Stage Ia1 Minimal microscopically evident stromal invasion
  - Stage Ia2 Lesions detected microscopically that can be measured
    - (i) Tumor with invasive component 3 mm or less in depth, taken from the base of the epithelium, *and* 7 mm or less in horizontal spread
    - (ii) Tumor with invasive component more than 3 mm but not more than 5 mm in depth, taken from the base of the epithelium, *and* 7 mm or less in horizontal spread.
- Stage Ib Lesions of greater dimensions than Stage Ia2 whether seen clinically or not. Preformed space involvement should not alter the stag ing but should be specifically recorded to determine whether it should affect treatment decisions in the future.

Stage II The carcinoma extends beyond the cervix but has not extended to the pelvic wall. The carcinoma involves the vagina, but not as far as the lower third.

- Stage IIa No obvious parametrial involvement
- Stage IIb Obvious parametrial involvement

Stage III The carcinoma has extended to the pelvic wall. On rectal examination, there is no cancer-free space between the tumor and the pelvic wall. The tumor involves the lower third of the vagina. All cases with hydronephrosis or nonfunctioning kidney are included, unless they are due to another cause.

- Stage IIIa No extension to the pelvic wall
- Stage IIIb Extension to the pelvic wall, hydronephrosis, or nonfunctioning kidney

Stage IV The carcinoma has extended beyond the true pelvis or has clinically involved the mucosa of the bladder or rectum. A bullous edema as such does not permit a case to be allotted to Stage IV.

- Stage IVa Spread of the growth to adjacent organs
- Stage IVb Spread to distant organs

Notes to the FIGO Staging

Stage 0 comprises those cases with full-thickness involvement of epithelium with atypical cells but with no signs of invasion in to the stroma.

Stage Ia carcinoma should include minimal microscopically evident stromal invasion as well as small cancerous tumors of measurable size. Stage Ia should be subdivided into those lesions with minute foci or invasion visible only microscopically as Stage Ia1, and the macroscopically measurable microcarcinomas as Stage Ia2, in order to gain further knowledge of the clinical behavior of these lesions. The term Ib occult should be omitted.

The diagnosis of both Stage Ia1 and Stage Ia2 should be based on microscopic examination of removed tissue, preferably a cone, which must include the entire lesion. As noted above, the lower limit of Stage Ia2 should be that it can be measured macroscopically (even if dots need to be placed on the slide before measurement), and the upper limit of Ia2 is given by measurement of the two largest dimensions in any given section. The depth of invasion should not be more than 5 mm taken from the base of the epithelium, either surface or glandular, from which it originates. The second dimension, the horizontal spread, must not exceed 7 mm. Lesions of greater size should be staged as Ib. Vascular space involvement, either venous or lymphatic, should not alter the staging but should be specifically recorded, as it may affect treatment decisions in the future. As a rule, it is impossible to estimate clinically whether cancer of the cervix has extended to the corpus. Extension to the corpus should therefore be disregarded.

A patient with a growth fixed to the pelvic wall by a short and indurated, but not nodular, parametrium should be allotted to Stage IIb. The presence of tumor cells in lymphatics of the parametrium does not qualify for T2b. T2b is used only for grossly evident continuous invasion beyond the myometrium. It is impossible at clinical examination to decide whether a smooth and indurated parametrium is truly cancerous or only inflammatory. Therefore, the case should be placed in Stage III even if according to other findings the case should be allotted to Stage I or Stage II. "Frozen pelvis" is a clinical term meaning that tumor extends to the pelvic wall(s), i.e., T3b. Invasion of the rectal wall or bladder wall (not mucosa) is classified as T3a. Mucosal involvement is T4.

The presence of bullous edema as such should not qualify a case to be allotted to Stage IV. Ridges and furrows into the bladder wall should be interpreted as signs of submucous involvement of the bladder if they remain fixed to the growth at palpation (i.e., examination from the vagina or the rectum during cystoscopy). A cytologic finding of malignant cells in washings from the urinary bladder requires further examination and a biopsy from the wall of the bladder.

The Bethesda System for Reporting Cervical/Vaginal Cytologic Diagnoses[6]

Adequacy of the Specimen
- Satisfactory for evaluation
- Satisfactory for evaluation but limited by . . . (specify reason)
- Unsatisfactory for evaluation . . . (specify reason)

General Categorization (optional)
- Within normal limits
- Benign cellular changes: See descriptive diagnosis
- Epithelial cell abnormality: See descriptive diagnosis

Descriptive Diagnoses
Benign Cellular Changes
INFECTION
- *Trichomonas vaginalis*
- Fungal organisms morphologically consistent with *Candida* spp.
- Predominance of coccobacilli consistent with shift in vaginal flora
- Bacteria morphologically consistent with *Actinomyces* spp.
- Cellular changes associated with herpes simplex virus
- Other

REACTIVE CHANGES
- Reactive cellular changes associated with
  - Inflammation (includes typical repair)
  - Atrophy with inflammation ("atrophic vaginitis")
  - Radiation
  - Intrauterine contraceptive device (IUD)
  - Other

Epithelial Cell Abnormalities
SQUAMOUS CELL
- Atypical squamous cells of undetermined significance: Qualify[1]
- Low-grade squamous intraepithelial lesion (LSIL)
  - Encompassing HPV[2] mild dysplasia/CIN 1
- High-grade squamous intraepithelial lesion (HSIL)
  - Encompassing moderate dysplasia, severe dysplasia, and carcinoma inn situ (CIN 2 and 3)
- Squamous cell carcinoma

GLANDULAR CELL
- Endometrial cells, cytologically benign, in a postmenopausal woman
- Atypical glandular cells of undetermined significance: Qualify[1]
- Endocervical adenocarcinoma
- Endometrial adenocarcinoma
- Extrauterine adenocarcinoma
- Adenocarcinoma, not otherwise specified

Other Malignant Neoplasms: Specify

Hormonal Evaluation (applies to vaginal smears only)
- Hormonal pattern compatible with age and history
- Hormonal pattern incompatible with age and history: Specify
- Hormonal evaluation not possible due to: Specify

[1]Atypical squamous or glandular cells of undetermined significance should be further qualified as to whether a reactive or a premalignant/malignant process is favored.

[2]Cellular changes of human papillomavirus (HPV)—previously termed koilocytosis, koilocytotic atypia, or condylomatous atypia—are included in the category of low-grade squamous intraepithlial lesion.

Definitions and Criteria for Specimen Adequacy

"Satisfactory for evaluation" indicates that the specimen has all of the following:
- Appropriate labeling and identifying information
- Relevant clinical information
- Adequate numbers of well-preserved and well-visualized squamous epithelial cells
- An adequate endocervical/transformation zone component (from a patient with a cervix)

Well-preserved and well-visualized squamous epithelial cells should be spread over more than 10% of the slide surface. An adequate endocervical/transformation zone component should, as a minimum, consistent of two clusters of well-preserved endocervical and/or squamous metaplastic cells, each cluster composed of a minimum of five appropriate cells. This definition applies to specimens from both premenopausal and postmenopausal women with a cervix except in the situation of marked atrophy in which metaplastic and endocervical cells often cannot be distinguished from parabasal cells. In cases of marked atrophic changes, the absence of an identifiable endocervical/transformation zone component does not affect the specimen adequacy categorization of a specimen otherwise determined to be "satisfactory for evaluation."

A specimen is "satisfactory for evaluation but limited by . . ." if any of the following apply:
- Lack of pertinent clinical patient information (age, LMP as a minimum; additional information as appropriate)
- Partially obscuring blood, inflammation, thick areas, poor fixation, air-drying artifact, contamination, etc., which precludes interpretation of approximately 50% to 75% of the epithelial cells
- Lack of endocervical/transformation zone component as defined above

"Satisfactory for evaluation but limited by . . ." indicates that the specimen provides useful information; however, interpretation may be compromised. A report of "satisfactory for evaluation but limited by an absence of endocervical cells/transformation zone component" does not necessarily require a repeat smear. Patient factors, such as location of transformation zone, age, pregnancy, and previous therapy, may limit the clinician's ability to obtain an endocervical sample. The ultimate determination of specimen adequacy rests with the clinician, who must correlate the findings described in the cytopathology report with the clinical knowledge of the individual patient.

A specimen is "unsatisfactory for evaluation" if any of the following apply:

- Lack of patient identification on the specimen and/or requisition
- A technically unacceptable slide defined as
  - One that is broken and cannot be repaired, or cellular material that is inadequately preserved
  - Scant squamous epithelial component (well-preserved and well-visualized squamous epithelial cells spread over less than 10% of the slide surface)
  - Obscuring blood, inflammation, thick areas, poor fixation, air-drying artifact, contamination, etc., which precludes interpretation of approximately 75% or more of the epithelial cells

The "unsatisfactory . . ." designation indicates that the specimen is unreliable for the detection of cervical epithelial abnormalities.

Specimen adequacy is evaluated in all cases. However, any epithelial abnormality is of paramount importance and must be reported regardless of compromised specimen adequacy. **If abnormal cells are detected, the specimen is never categorized as "unsatisfactory."** Such cases may be considered "satisfactory" or "satisfactory but limited by . . ." based on the above-outlined criteria.

BIBLIOGRAPHY

General Reading

1. Clement PB, Young RH: *Tumors and tumorlike lesions of the uterine corpus and cervix,* New York, 1993, Churchill Livingstone.
2. Crum CP, Nuovo GJ: *The cervix.* In Sternberg SS, editor: *Diagnostic surgical pathology,* ed 2, New York, 1994, Raven Press.
3. Fu Y, Reagan J: *Pathology of the uterine cervix, vagina, and vulva,* Philadelphia, 1989, WB Saunders.
4. Kurman RJ, editor: *Blaustein's pathology of the female genital tract,* ed 4, New York, 1994, Springer-Verlag.
5. Kurman RJ, Norris HJ, Wilkinson EJ: *Tumors of the cervix, vagina, and vulva. Atlas of tumor pathology,* 3rd series, fascicle 4, Washington, DC, 1992, Armed Forces Institute of Pathology.
6. Kurman RJ, Solomon D: The Bethesda System for reporting Cervical/Vaginal Cytology Diagnoses. New York: Springer-Verlag, 1994.
7. Lawrence WD: Advances in the pathology of the uterine cervix, *Hum Pathol* 22:792-806, 1991.
8. Scully RE, Bonfiglio TA, Kurman RJ, Silverberg SG, Wilkinson EJ: *World Health Organization. Histological classification of tumors of the female genital tract,* New York, 1994, Springer-Verlag.

References

9. Abeler VM, Holm R, Nesland JM, Kjorstad KE: Small cell carcinoma of the cervix, *Cancer* 73:672-677, 1994.
10. Aozasa K, Sacki K, Ohsawa M, Horiuchi K, Mishima K, Tsujimoto M: Malignant lymphoma of the uterus, *Cancer* 72:1959-1964, 1993.
11. Ayre JE: The vaginal smear: "precancer" cell studies using a modified technique, *Am J Obstet Gynecol* 58:1205-1219, 1949.
12. Ayre JE: Role of the halo cell in cervical cancerigenesis: a virus manifestation in premalignancy, *Obstet Gynecol* 17:175-182, 1960.
13. Bergeron C, Barrasso R, Beaudenon S, Flamant P, Croissant O, Orth G: Human papillomaviruses associated with cervical intraepithelial neoplasia, *Am J Surg Pathol* 16:641-649, 1992.
14. Bernstein SG, Voet RL: *Human papillomavirus infections of the female genital tract.* In Seiarra JJ, editor: *Gynecology and obstetrics,* vol 4, *Gynecologic oncology,* Hagerstown, MD, 1984, Harper & Row.
15. Bernstein SG, Voet RL, Guzick DS, Melancon JT, Ronan-Cowen L, Lifshitz S, Buchsbaum HJ: Prevalence of papillomavirus infection in colposcopically directed cervical biopsies in 1972 and 1982, *Am J Obstet Gynecol* 151:577-581, 1985.

16. Casas-Cordero M, Morin C, Roy M, Fortier M, Meisels A: Origin of the koilocyte in condylomata of the human cervix, *Acta Cytol* 25:383-392, 1981.
17. Crum CP, Ikenberg H, Richart RM, Gissman L: Human papillomavirus type 16 and early cervical neoplasia. *N Engl J Med* 310:880-883, 1984.
18. Crum CP, Mitao M, Levine RU, Silverstein S: Cervical papillomaviruses segregate within morphologically distinct precancerous lesions, *J Virol* 54: 675-681, 1985.
19. Daya DA, Scully RE: Sarcoma botryoides of the uterine cervix in young women: a clinicopathological study of 13 cases, *Gynecol Oncol* 29:290-304, 1988.
20. Daya DA, Young RH: Florid deep glands of the uterine cervix, *Am J Clin Pathol* 103:614-617, 1995.
21. Duggan MA, Benoit JL, McGregor SE, Inoue M, Nation JG, Stuart GCE: Adenocarcinoma in situ of the endocervix: human papillomavirus determination by dot blot hybridization and polymerase chain reaction amplification, *Int J Gynecol Pathol* 3:143-149, 1994.
22. Ferry JA, Scully RE: "Adenoid cystic" carcinoma and adenoid basal carcinoma of the uterine cervix, *Am J Surg Pathol* 12:134-144, 1988.
23. Ferry JA, Scully RE: Mesonephric remnants, hyperplasia, and neoplasia in the uterine cervix, *Am J Surg Pathol* 14:1100-1111, 1990.
24. Gershell DJ, Mazoujian G, Mutch DG, Rudloff MA: Small-cell undifferentiated carcinoma of the cervix, *Am J Surg Pathol* 12:684-698, 1988.
25. Gilks CB, Young RH, Aguirre P, DeLellis RA, Scully RE: Adenoma malignum (minimal deviation adenocarcinoma) of the uterine cervix, *Am J Surg Pathol* 13:717-729, 1989.
26. Greeley C, Schroeder S, Silverberg SG: Microglandular hyperplasia of the cervix: a true "pill" lesion?, *Int J Gynecol Pathol* 14:50-54, 1995.
27. Hafiz MA, Kragel PJ, Toker C: Carcinoma of the uterine cervix resembling lymphoepithelioma, *Obstet Gynecol* 66:829-831, 1985.
28. Hasumi K, Sugano H, Sakamoto G, Masubuchi K, Kubo H: Circumscribed carcinoma of the uterine cervix, with marked lymphocytic infiltration, *Cancer* 39:2503-2507, 1977.
29. Hausen HZ: Papillomaviruses in human cancer, *Cancer* 59:1692-1696, 1987.
30. Jones MW, Lefkowitz M: Adenosarcoma of the uterine cervix: a clinicopathological study of 12 cases, *Int J Gynecol Pathol* 14:223-229, 1995.
31. Jones MW, Silverberg SG, Kurman RJ: Well-differentiated villoglandular adenocarcinoma of the uterine cervix: a clinicopathological study of 24 cases, *Int J Gynecol Pathol* 12:1-7, 1993.
32. Kapp DS, LiVolsi VA: Intense eosinophilic stromal infiltration in carcinoma of the uterine cervix: a clinicopathologic study of 14 cases, *Gynecol Oncol* 16:19-30, 1983.
33. Lemoine NR, Hall PA: Epithelial tumors metastatic to the uterine cervix. A study of 33 cases and review of the literature, *Cancer* 57:2002-2005, 1986.
34. Leung KM, Chan WY, Hui PK: Invasive squamous cell carcinoma and cervical intraepithelial neoplasia III of uterine cervix, *Am J Clin Pathol* 101:508-513, 1994.
35. Meisels A: The story of a cell, *Acta Cytol* 7:584-596, 1983.
36. Meisels A, Roy M, Fortier M, Casas-Cordero M, Shan R, Turgeion H: Human papillomavirus infection of the cervix. The atypical condyloma, *Acta Cytol* 25:7-16, 1981.
37. Mills SE, Austin MB, Randall ME: Lymphoepithelioma-like carcinoma of the uterine cervix, *Am J Surg Pathol* 9:883-889, 1985.
38. Moberg PJ, Einhorn N, Silfversward C, Soderberg G: Adenocarcinoma of the uterine cervix, *Cancer* 57:407-410, 1986.
39. Moller BR, Johannesen P, Osther K, Ulmsteen U, Hastrup J, Berg K: Treatment of dysplasia of the cervical epithelium with an interferon gel, *Obstet Gynecol* 62:625-629, 1983.
40. Mordel N, Mor-Yosef S, Ben-Baruch N, Anteby SO: Malignant melanoma of the uterine cervix: case report and review of the literature, *Gynecol Oncol* 32:375-380, 1989.
41. Oliva E, Clement PB, Young RH: Tubal and tuboendometrioid metaplasia of the uterine cervix, *Am J Clin Pathol* 103:618-623, 1995.
42. Ostor AG, Pagano R, Davoren AM, Fortune DW, Chanen W, Rome R: Adenocarcinoma in situ of the cervix, *Int J Gynecol Pathol* 3:179-190, 1984.
43. Prasad CJ, Genest DR, Crum CP: Nondiagnostic squamous atypia of the cervix (atypical squamous epithelium of undetermined significance): histologic and molecular correlates, *Int J Gynecol Pathol* 13:220-227, 1994.
44. Qizilbash AH: In situ and microinvasive adenocarcinoma of the uterine cervix, *Am J Clin Pathol* 64:155-170, 1975.
45. Randall ME, Andersen WA, Mills SE, Kim JC: Papillary squamous cell carcinoma of the uterine cervix: a clinicopathologic study of nine cases, *Int J Gynecol Pathol* 5:1-10, 1986.

46. Reid R, Crum CP, Herschman BR, Fu YS, Braun L, Shah KV, Agronow SJ, Stanhope CR: Genital warts and cervical cancer. Subclinical papillomaviral infection and cervical neoplasia are linked by a spectrum of continuous morphologic and biologic change, *Cancer* 53:943-953, 1984.
47. Reid R, Fu YS, Herschman BR, Crum CP, Braun L, Shah KV, Agronow SJ, Stanhope CR: Genital warts and cervical cancer. VI. The relationship between aneuploid and polyploid cervical lesions, *Am J Obstet Gynecol* 150:189-199, 1984.
48. Reid R, Herschman BR, Crum CP, Fu YS, Braun L, Shah KV, Agronow SJ, Stanhope CR: Genital warts and cervical cancer. V. The tissue basis of colposcopic change, *Am J Obstet Gynecol* 149:293-303, 1984.
49. Rhatigan RM: Endocervical gland atypia secondary to Arias-Stella change, *Arch Pathol Lab Med* 116:943-946, 1992.
50. Richart RM: Cervical intraepithelial neoplasia, *Pathol Annu* 8:301-363, 1973.
51. Segal GH, Hart WR: Cystic endocervical tunnel clusters, *Am J Surg Pathol* 14:895-903, 1990.
52. Silverberg SG, Hurt WG: Minimal deviation adenocarcinoma ("adenoma malignum") of the cervix: a reappraisal, *Am J Obstet Gynecol* 121:971-975, 1975.
53. Steeper TA, Wick MR: Minimal deviation adenocarcinoma of the uterine cervix ("adenoma malignum"). An immunohistochemical comparison with microglandular endocervical hyperplasia and conventional endocervical adenocarcinoma, *Cancer* 58:1131-1138, 1986.
54. Syrjanon KJ: Current views on the condylomatous lesions in uterine cervix and their possible relationship to cervical squamous cell carcinoma, *Obstet Gynecol Surv* 35:685-694, 1980.
55. Tobon H, Dave H: Adenocarcinoma in situ of the cervix, *Int J Gynecol Pathol* 7:139-151, 1988.
56. Tsokos, M: The diagnosis and classification of childhood rhabdomyosarcoma, *Semin Diagn Pathol* 11:26-38, 1994.
57. Turner RJ, Cohen RA, Voet RL, Stephens SR, Weinstein SA: Analysis of the tissue margins of cone biopsy specimens obtained with "cold knife," CO_2 and Nd:Yag lasers and a radiofrequency surgical unit, *J Reprod Med* 37:607-610, 1992.
58. Ulbright TM, Gersell DJ: Glassy cell carcinoma of the uterine cervix, *Cancer* 51:2255-2263, 1983.
59. Van Nagel JR, Powell DE, Gallion HH, Elliott DG, Donaldson ES, Carpenter AE, Higgins RV, Kryscio R, Pavlik EJ: Small cell carcinoma of the cervix, *Cancer* 62:1586-1593, 1988.
60. Voet RL, Waisman J, Ballon SC: Intraepithelial epidermoid carcinoma of the cervix, endometrium and a fallopian tube, *Gynecol Oncol* 8:349-352, 1979.
61. Weiss RJ, Lucas WE: Adenocarcinoma of the uterine cervix, *Cancer* 57:1996-2001, 1986.
62. Wijnaendts LCD, Van Der Linder JC, Van Unnik AJM, Delemarre JFM, Voute PA, Meijer CJLM: Histopathological classification of childhood rhabdomyosarcomas, *Hum Pathol* 25:900-907, 1994.
63. Wilczynski SP, Walker J, Liao S-Y, Bergen S, Berman M: Adenocarcinoma of the cervix associated with human papillomavirus, *Cancer* 62:1331-1336, 1988.
64. Wilkinson E, DuFour DR: Pathogenesis of microglandular hyperplasia of the cervix uteri, *Obstet Gynecol* 47:189-195, 1976.
65. Willett GD, Kurman RJ, Reid R, Greenberg M, Jenson AB, Lorincz AT: Correlation of the histologic appearance of intraepithelial neoplasia of the cervix with human papillomavirus types, *Int J Gynecol Pathol* 8:18-25, 1989.
66. Yee C, Krishnan-Hewlett I, Baker CC, Schlegel R, Howley PM: Presence and expression of human papillomavirus sequences in human cervical carcinoma cell lines, *Am J Pathol* 119:361-366, 1985.
67. Young RH, Harris NL, Scully RE: Lymphoma-like lesions of the lower female genital tract: a report of 16 cases, *Int J Gynecol Pathol* 4:289-299, 1985.
68. Young RH, Scully RE: Atypical forms of microglandular hyperplasia of the cervix simulating carcinoma, *Am J Surg Pathol* 13:50-56, 1989.
69. Young RH, Scully RE: Villoglandular papillary adenocarcinoma of the uterine cervix. A clinicopathologic analysis of 13 cases, *Cancer* 63:1773-1779, 1989.
70. Young RH, Scully RE: Uterine carcinomas simulating microglandular hyperplasia, *Am J Surg Pathol* 16:1092-1097, 1992.
71. Young RH, Scully RE: Minimal-deviation endometrioid adenocarcinoma of the uterine cervix, *Am J Surg Pathol* 17:660-665, 1993.

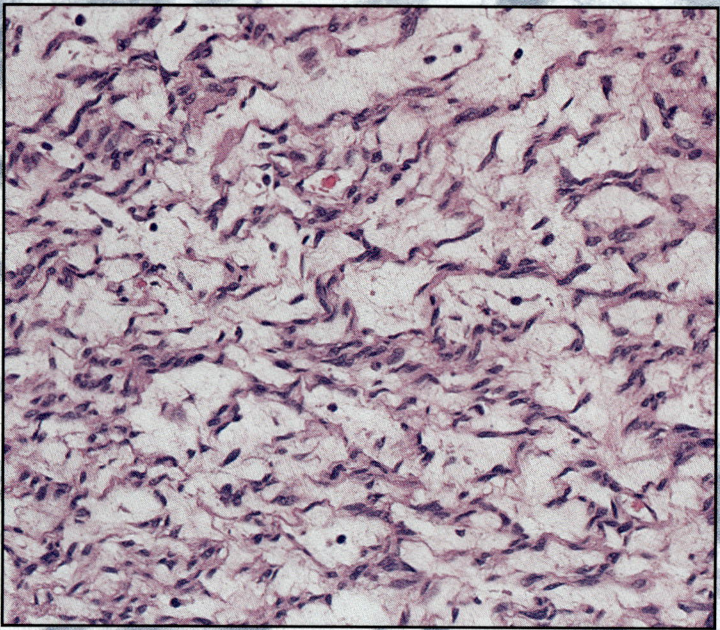

Chapter 4

Pathology of the Uterine Corpus

INFLAMMATION

Acute endometritis is usually associated with pregnancy or abortion (Figure 4-1). A variety of aerobic and anaerobic organisms can be involved in this process, which may lead to marked tissue destruction and necrosis. Chronic endometritis[29,42] is many times asymptomatic but may present with menometrorrhagia. Since lymphocytes and lymphoid follicles are often seen in normal endometrium, the diagnosis of chronic endometritis requires the identification of plasma cells in histologic sections (Figure 4-2). Chronic endometritis may be associated with pelvic inflammatory disease, intrauterine devices, or recent spontaneous or induced abortions.

Tuberculous endometritis is characterized by the presence of granulomatous inflammation with the typical Langhans giant cells. As in the cervix, tuberculous endometritis is usually a part of a systemic infection, especially that in the fallopian tubes and peritoneal cavity. Tuberculous endometritis may be found during evaluation of infertility, since these patients are usually sterile. Actinomycosis (Figure 4-3) has an increased incidence in patients who have intrauterine devices.[54] Whenever an intrauterine device is removed, it should be examined for any adherent tissue fragments, and these fragments should be examined by culture and histologically for evidence of actinomycosis or other organisms.

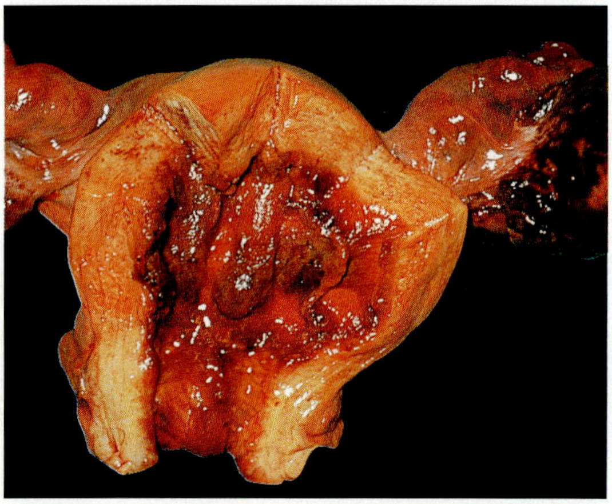

4.1 Gross view of a uterus showing acute endometritis due to a septic incomplete abortion.

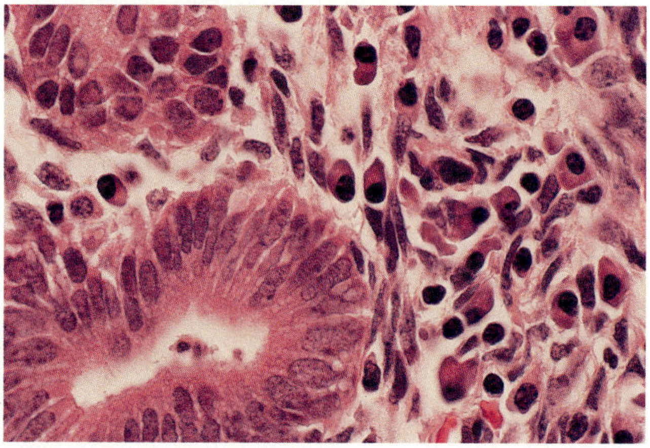

4.2 Chronic endometritis with numerous plasma cells.

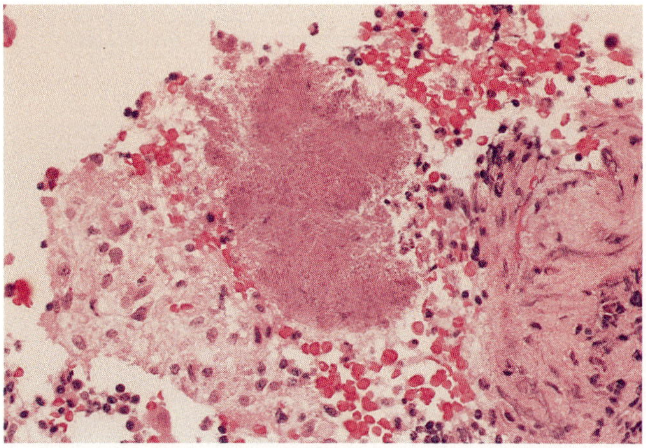

4.3 Actinomycosis of the endometrium demonstrating a cluster of filamentous bacteria (sulfur granule) characteristically seen with this infection.

FUNCTIONAL STATES OF THE ENDOMETRIUM

Proliferative endometrium is characterized by straight tubular glands (Figure 4-4). In the early proliferative stage the glands are small and widely spaced. Mitoses are present throughout all proliferative phases. In the middle to late proliferative phases the glands become increasingly crowded and develop slight tortuosity. The nuclei become pseudostratified (Figure 4-5) and mitotic figures are increased. The stroma becomes dense and also contains mitotic figures. One of the key features of the proliferative phase is the shape of the nuclei, which are oval and pseudostratified. Adenomyosis consists of the presence of endometrial glands and stroma in the myometrium (Figures 4-6 and 4-7).

The secretory phase begins at the time of ovulation, usually at day 14 (Table 4-1). The immediate postovulatory phase shows little change for the first 48 hours. On day 16, small subnuclear vacuoles begin to appear, which increase in number and uniformity (Figure 4-8). These vacuoles eventually assume a supranuclear position and disappear into the midsecretory phase, which the vacuoles are absent and secretions appear in the glandular lumen (Figure 4-9). The nuclei at this point are round and basally oriented. There is a virtual absence of mitotic figures, and stromal edema is present. Secretions of stromal edema increase into the late secretory phase. During the late secretory phase, predecidual changes begin to occur around spiral arteries (Figure 4-10). Into the middle of the late secretory phase, these predecidual islands begin to increase and start to coalesce (Figure 4-11). Toward the end of the late secretory phase, the predecidua becomes confluent and granulocytes appear in the endometrium. Blood begins to dissect through the stroma in the premenstrual phase (Figure 4-12). The stromal dissolution increases into the menstrual phase and then the cycle repeats itself.

Abnormal secretory states can be endogenous or exogenous. An inadequate luteal phase results from early regression of the corpus luteum with decreased progesterone secretion. The endometrium of the luteal-phase deficiency may have a normal secretory appearance, but it will not coincide with the dating by basal

TABLE 4-1 Endometrial Dating Criteria

MENSTRUAL (Days 1-3)	
Stellate secretory glands (secretory exhaustion)	
Crumbling of stroma, PMN infiltration, hemorrhage	
Beginning regeneration	
PROLIFERATIVE (Days 4-14) Proliferative glands, spindled nonpredecidualized stroma	
Early proliferative (days 4-7): glands noncoiled	
Midproliferative (days 7-10): glands coiled, stroma edematous	
Late proliferative (days 10-14): glands coiled, stroma compact	
SECRETORY (Days 14-28)	
Early Secretory: Vacuolated cells, nonpredecidualized stroma	
POD 1:	Irregular, nonuniform subnuclear vacuolization; otherwise has appearance of late proliferative endometrium
POD 2:	Uniform subnuclear vacuolization, causing an exaggerated nuclear pseudostratification; mitotic figures present
POD 3:	Subnuclear vacuoles uniformly aligned
POD 4:	Vacuoles slip around nucleus to assume luminal position
POD 5:	Vacuoles infrequent; secretion appears in lumen
Midsecretory: Nonvacuolated cells, nonpredecidualized stroma	
POD 6:	Vacuoles largely absent, secretion prominent
POD 7:	Stroma becomes edematous
POD 8:	Maximal stromal edema, maximal glandular secretion
Late secretory: Nonvacuolated secretory cells, stroma predecidualized	
POD 9:	Spiral arteries become prominent by virtue of early periaterial predecidual change
POD 10:	Thick periarterial cuffs of predecidua
POD 11:	Appearance of surface islands of predecidua
POD 12:	Increasing prominence of surface islands of predecidua
POD 13:	Confluence of surface islands of predecidua, number of stromal granulocytes increase
POD 14:	Extravasation of red blood cells, stromal granulocytes prominent

From: Kempson RL, Hendrickson MR. The Female Reproductive System. In: *Surgical Pathology,* Coulson WF (ed.). Philadelphia: JB Lippincott, 1978, with permission.

PMN, Polymorphonuclear neutrophil leukocytes; POD, postovulatory day.

body temperature or day of the menstrual cycle. Irregular shedding is characterized by prolonged bleeding at the time of menses and appears to be caused by a persistent corpus luteum with continued secretion of progesterone. The endometrial changes in this entity are less well defined, showing an admixture of advanced secretory changes and early proliferative glands. There is focal decidual change within the stroma, and degeneration of the stroma may be characterized by hemorrhage.

Hypersecretory changes may be the result of an ectopic pregnancy. In this situation the endometrial glands continue to proliferate and display a characteristic pattern that has been termed the Arias-Stella reaction[8,36] (Figure 4-13). The glands become vacuolated with nuclei protruding into the lumen, showing the so-called hobnail pattern. There is marked decidualization of the stroma and absence of chorionic villi. This pattern can also be present with a coexisting intrauterine pregnancy and does not necessarily indicate an ectopic pregnancy. The pattern can also be seen with early abortions in which the glands have not yet undergone secretory exhaustion. A decidual cast (Figure 4-14) of the uterine cavity may form from the abundant decidua. Occasionally, nuclear clearing may be seen in gestational endometrium, which may give rise to a pseudoherpetic pattern[51,72] (Figure 4-15).

Progesterone therapy initially gives a hypersecretory pattern; however, after several weeks of therapy the glands undergo secretory exhaustion in which they become essentially atrophic. The stroma continues to show a marked decidual change (Figure 4-16). It is the progesterone-only therapy that most closely resembles the pregnancy state of the endometrium.

Changes associated with oral contraceptive use are dependent on the type and duration of the agent. In the typical combined oral contraceptive use, the first few months of therapy show somewhat normal cycling of the endometrium with a more hypersecretory state toward the end of the cycle. After several months of therapy, the endometrial changes resemble those that are caused by progesterone only. The glands show atrophic changes, but the stroma does not show the marked decidual change as in progesterone-only therapy. It is this somewhat atrophic pattern with mild secretory changes that is typical of the oral contraceptive pattern (Figure 4-17).

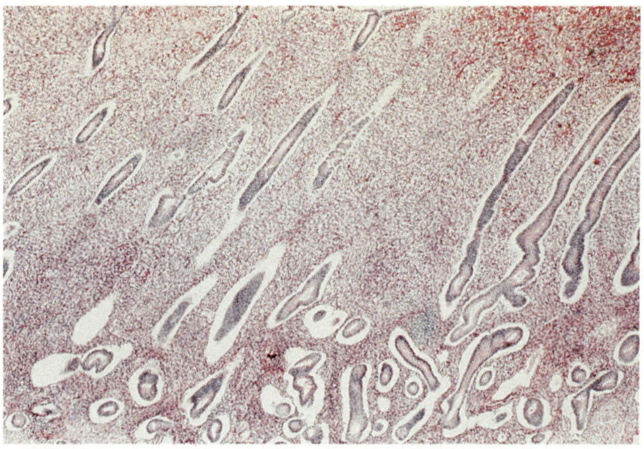

4.4 Proliferative endometrium demonstrating irregular tubular glands with an underlying basal layer showing mild architectural disarray.

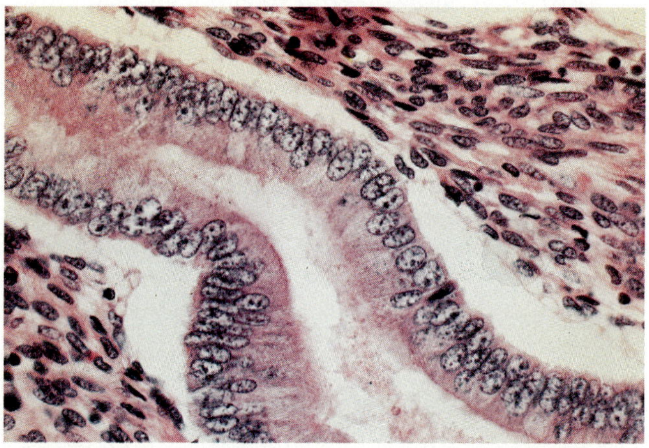

4.5 Proliferative endometrium demonstrating overlapping oval nuclei.

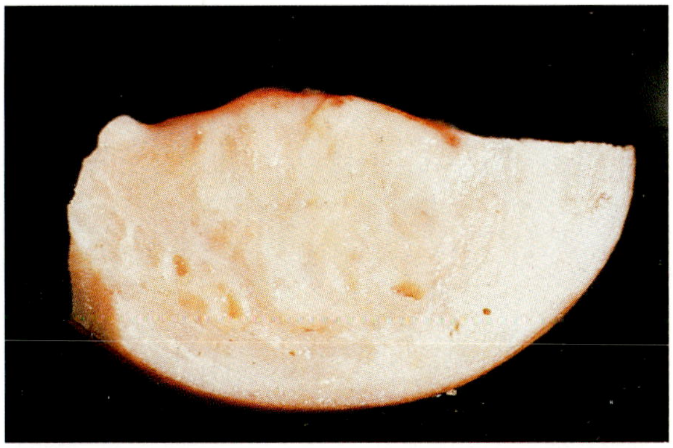

4.6 Gross view of adenomyosis showing irregular trabeculation of the myometrium with scattered small cystic areas.

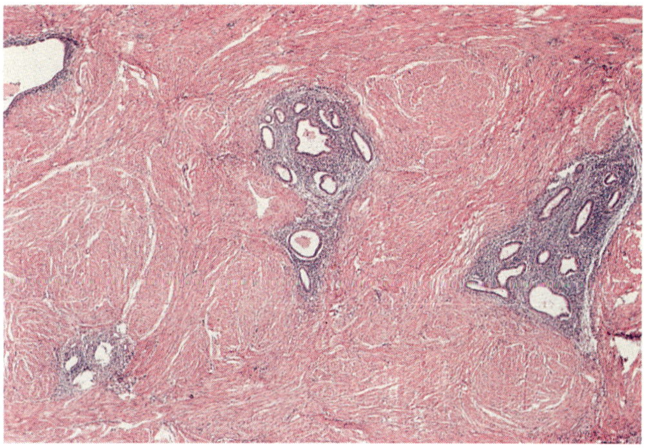

4.7 Adenomyosis demonstrating endometrial glands and stroma embedded in the myometrium.

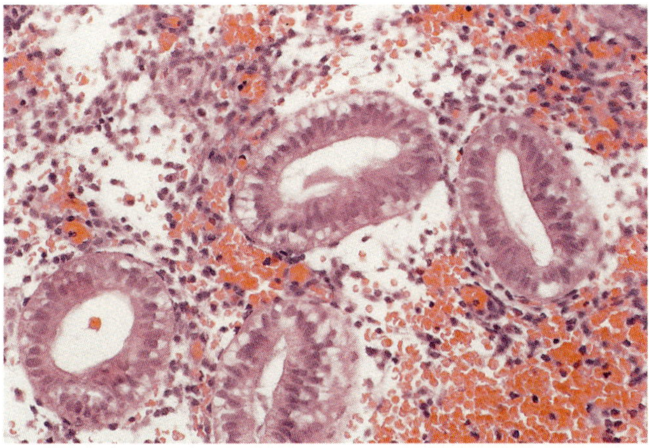

4.8 Early secretory endometrium characterized by uniform subnuclear vacuoles.

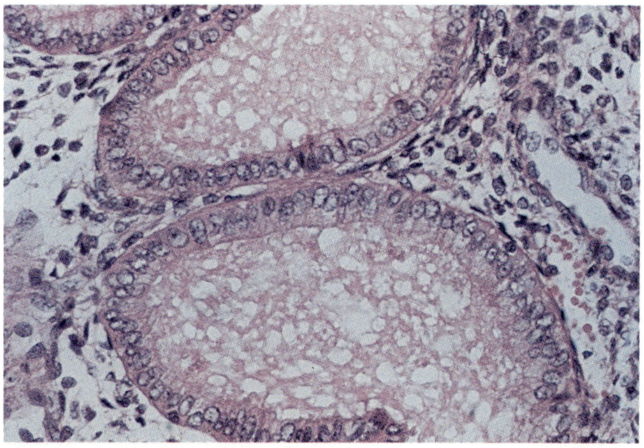

4.9 Midsecretory endometrium with abundant luminal secretions and an edematous stroma.

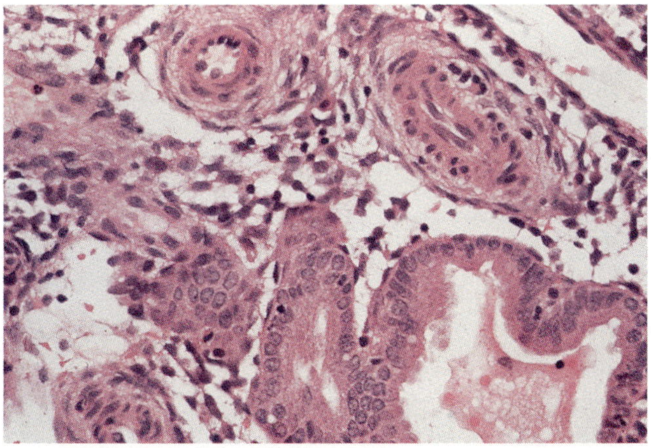

4.10 Late secretory endometrium with prominent periarterial tufts of predecidua.

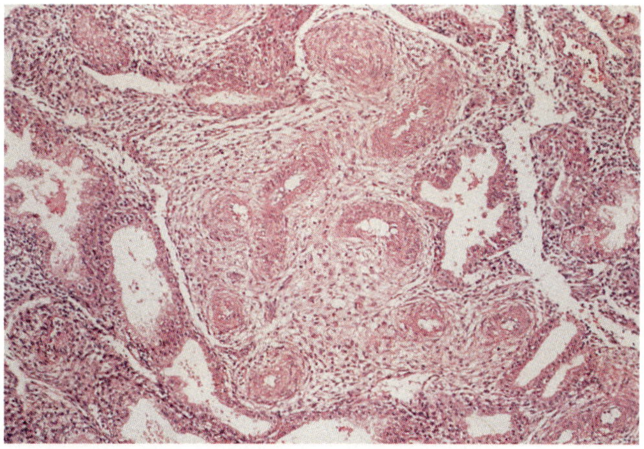

4.11 Late secretory endometrium showing confluence of predecidua surrounding several spiral arterioles.

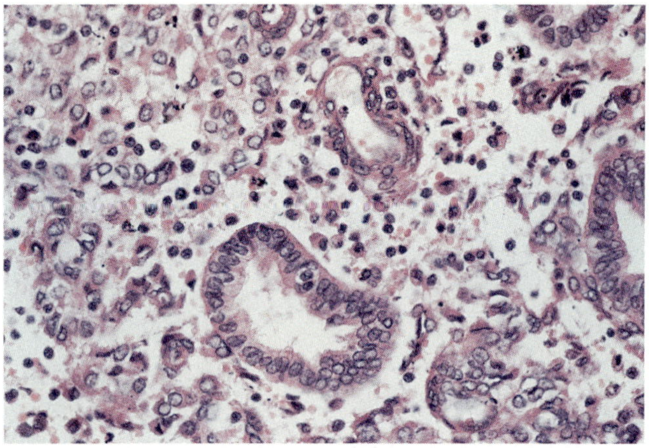

4.12 Premenstrual endometrium demonstrating a lytic stroma with scattered endometrial granulocytes and early extravasation of blood.

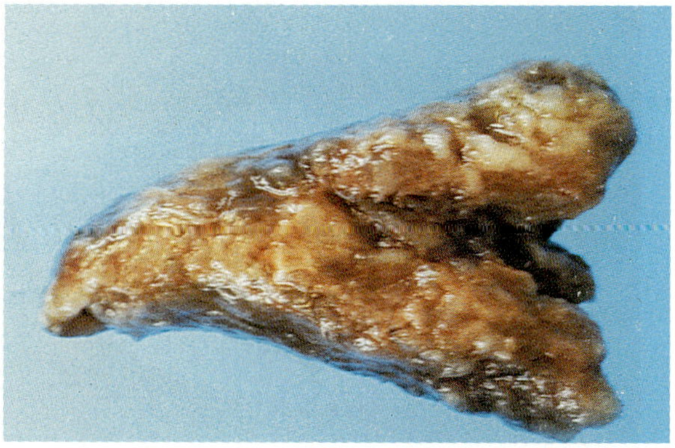

4.13 Gross view of a decidual cast from the endometrium.

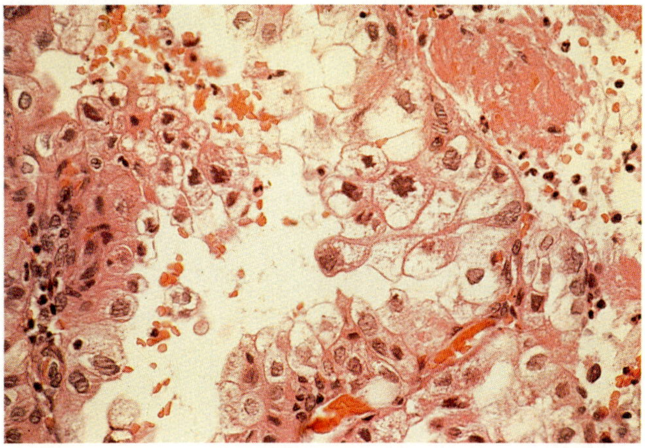

4.14 Hypersecretory endometrium (Arias-Stella reaction) with vacuolated cells containing irregular nuclei and retraction of the cytoplasm (hobnail cells).

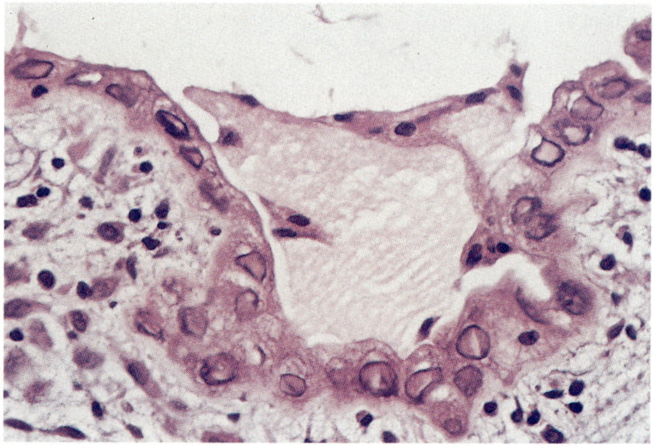

4.15 Endometrial glands from a gestational endometrium demonstrating pseudoherpetic nuclear inclusions.

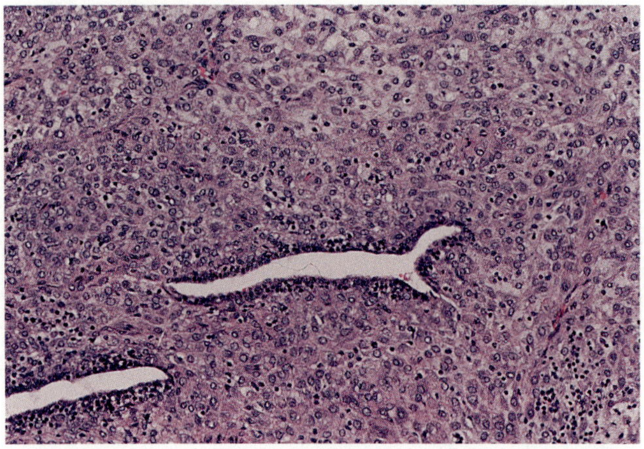

4.16 Exogenous progesterone effect on an endometrium showing inactive glands surrounded by a markedly decidualized stroma.

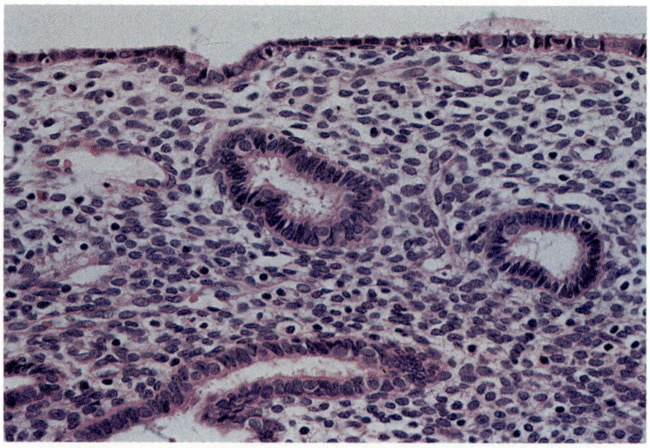

4.17 Endometrium from a patient on combination oral contraceptive therapy. The glands are mildly inactive and embedded in a stroma showing mild predecidual change in the individual stromal cells.

ABNORMAL PROLIFERATIVE STATES

Atrophic endometrium is the result of decreased circulating estrogen. Atrophic patterns are found in prepubertal and postmenopausal patients. They can also be transiently found during the reproductive years, in the immediate postpartum period, and as the result of abnormal hormonal states.

Disordered proliferative endometrium is the term that has been introduced by Kempson and Hendrickson to refer to that functional state of the endometrium that lies between normal proliferative endometrium and hyperplasia (Figure 4-18). It is caused by unopposed estrogen, which can be exogenous or endogenous. Endogenous unopposed estrogen is usually the result of anovulatory cycles. This is usually a transient phenomenon, but in some cases it can extend into hyperplasia. With exogenous estrogen therapy, the disordered proliferative pattern shows similar findings, and the distinction between disordered proliferative endometrium and hyperplasia becomes more difficult, resting generally on the amount of tissue obtained at the time of the curettage. This diagnosis is more difficult with endometrial biopsy and is usually more reassuring when a formal curettage has been performed.

Hyperplasia of the endometrium is a confusing term and various classifications have been proposed.[35,45] The traditional classification has separated cystic from adenomatous hyperplasia; however, these two are linked by a spectrum, with cystic hyperplasia more often present at the lower end near disordered proliferative, and adenomatous hyperplasia more on the opposite end near carcinoma. Admixtures of the two can occur and frequently do, and these two entities should not be thought of as separate but as various points on a spectrum. The endometrial stroma is also usually hyperplastic. Occasionally the stroma contains lipid-laden macrophages, often referred to as foamy macrophages (Figure 4-19). The most recent World Health Organization (WHO) classification for endometrial hyperplasia is simple (which includes cystic), complex, and atypical hyperplasia. Simple hyperplasia (Figure 4-20) refers to mild architectural crowding with or without cystic hyperplasia. Complex hyperplasia (Figure 4-21) refers to adenomatous hyperplasia without atypia. Atypical hyperplasia (Figure 4-22) refers to hyperplastic endometrium with cytologic atypia. Endometrial polyps (Figures 4-23 and 4-24) consist of polypoid projections of simple hyperplasia[69, 71] that may represent focal areas of the endometrium that are unresponsive to progesterone.

Various müllerian metaplasias may occur in hyperplastic endometrium.[30] Metaplasias can take a variety of forms, including squamous (Figure 4-25), tubal (Figure 4-26), clear cell, papillary (Figure 4-27), and mucinous metaplasia. These patterns may occur in hyperplasia and in adenocarcinoma. The presence or absence of metaplastic foci does not indicate whether the lesion is benign or malignant. However, metaplastic foci can occasionally be confused with adenocarcinoma. This is particularly true of squamous and mucinous metaplasia.

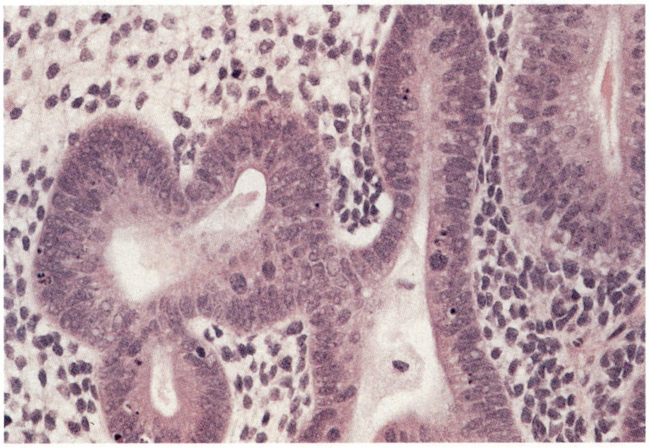

4.18 Endometrium from an anovulatory patient showing disordered proliferative endometrium characterized by mild architectural complexity and disarray. There is insufficient volume and complexity to warrant a diagnosis of hyperplasia in this patient.

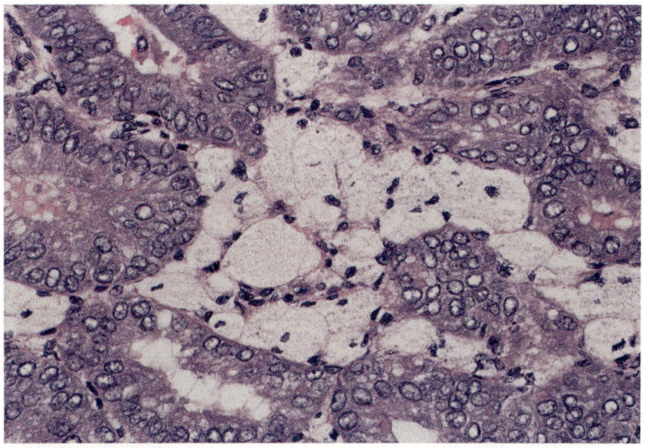

4.19 Endometrium containing lipid-laden stromal cells (often referred to as foamy histiocytes).

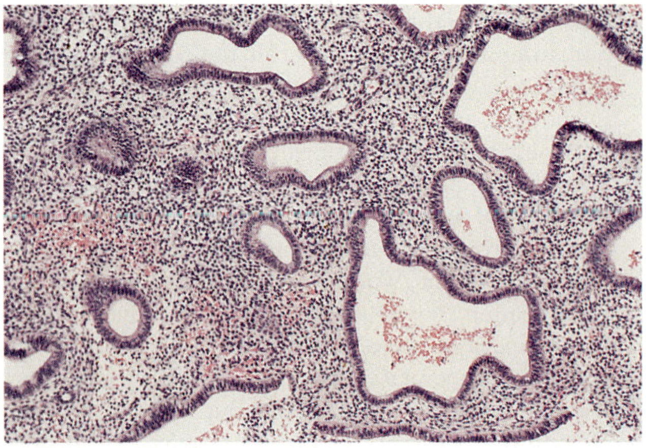

4.20 Simple hyperplasia showing mild architectural disarray and early cystic change within the glands.

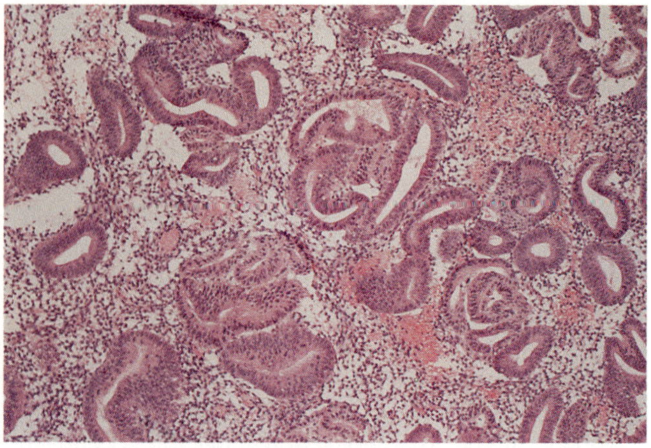

4.21 Complex hyperplasia characterized by architectural disarray and crowding without cytologic atypia.

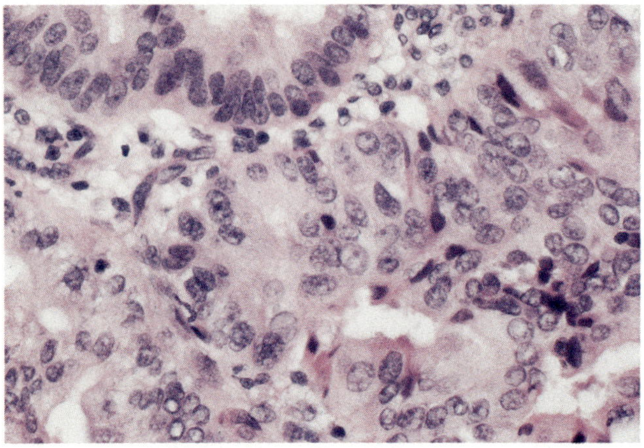

4.22 Atypical hyperplasia showing cytologic atypia without invasion.

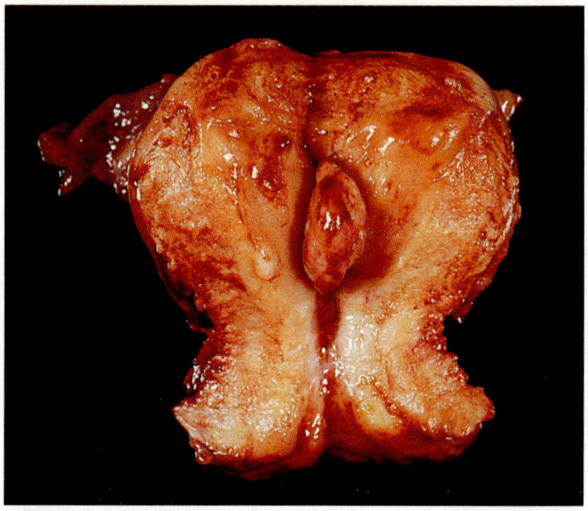

4.23 Gross view of an endometrial polyp.

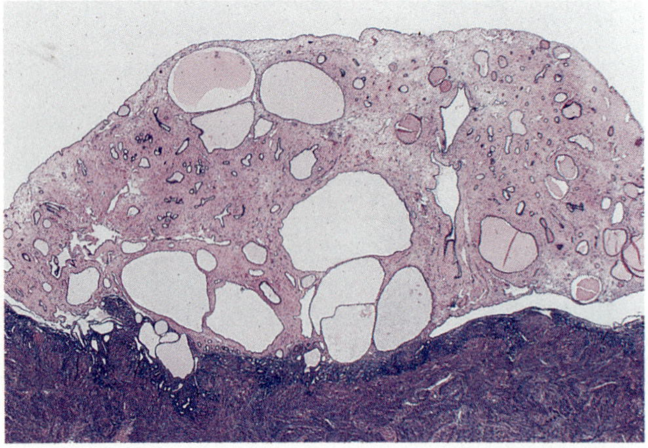

4.24 Endometrial polyp demonstrating simple (cystic) hyperplasia.

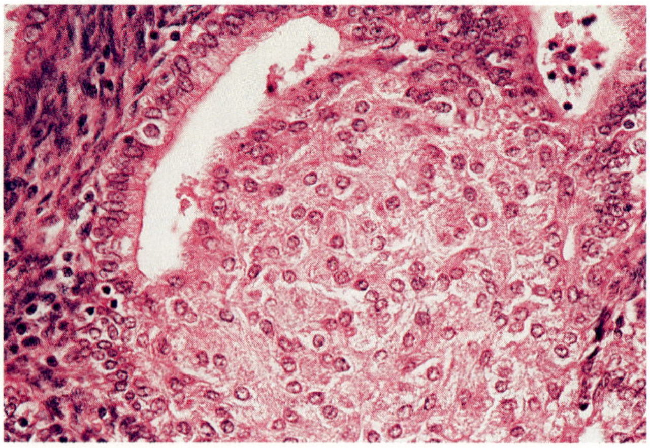

4.25 Squamous metaplasia of the endometrium forming a squamous morule.

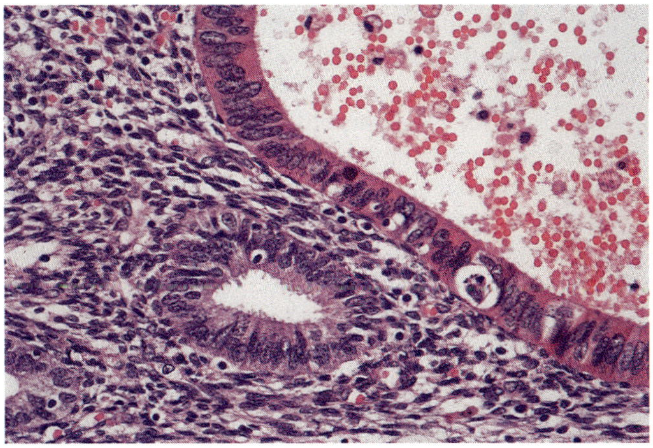

4.26 Tubal metaplasia of the endometrium with eosinophilic cytoplasm and cilia.

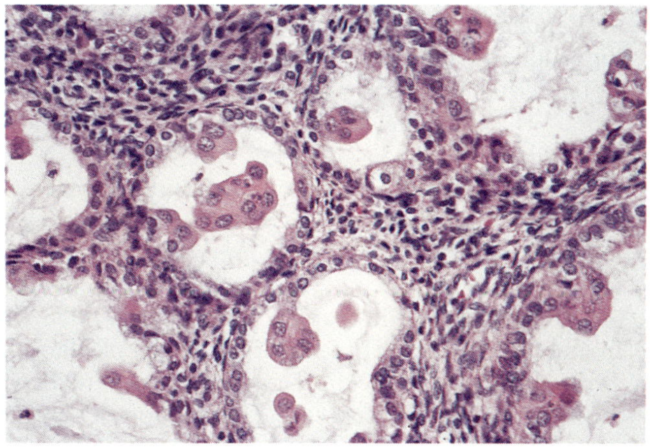

4.27 Papillary metaplasia of the endometrium with intraluminal epithelial tufts.

ENDOMETRIAL CARCINOMA

The distinction between atypical hyperplasia and adenocarcinoma is difficult and has been the subject of much controversy.* It has been the general feeling of many investigators that endometrial carcinoma has been overdiagnosed in the past, and more precise histologic criteria have been sought in order to determine which lesions will be biologically aggressive. Kurman and Norris[44] stress the stromal response to the glands as being indicative of their invasive nature. When the tumor invades the stroma, there is a desmoplastic reaction. This, along with the complexity of the glands, the amount within a microscopic field, and necrosis between glands, has given some additional guidelines to help select the truly malignant lesions.

The grading of endometrial carcinoma by the International Federation of Gynecology and Obstetrics (FIGO) is that of a well-, moderately, and poorly differentiated classification. Well-differentiated adenocarcinoma (Figure 4-28) is predominantly glandular, containing less than 5% solid areas. Moderately differentiated adenocarcinoma (Figure 4-29) contains between 6% and 50% solid growth pattern. Poorly differentiated adenocarcinoma (Figure 4-30) contains more than 50% solid growth pattern. Notable nuclear atypia, inappropriate for the architectural grade, raises the Grade 1 or Grade 2 tumor by 1. In serous adenocarcinomas, clear cell adenocarcinomas, and squamous cell carcinomas, nuclear grading takes precedence. The depth of invasion (Figures 4-31, 4-32 and 4-33) and cervical involvement (Figures 4-34 and 4-35) also contribute to the stage (see boxes on p. 97).

Adenocarcinomas with squamous differentiation (Figure 4-36) are graded according to the nuclear grade of the glandular component.[80] A solid focus of tumor in an endometrioid-type carcinoma should be considered glandular unless at least one of the following criteria suggesting squamous differentiation is present:

A. Keratinization demonstrated with standard (e.g., hematoxylin and eosin) staining techniques
B. Intercellular bridges
C. Three or more of the following 4 criteria:
   1. Sheetlike growth without gland formation or palisading
   2. Sharp cell margins
   3. Eosinophilic, and thick or glassy, cytoplasm
   4. A decreased (compared with other foci of the same tumor) nuclear-cytoplasmic ratio

Squamous differentiation can occur in hyperplasia and well-differentiated adenocarcinoma as squamous morulae. These morulae can also differentiate and be more readily recognized as squamous differentiation. The latter is usually not a problem in well-differentiated lesions; however, the moderate and poorly differentiated tumors give increasing atypia to the squamous cells, and the point at which the squamous differentiation becomes squamous carcinoma is not always clear. Squamous cells are classified as histologically malignant (adenosquamous carcinoma) (Figure 4-37) as opposed to histologically benign (adenocarcinoma with squamous metaplasia, adenoacanthoma) if they satisfy one or more of the following criteria:

A. Standard cytologic criteria of malignancy
B. Mitoses in the indisputably squamous component
C. Destructive stromal infiltration by the squamous elements

*References 23, 31, 33, 47, 56, 75.

Malignant squamous elements in adenosquamous carcinoma do not need to be graded or characterized further. If the term "adenocarcinoma with squamous differentiation" is used alone, only the glandular element should be graded.

Serous carcinoma of the endometrium (Figures 4-38 and 4-39) is a special subtype that has a more aggressive clinical course than typical endometrial adenocarcinoma.[28,32,38] This tumor resembles that of the ovary in which there are serous papillary projections, often with psammoma bodies. The nuclei are quite pleomorphic with prominent nucleoli. The tumor tends to invade myometrial vascular spaces and extend to the serosa. It then spreads intraperitoneally and covers serosal surfaces in the same fashion as ovarian carcinoma. This tumor can also secondarily involve the ovary, making it difficult to determine whether it is a metastasis or synchronous primary tumors. Serous carcinoma needs to be distinguished from the more bland villoglandular pattern (Figure 4-40) of adenocarcinoma.[7,15]

Clear cell carcinoma of the endometrium[46,48] (Figure 4-41) can present in three basic patterns. The solid clear cell component (from which it receives its name) is one pattern; the other two are papillary and tubulocystic. The papillary component of clear cell carcinoma can also lead to confusion in determining whether there is a coexistent papillary serous carcinoma. Clear cell carcinoma can occur either exclusively or in combination with other cell types, such as those with a typical endometrioid pattern. It has been considered an aggressive tumor with a worse prognosis than typical endometrioid carcinoma. Recent studies[12] demonstrate a prognosis similar to that of Grade 3 endometrioid carcinoma but better than that of papillary serous carcinoma.

Mucinous carcinoma of the endometrium[68] (Figure 4-42) is another variant, but this has not been shown to significantly alter the prognosis from that of a more typical endometrial carcinoma. Mucinous carcinoma can occur in combination with typical endometrial carcinoma or as a pure tumor itself. The major problem with this cell type lies in distinguishing it from a primary adenocarcinoma of the endocervix.[21]

Squamous carcinoma of the endometrium[78] is rare (Figures 4-43 and 4-44) and is sometimes the result of upward extension of carcinoma of the cervix. Secretory carcinoma has been occasionally referred to in the literature. This entity has usually been described as a well-differentiated endometrial adenocarcinoma that shows subnuclear vacuoles and other evidence of secretory function. Most of these cases are probably superimposed progesterone changes on an otherwise typical endometrioid adenocarcinoma. Small cell neuroendocrine carcinomas of the endometrium have also been described.[34,37]

A carcinoma is classified as mixed if two or more subtypes are present, with each pattern making up at least 10% of total tumor volume. Ideally, this decision is best made on the basis of a hysterectomy specimen, but if only a smaller specimen is available, any amount of a second tumor category will suffice for the diagnosis of mixed carcinoma. When a carcinoma is classified as mixed, the major and minor types and their relative proportions should be specified.

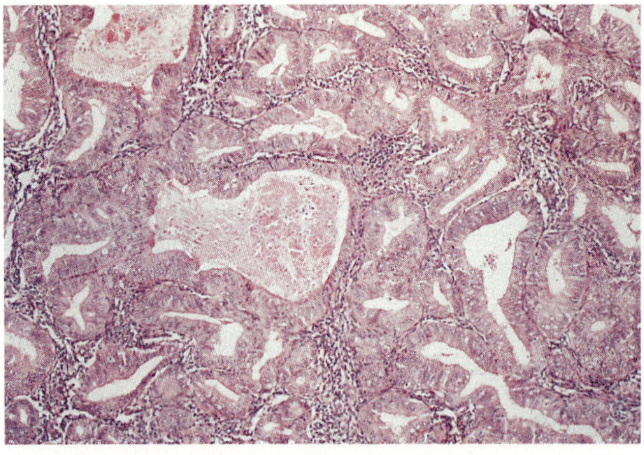

4.28 Well-differentiated (Grade I) adenocarcinoma of the endometrium showing a predominantly glandular pattern.

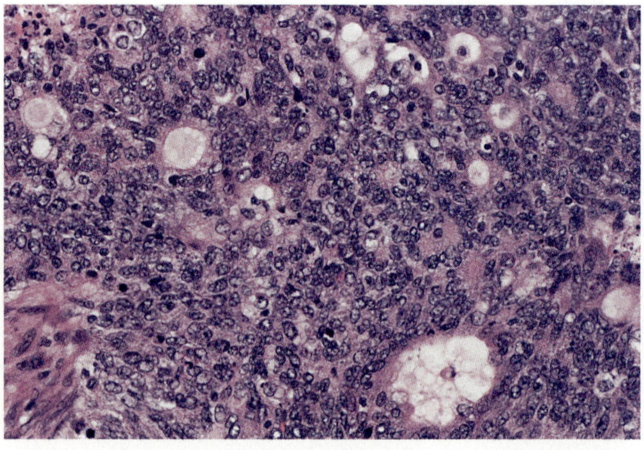

4.29 Moderately differentiated (Grade II) adenocarcinoma of the endometrium showing a mixture of glandular and solid differentiation.

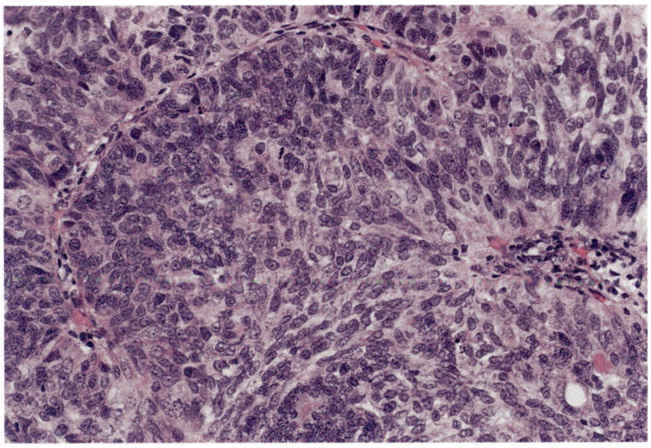

4.30 Poorly differentiated adenocarcinoma of the endometrium (Grade III) showing a predominant solid component to the adenocarcinoma.

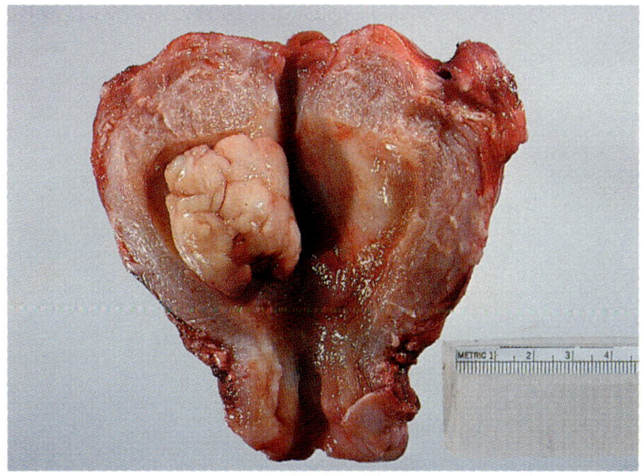

4.31 Gross view of polypoid adenocarcinoma of the endometrium showing no gross evidence of myometrial invasion.

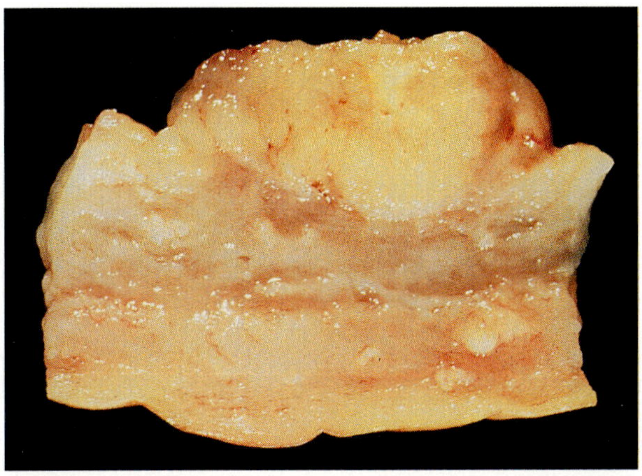

4.32 Adenocarcinoma of the endometrium showing superficial myometrial invasion.

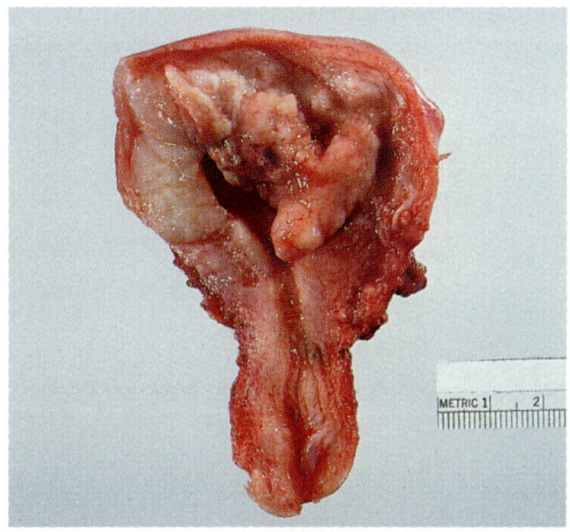

4.33 Endometrial adenocarcinoma demonstrating deep myometrial invasion.

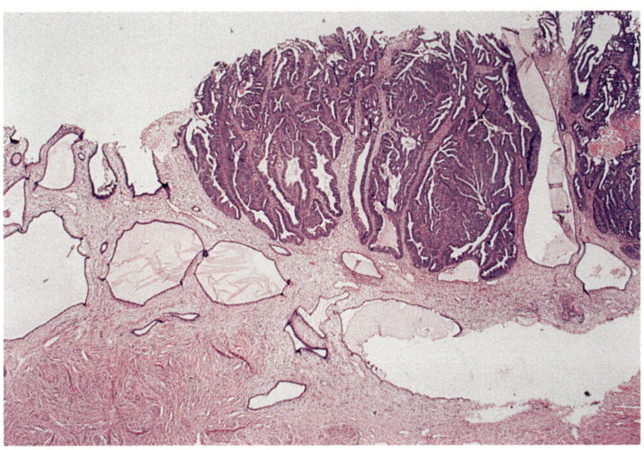

4.34 Adenocarcinoma of the endometrium with mucosal extension to the endocervix (FIGO Stage IIA).

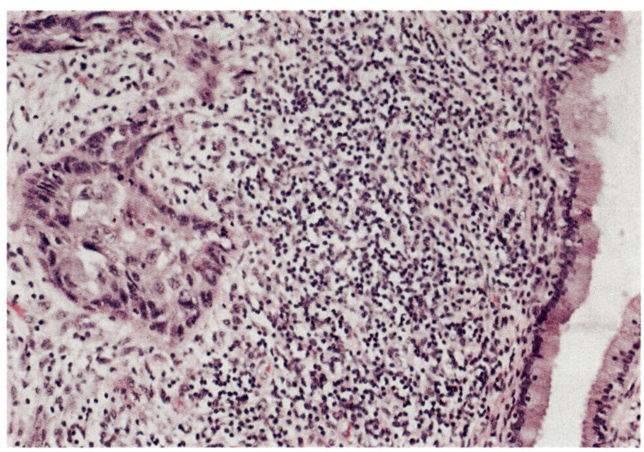

4.35 Endometrial adenocarcinoma extending to the cervix with evidence of stromal invasion (FIGO Stage IIB).

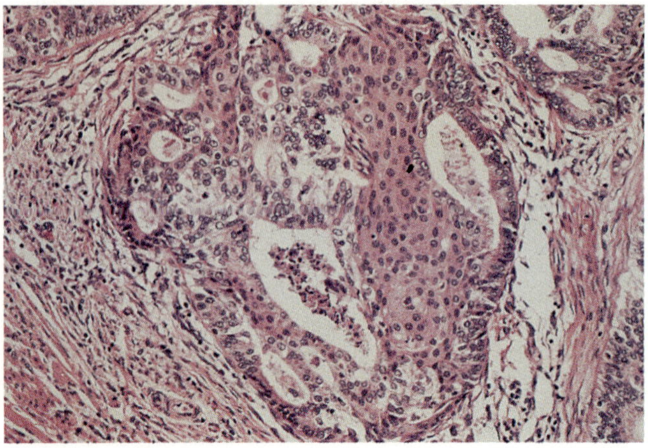

4.36 Adenocarcinoma of the endometrium with squamous differentiation. The squamous component is confined to the glandular component and shows no significant cytologic atypia or evidence of destructive invasion.

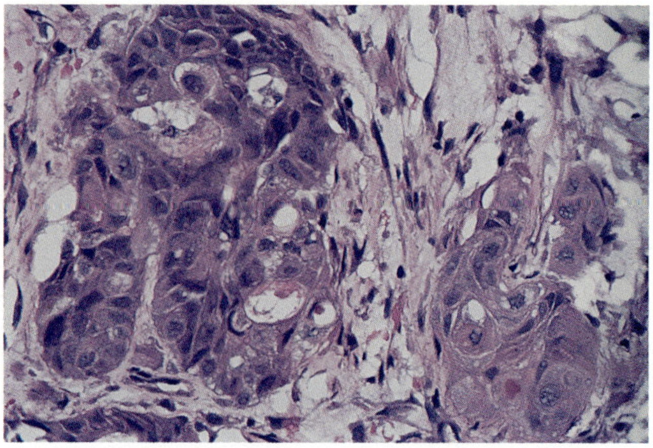

4.37 Mixed adenosquamous carcinoma of the endometrium revealing cytologic atypia in the squamous component. The squamous component also shows destructive invasion of the surrounding stroma.

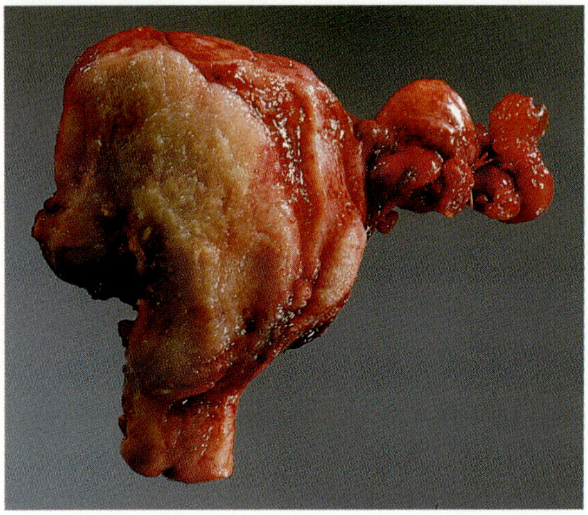

4.38 Primary squamous carcinoma of the endometrium with deep myometrial invasion.

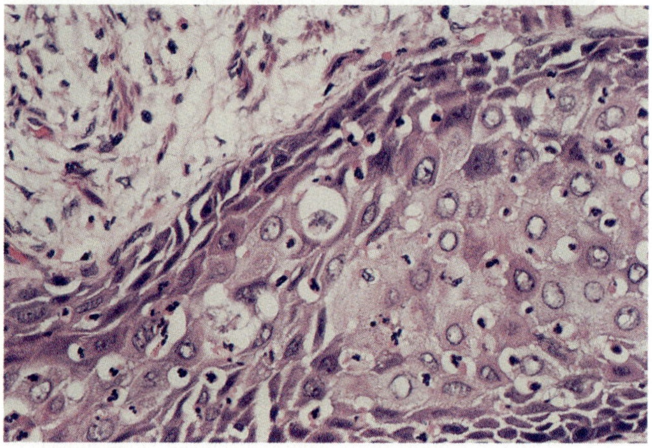

4.39 Primary squamous carcinoma of the endometrium.

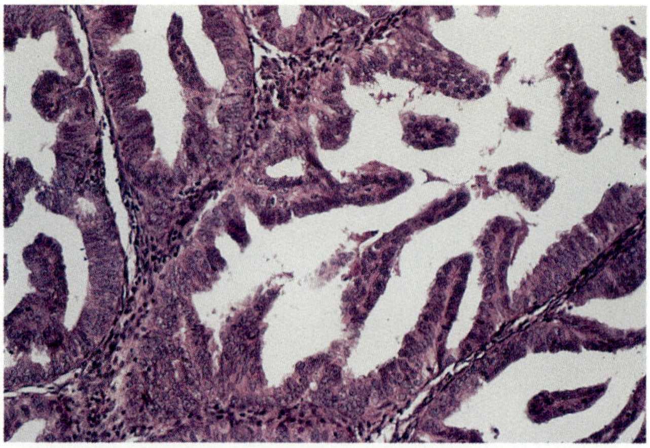

4.40 Endometrial adenocarcinoma demonstrating a villoglandular pattern with finger-like projections.

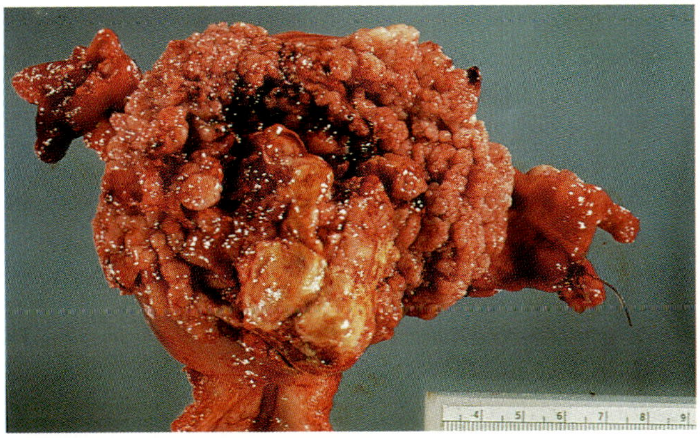

4.41 Gross view of papillary serous carcinoma of the endometrium.

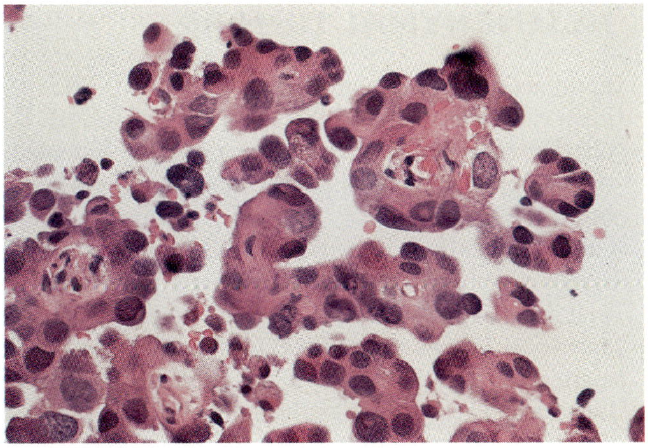

4.42 Papillary serous carcinoma of the endometrium with marked nuclear atypia and features similar to those seen in ovarian serous carcinoma.

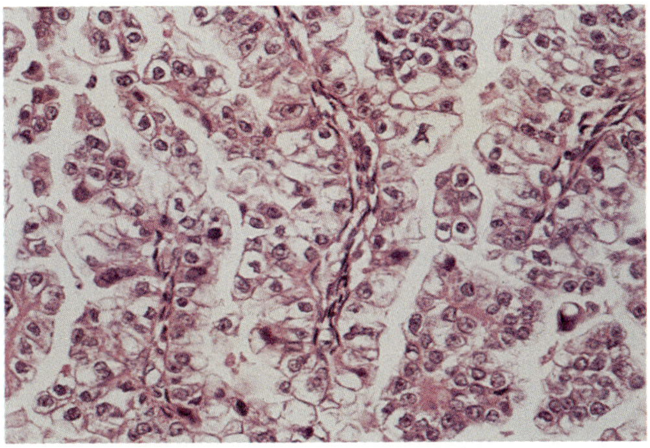

4.43 Clear cell adenocarcinoma of the endometrium.

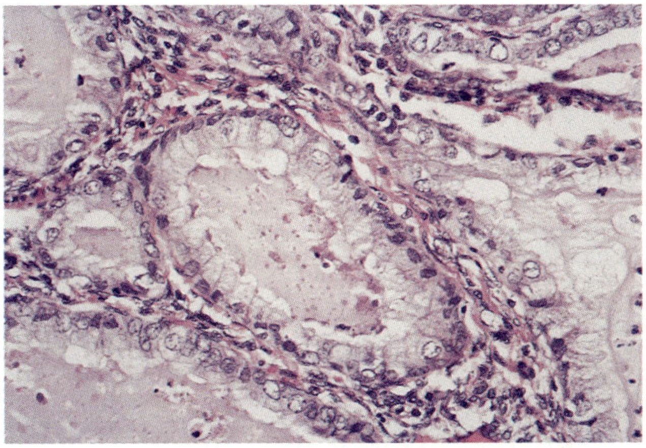

4.44 Mucinous adenocarcinoma of the endometrium.

MESENCHYMAL TUMORS

Endometrial stromal tumors[14,26,57] are divided into four main categories (Table 4-2). The first is the stromal nodule (Figure 4-45). This is a proliferation of endometrial stroma that is usually an isolated nodule, although it can occur in multiple foci. It usually occurs within the endometrium but can extend into the myometrium. It is a well-circumscribed lesion composed of bland endometrial stromal cells with a mitotic activity of less than ten mitoses in 10 high-power fields (HPF). There is a pushing margin, and no lymphatic or vascular invasion can be identified. These lesions are benign.

The second category of stromal tumors is low-grade stromal sarcoma[65] (endolymphatic stromal myosis) (Figures 4-46 to 4-49). This is a proliferation of bland endometrial stromal cells that resemble proliferative endometrium. Hyalinization, plexiform, and sex cord–like patterns are common. Infiltration of the myometrium and vascular lymphatic invasion can be extensive, giving rise to a distinctive gross and microscopic pattern. This lesion may extend beyond the uterus and can metastasize. Up to 15 normal mitoses in 10 HPF may be seen. This tumor is more common in patients under the age of 50. Both stromal nodules (tumors with pushing borders) and low-grade endometrial stromal sarcomas (tumors with infiltrating borders) may contain areas of glandular or sex cord–like growth, which should not alter the diagnosis. Uterine sex cord–like tumors[19] (Figure 4-50) produce a predominant sex cord pattern.

The third major category of endometrial stromal tumors is the high-grade stromal sarcoma[24] or undifferentiated uterine sarcoma (Figures 4-51 and 4-52). This tumor has significant cellular atypia resembling the sarcomatous portion of a malignant mixed müllerian tumor. It is usually a bulky lesion filling the endometrial cavity and invading the myometrium. There are more than ten mitoses per 10 HPF, and nuclear pleomorphism is common. Vascular lymphatic invasion is usually present but is less often grossly visible. This is an aggressive tumor that frequently extends beyond the uterus and often metastasizes. It is more common in patients over the age of 50. These tumors are currently of uncertain histogenesis. It is possible that some, most, or even all of these tumors may be proved eventually not to be of endometrial stromal type.

TABLE 4-2 Pathologic Characteristics of Endometrial Stromal Tumors

I. STROMAL NODULE

- A. Bland stromal cells resembling normal proliferative phase
- B. Circumscribed with pushing margins
- C. Less than 10 mitoses per 10 HPF
- D. Confined to uterus
- E. No lymphatic or vascular intrusion

II. LOW-GRADE STROMAL SARCOMA (ENDOLYMPHATIC STROMAL MYOSIS)

- A. Bland stromal cells resembling normal proliferative phase
- B. Hyalin, plexiform, and sex cord–like patterns common
- C. Up to 15 normal mitoses per 10 HPF
- D. Infiltration of myometrium
- E. Vascular and lymphatic invasion, which may be massive, is common, giving rise to distinctive gross and microscopic patterns
- F. May extend beyond uterus and can metastasize
- G. Patients usually under age 50 years

III. HIGH-GRADE STROMAL SARCOMA (UNDIFFERENTIATED UTERINE SARCOMA)

- A. Cellular atypia resembling MMMT
- B. Greater than 10 mitoses per 10 HPF
- C. Infiltrating margins, usually with extensive myometrial infiltration
- D. Vascular and lymphatic invasion less often grossly visible
- E. Frequently extends beyond uterus, and metastases are common
- F. Patients usually over age 50 years

IV. UTERINE TUMOR RESEMBLING OVARIAN SEX CORD TUMOR

- A. Predominantly or exclusively composed of cells arranged in cords, trabeculae, or tubules resembling structures found in ovarian sex cord stromal tumors
- B. Aggressive potential to be evaluated by using criteria listed above

HPF, High-power fields; MMMT, malignant mixed müllerian tumor.
Modified from Hendrickson MR, Kempson RL: *Surgical Pathology of the Uterine Corpus*, Bennington JL (ed) Philadelphia, WB Saunders, 1980.

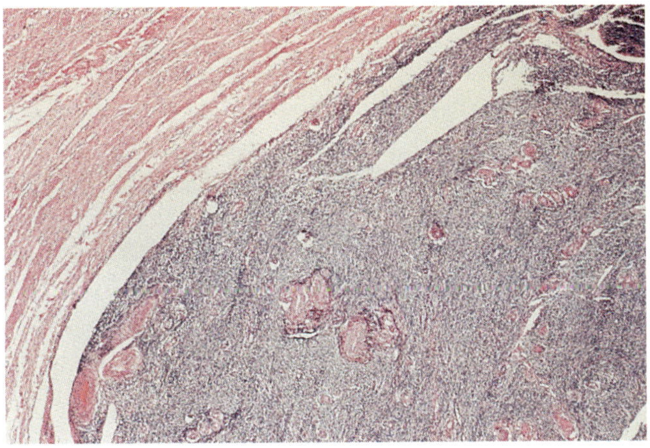

4.45 Endometrial stromal nodule with a well-circumscribed margin showing no evidence of invasion.

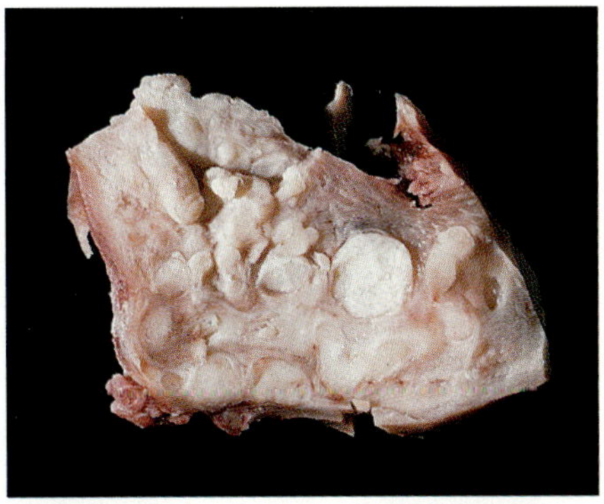

4.46 Low-grade endometrial sarcoma (endolymphatic stromal myosis) demonstrating on gross view numerous vascular channels infiltrated by tumor.

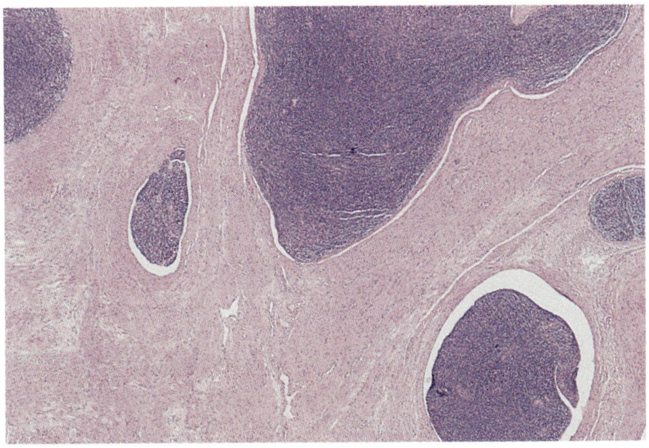

4.47 Low-grade endometrial stromal sarcoma showing the vascular space involvement and irregular margins on low power.

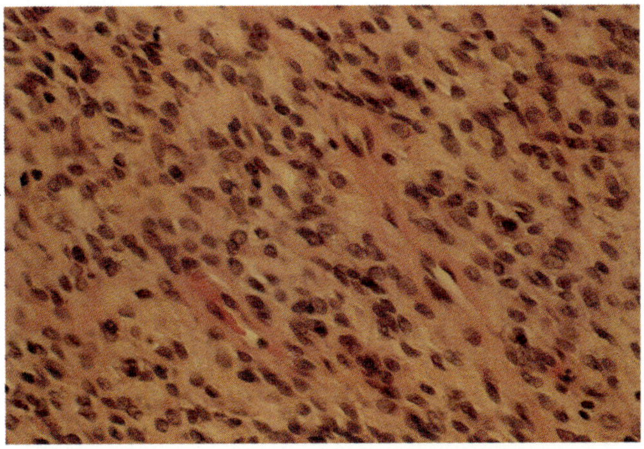

4.48 Low-grade endometrial stromal sarcoma demonstrating scattered blood vessels similar to those seen in proliferating endometrium.

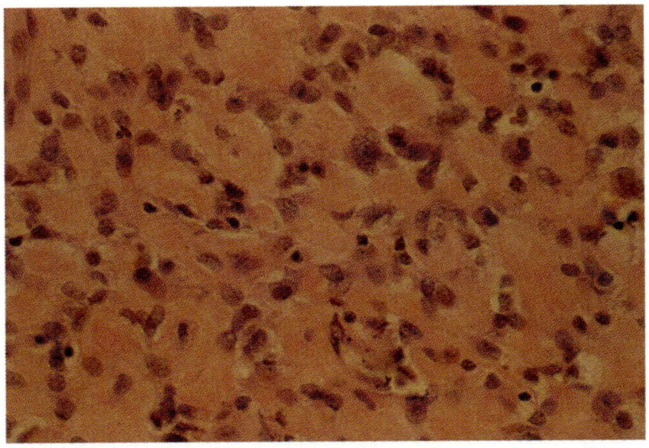

4.49 Low-grade endometrial stromal sarcoma with areas of hyalinization.

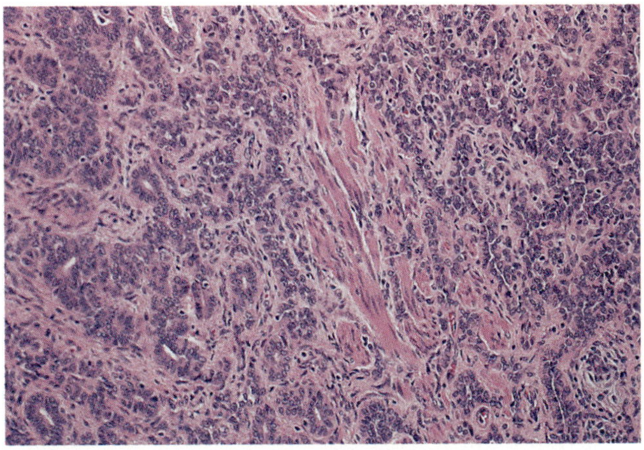

4.50 Uterine tumor resembling an ovarian sex cord stromal tumor.

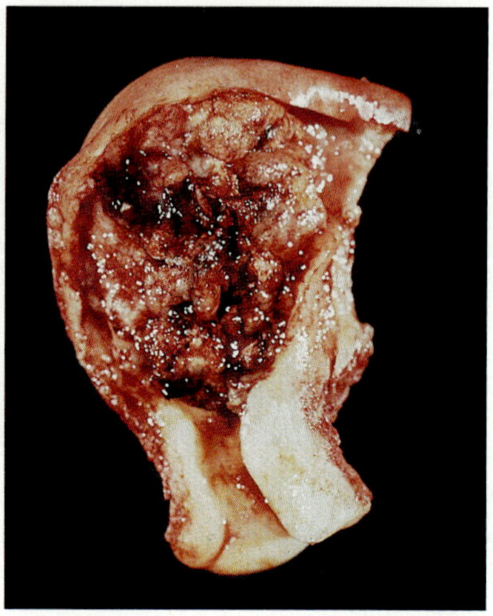

4.51 Gross view of a high-grade endometrial stromal sarcoma showing areas of necrosis, hemorrhage, and deep myometrial invasion.

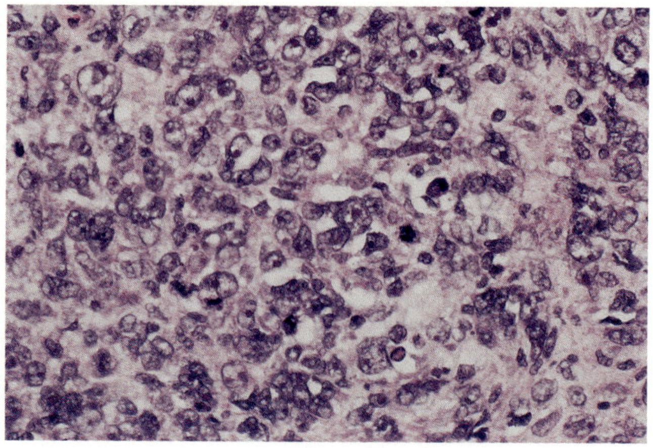

4.52 High-grade endometrial stromal sarcoma with marked cytologic atypia and numerous mitotic figures.

SMOOTH MUSCLE TUMORS

Leiomyomas are the most common benign mesenchymal tumor of the uterus. They have a characteristic gross appearance composed of well-circumscribed nodules of white, whorled, firm tissue (Figures 4-53 and 4-54). There may be central necrosis and degeneration with infarction (Figure 4-55). Myxoid change is occasionally seen (Figures 4-56 and 4-57) and needs to be distinguished from myxoid leiomyosarcoma. Leiomyomas can be subclassified into histologic variants and those with unusual growth patterns. Adenomatoid tumors of the uterus[13] may resemble leiomyomas grossly.

The histologic variants include the epithelioid leiomyoma[43] (Figures 4-58 and 4-59). This form of leiomyoma contains polygonal cells resembling epithelial cells. There can also be a clear cell component and a plexiform variant[40] (Figures 4-60 and 4-61). A cellular leiomyoma is defined as a leiomyoma that is more cellular than the surrounding myometrium (Figure 4-62). Some of these tumors may be difficult to distinguish from endometrial stromal tumors.[61] A comparison is seen in Table 4-3. The symplastic or bizarre cellular leiomyoma is a markedly pleomorphic variant that contains bizarre multinucleated

TABLE 4-3 Comparative Features of Highly Cellular Leiomyomas and Endometrial Stromal Nodules

	Highly Cellular Leiomyomas	Endometrial Stromal Nodules
Fascicular pattern	Usual	Infrequent
Large vessels with thick muscular walls	Common	Rare
Arterioles	Occasional	Numerous
Cleftlike spaces	Frequent	Absent
Foam cells	Rare	Frequent
Desmin positivity	Almost always	Rare, focal

From Olivia E, Young RH, Clement PB, Bhan AK, Scully RE: *Am J Surg Pathol,* 19:757-768, 1995, with permission.

giant cells but a virtual absence of mitotic activity (Figure 4-63). It is a benign lesion that rarely, if ever, metastasizes and appears to be associated with either pregnancy or oral contraceptive use. There are several other patterns of leiomyomas, including those that resemble a neurilemoma (Figure 4-64) and those that contain tubules.[52] A lipoleiomyoma contains adipose tissue and is considered a benign heterologous mesenchymal tumor (Figures 4-65 and 4-66).

The unusual growth patterns of leiomyomas can cause some confusion clinically.[20,25] Leiomyomas can have vascular invasion focally (Figure 4-67), and if the mitotic activity is low, the vascular involvement does not appear to have any predictive value. The vascular invasion can be extensive and can be viewed grossly; this is referred to as intravenous leiomyomatosis[17,55] (Figure 4-68). This condition can extend outside the uterus into the pelvic vessels and up the vena cava in extreme circumstances. A condition known as benign metastasizing leiomyoma has been reported rarely and usually presents with multiple bland lung nodules. There are several possible theories for this condition. One is that it is obviously a low-grade leiomyosarcoma. Another is that there is a field effect for multifocal proliferation of smooth muscle, and the lung lesions are not actually metastatic. Another theory is that some of these patients have undergone previous manipulation of the uterus, by cesarean section delivery or by dilatation and curettage. It is possible that fragments of the smooth muscle neoplasm were dislodged, entered the bloodstream, and reside in the lung. This would be similar to trophoblastic embolization in trophoblastic disease. Parasitic leiomyomas occur when a pedunculated leiomyoma is parasitized, usually by the omentum or another pelvic structure. Infiltrating leiomyoma is the term used for a locally infiltrating smooth muscle tumor that is bland and not well encapsulated. If the mitotic activity is low, this infiltrating margin is also not predictive of a poor prognosis. The term disseminated peritoneal leiomyomatosis[76] has been given to an unusual condition of proliferating smooth muscle nodules that are present throughout the serosal surfaces in the peritoneal cavity. This condition is usually found at the time of cesarean section and is thought to be a metaplastic process of the subcoelomic mesenchymal tissue differentiating toward smooth muscle.

The term smooth muscle tumors of uncertain malignant potential has been applied to tumors in which the histologic pattern and/or mitotic activity[70] is greater than that seen in the benign condition, but not yet that of a leiomyosarcoma (Table 4-4). In an otherwise typical leiomyoma, a mitotic count of up to five mitoses per 10 HPF can be tolerated. If there is epithelioid cell differentiation or mild to moderate nuclear atypia, less than two mitotic figures per 10 HPF must be found to classify it as benign. In an otherwise typical leiomyoma, a mitotic count of five to nine mitoses per 10 HPF would place this tumor in a category with uncertain malignant potential. If there is epithelioid cell differentiation or mild to moderate nuclear atypia, two to four mitoses per 10 HPFs would represent a tumor of uncertain malignant potential. This category is, as it states, of uncertain malignant potential. Although most of these lesions will not metastasize, their ultimate behavior is not known at this time. Some authors suggest terms such as "mitotically active leiomyomas" for some of the smooth muscle tumors that fall into this category.[9,60,63,66]

Leiomyosarcomas[11,39] are defined (Table 4-4) as cellular smooth muscle tumors containing more than 10 mitoses per 10 HPF, or tumors with cellular pleomorphism or of an epithelioid cell type containing five to 10 mitoses per 10 HPF. Most leiomyosarcomas are tumors that have a distinctive gross appearance. They are tumors that arise in the myometrium, have a soft, irregular consistency (Figure 4-69), and are not well circumscribed or firm and whorled like leiomyomas. The surrounding myometrium is infiltrated (Figure 4-70) and the nuclei are atypical (Figure 4-71). Tumor cell necrosis is present (Figure 4-72) that differs from the hyaline necrosis (Figure 4-73) sometimes seen in leiomyomas. Myxoid leiomyosarcomas[41] show deceptively bland nuclei and a relative paucity of mitotic figures (Figures 4-74 and 4-75). These lesions are aggressive tumors with a poor prognosis. Leiomyosarcomas sometimes produce osteoclastic-like giant cells[49,53] (Figure 4-76).

TABLE 4-4 Definitions of Uterine Smooth Muscle Tumors

I. LEIOMYOMA (with or without usual histologic pattern or growth pattern)

A. Fewer than two mitotic figures per 10 HPF with no abnormal mitotic figures, no tumor cell necrosis, no myxoid stroma, and no anaplastic cells

B. Fewer than five mitotic figures per 10 HPF if tumor is composed of well-differentiated spindled smooth muscle cells without atypia or pleomorphism

II. SMOOTH MUSCLE TUMOR OF UNCERTAIN MALIGNANT POTENTIAL

A. More than 15 mitoses per 10 HPF if tumor is paucicellular without cytologic atypia or nuclear pleomorphism

B. Five to 10 mitoses per 10 HPF if tumor is composed of hypercellular, well-differentiated smooth muscle cells without atypia, anaplasia, or pleomorphism

C. Two to five mitoses per 10 HPF if tumor cells demonstrate nuclear atypia, cellular pleomorphism, giant cell transformation, an epithelioid pattern, or tumor cell necrosis.

D. Smooth muscle tumors with mitotic counts less than above but containing abnormal mitotic figures or tumor cell necrosis

III. LEIOMYOSARCOMA

A. Cellular smooth muscle tumor containing more than 10 mitoses per 10 HPF (most often tumor cell nuclei and some mitotic figures are abnormal)

B. Uterine smooth muscle tumor with cellular anaplasia, pleomorphism, and containing five to 10 mitoses per 10 HPF

C. Epithelioid smooth muscle tumor containing five or more mitoses per 10 HPF

IV. SMOOTH MUSCLE TUMOR WITH INCREASED NUMBERS OF MITOTIC FIGURES

Pauci- or normocellular or rarely hypercellular smooth muscle tumor composed of cells with bland nuclei and mitotic counts of five to 15 per 10 HPF; mitotic figures are not abnormal (almost always history of pregnancy or progestogen therapy or mitotically active cells in an area of regeneration)

V. CELLULAR LEIOMYOMA

Contains more cells per unit area than surrounding myometrium

VI. EPITHELIOID SMOOTH MUSCLE TUMORS

A. Epithelioid leiomyoma: epithelium-like, clear cell, leiomyoblastoma, or plexiform pattern containing less than two mitotic figures per 10 HPF

B. Epithelioid smooth muscle tumor of uncertain malignant potential: as in A, but with two to five mitoses per 10 HPF

C. Epithelioid leiomyosarcoma: as in A, but with more than five mitoses per 10 HPF

VII. SYMPLASTIC (ATYPICAL) LEIOMYOMA

Benign smooth muscle tumor as defined in I that contains giant cells, sometimes multinucleated or hyperlobated, and/or cells with hyperchromatic, often smudged nuclei or enlarged nuclei

Modified from Hendrickson MR, Kempson RL: *Surgical Pathology of the Uterine Corpus,* Bennington JL (ed), Philadelphia, WB Saunders, 1980.
HPF, High-power fields.

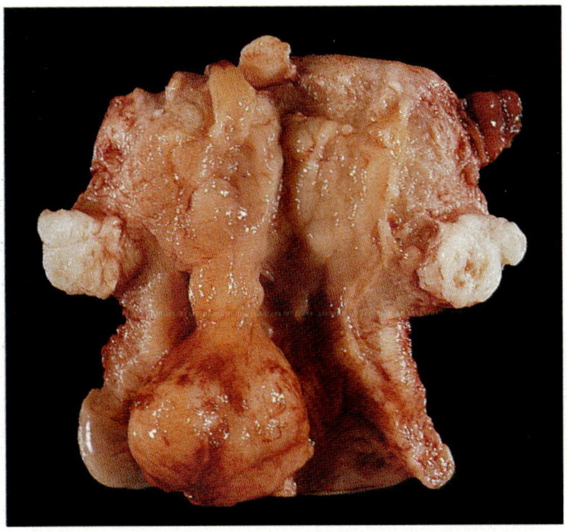

4.53 Uterus demonstrating numerous leiomyomas including subserosal, intramural, and submucosal patterns.

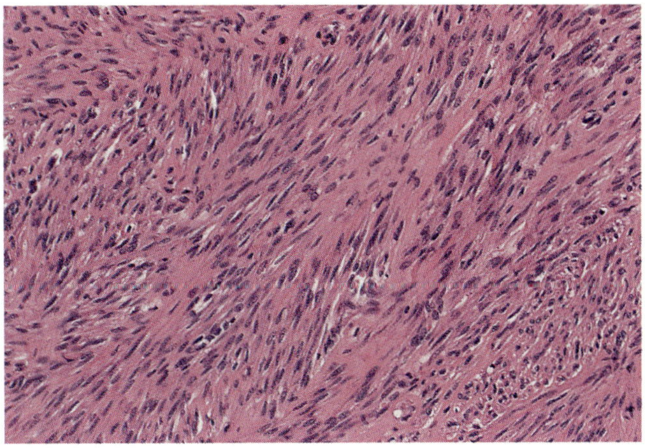

4.54 Leiomyoma demonstrating intertwining fascicles of smooth muscles with uniform oval nuclei and no pleomorphism.

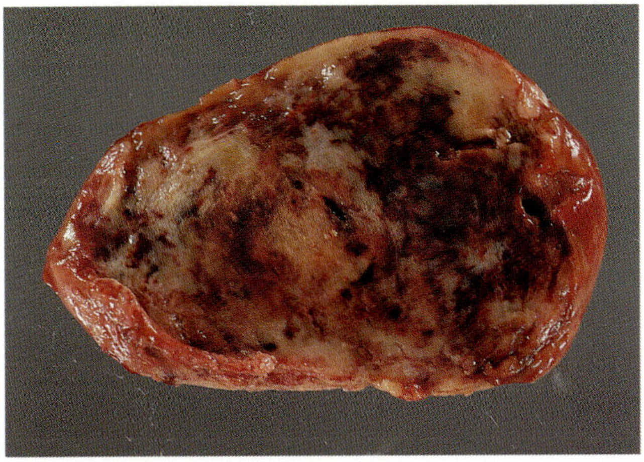

4.55 Gross view of an infarcted leiomyoma.

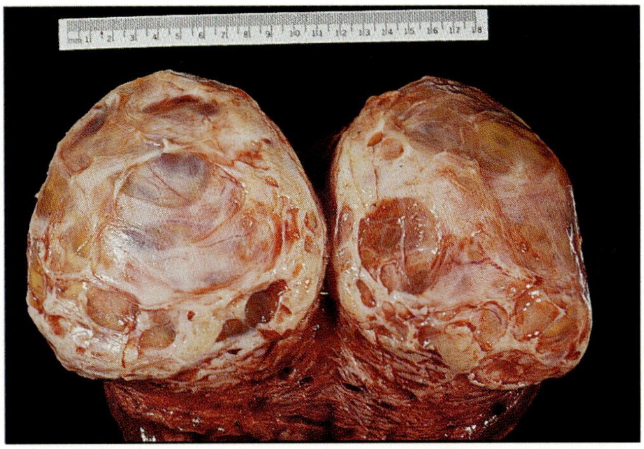

4.56 Leiomyoma demonstrating cystic and myxoid degeneration.

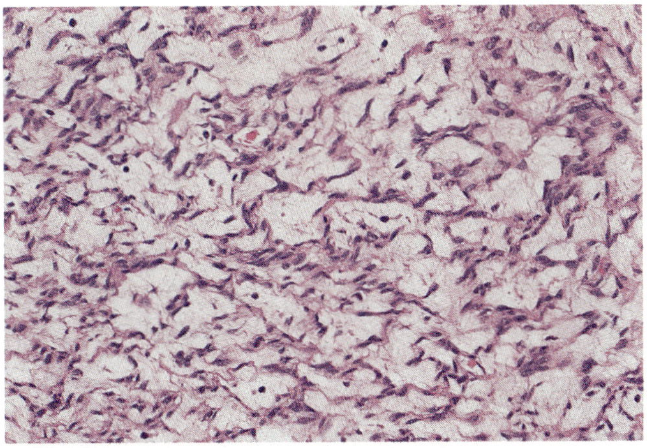

4.57 Myxoid degeneration within a leiomyoma.

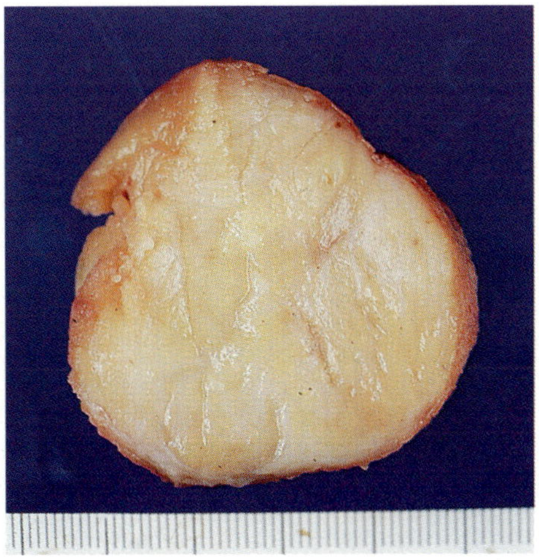

4.58 Gross view of an epithelioid leiomyoma (leiomyoblastoma).

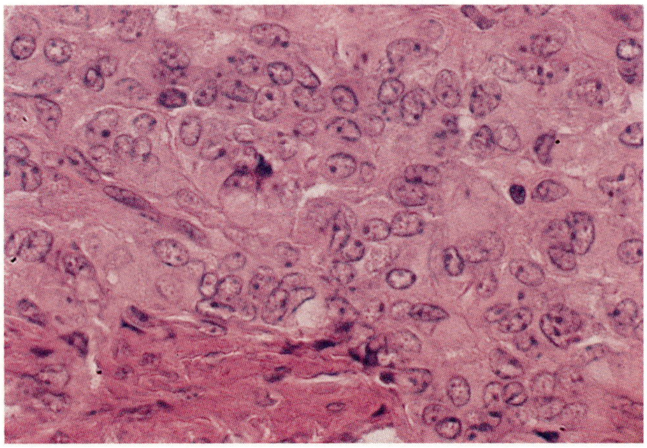

4.59 Epithelioid leiomyoma (leiomyoblastoma). The smooth muscle cells have a rounder nucleus and more cytoplasm, giving an epithelioid appearance.

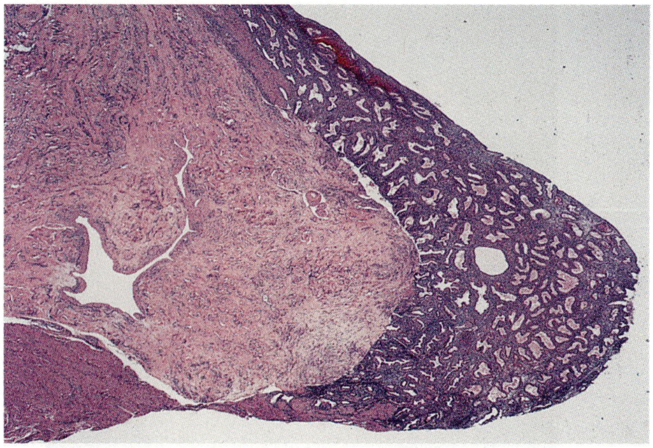

4.60 Plexiform tumor of the uterus demonstrating the characteristic submucosal position of this particular lesion.

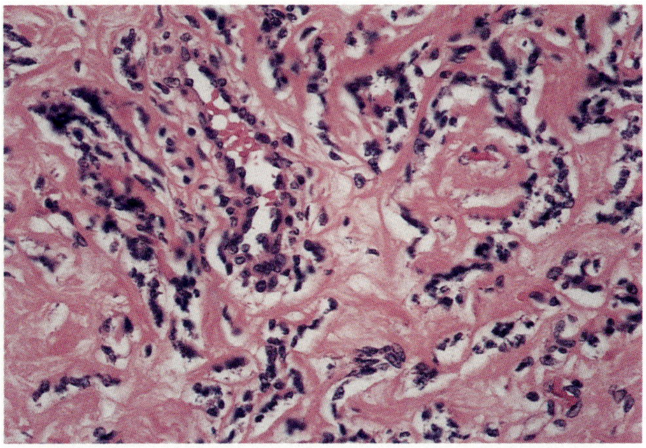

4.61 Higher-power view of a plexiform tumor showing epitheloid smooth muscle cords with surrounding hyalinization.

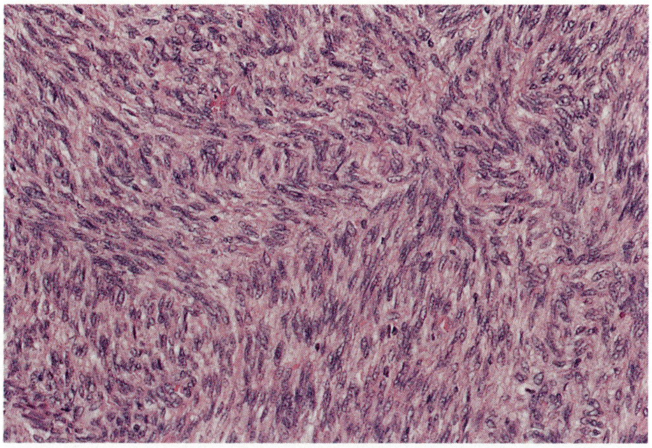

4.62 Cellular leiomyoma demonstrating an increased nuclear-to-cytoplasmic ratio but no cytologic atypia.

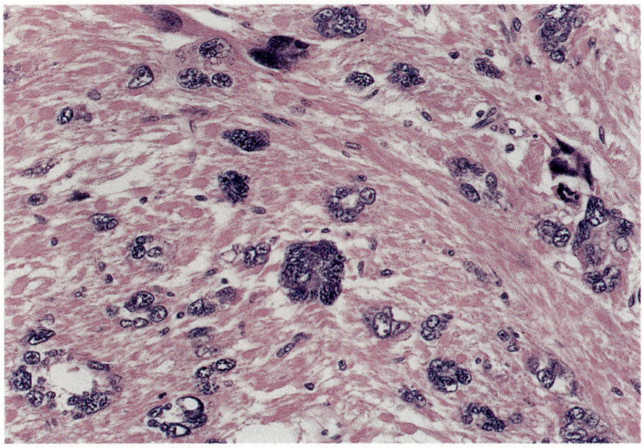

4.63 Bizarre cellular (symplastic) leiomyoma with multinucleated giant cells showing pleomorphic nuclei in the absence of mitotic figures.

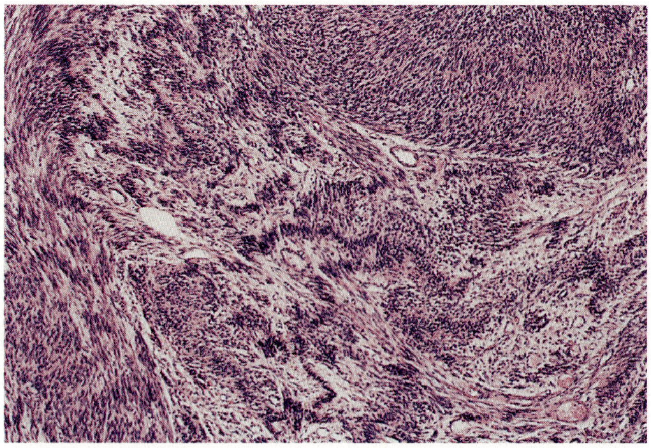

4.64 Leiomyoma with a neurilemoma-like pattern showing areas of palisading nuclei.

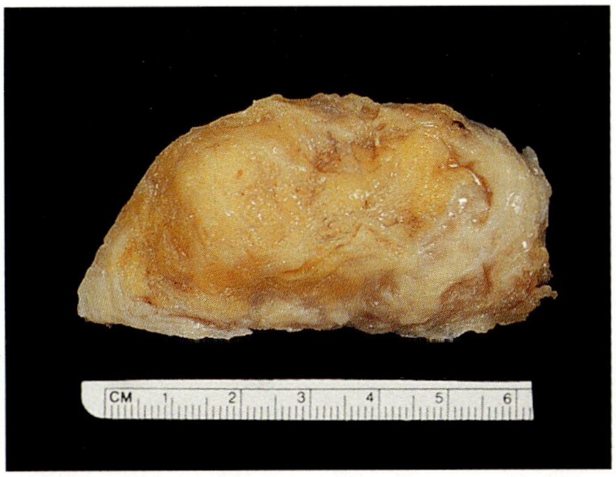

4.65 Gross view of a lipoleiomyoma.

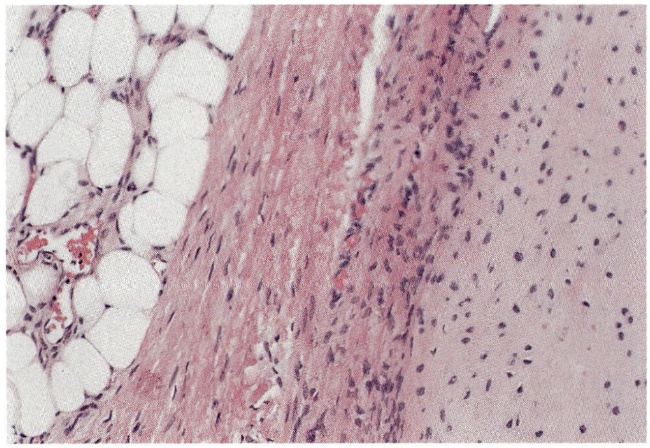

4.66 Lipoleiomyoma with focal cartilaginous differentiation.

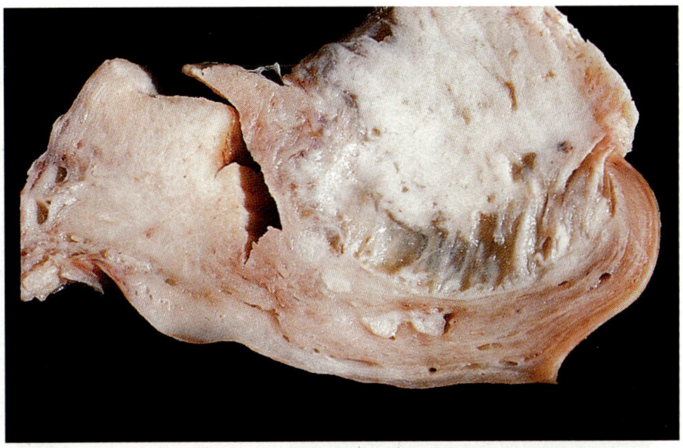

4.67 Leiomyoma with vascular involvement that can be seen grossly.

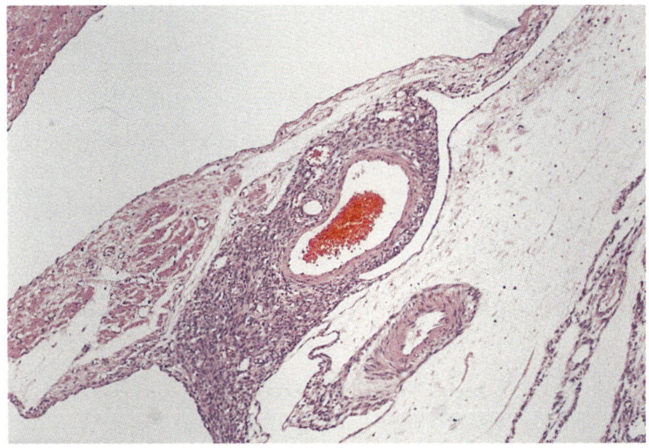

4.68 Intravenous leiomyoma.

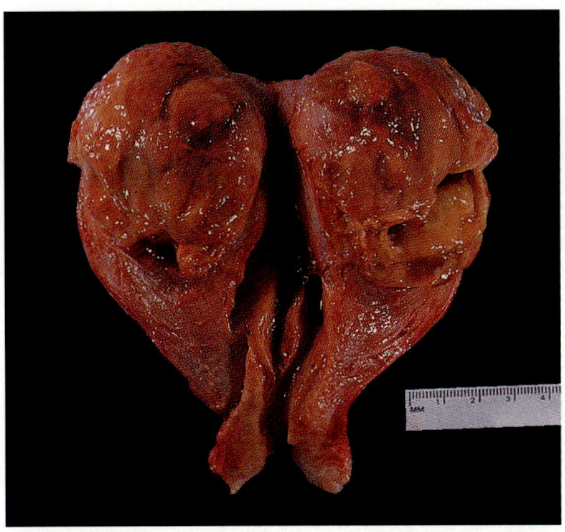

4.69 Gross view of leiomyosarcoma showing necrosis and irregular infiltration.

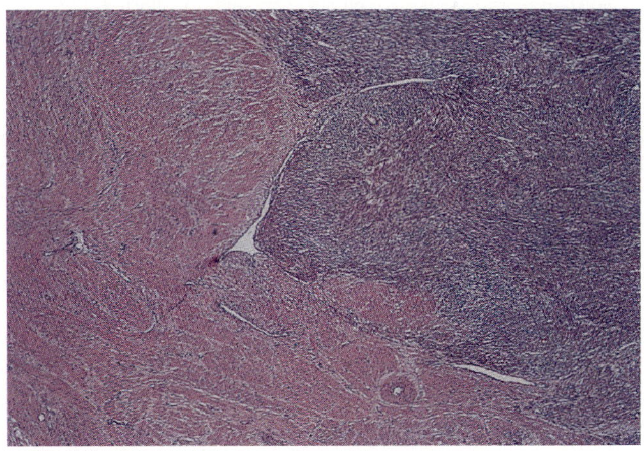

4.70 Leiomyosarcoma demonstrating a high cellularity and infiltration of the surrounding myometrium.

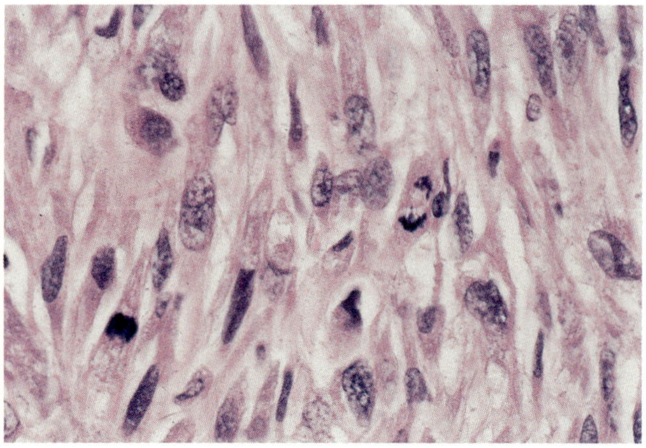

4.71 Leiomyosarcoma revealing numerous mitotic figures and nuclear pleomorphism.

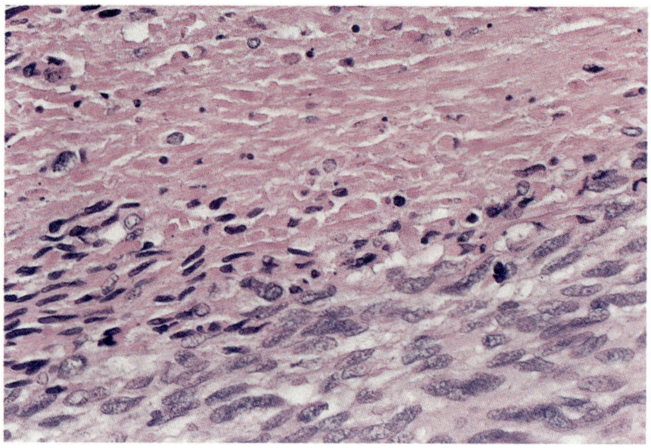

4.72 Leiomyosarcoma revealing tumor cell necrosis.

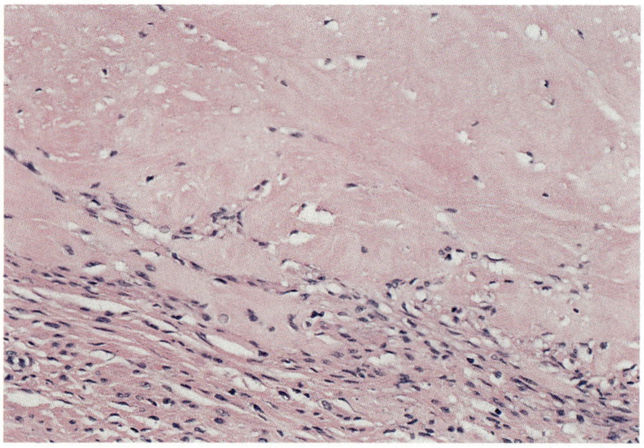

4.73 Leiomyoma with hyaline necrosis that should be distinguished from the tumor cell necrosis seen in Figure 4-72.

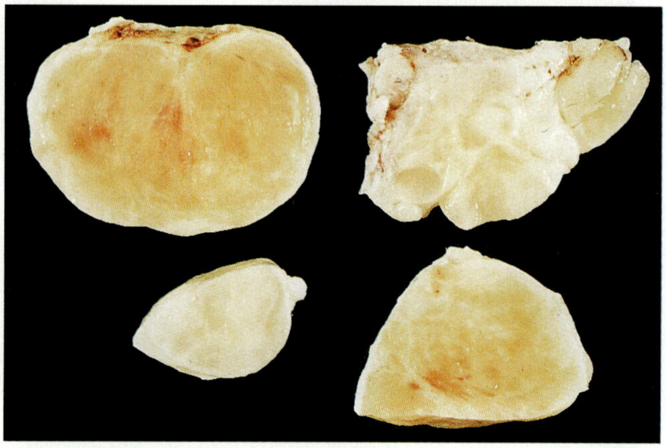

4.74 Myxoid leiomyosarcoma.

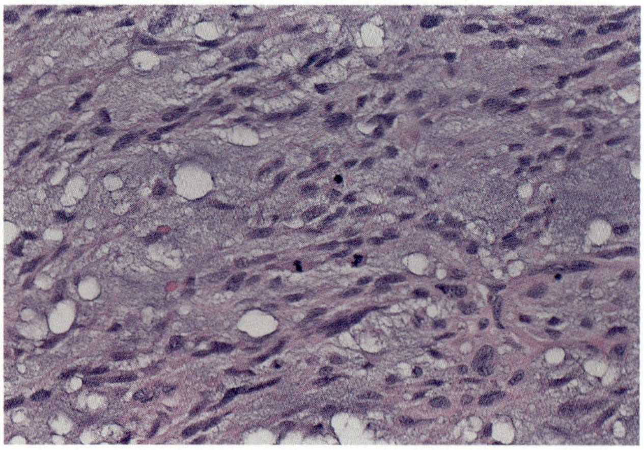

4.75 Myxoid leiomyosarcoma showing deceptively bland nuclei and a relative paucity of mitotic figures.

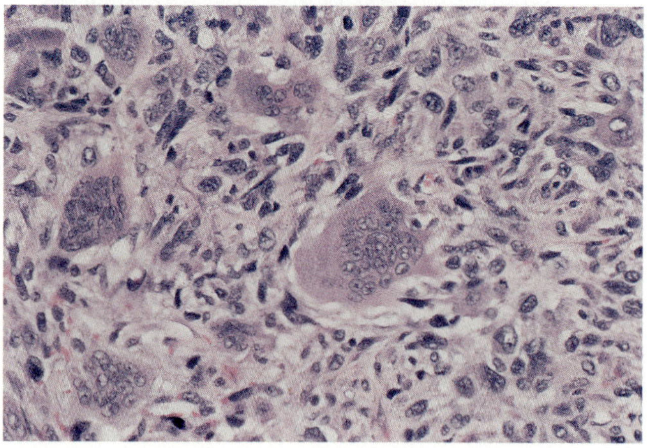

4.76 Leiomyosarcoma with osteoclastic-like giant cells.

MIXED EPITHELIAL AND MESENCHYMAL TUMORS

Adenofibroma[77] is characterized by blunt papillary processes lined usually by benign serous epithelium (Figures 4-77 and 4-78), although mucinous, endometrioid, and clear cell types of epithelium can occur. There is a fibrous stroma and the mitotic activity is less than four per 10 HPF. Atypical polypoid adenomyoma[50,79] (Figure 4-79) is a variant containing endometrioid glands with varying atypia, often with squamous differentiation, embedded in a muscular stroma.

The malignant counterpart of the adenofibroma is the adenosarcoma.[17,62,81] This is a proliferation of benign epithelial cells with a malignant stromal component (Figures 4-80 to 4-82). The stromal component is usually more fibrous than the endometrial stromal tumors. The mitotic activity is greater than four per 10 HPF. It is this amount of mitotic activity that correlates best with the myometrial invasion that in turn correlates with a worse prognosis. Stromal overgrowth[16] (Figure 4-83) is also a poor prognostic indicator.

The next category is carcinosarcoma (malignant mixed müllerian tumors).* These tumors contain both a malignant epithelial and a malignant mesenchymal component of the endometrium (Figures 4-84 and 4-85). They are categorized into two major areas; homologous and heterologous. Homologous and heterologous usually refer to the stromal component. If there is differentiation toward endometrial stromal sarcoma or leiomyosarcoma, the tumor is considered homologous; if there is differentiation toward other cell types, such as rhabdomyosarcoma (Figure 4-86), chondrosarcoma (Figure 4-87), and osteosarcoma (Figure 4-88), it is considered a heterologous type. The epithelial component[10] is often composed of a typical endometrial adenocarcinoma; however, papillary, clear cell, and squamous forms of adenocarcinoma have been described as components of the tumor. The homologous malignant mixed müllerian tumor is a variant that has been referred to as carcinosarcoma. These tumors, which are highly aggressive, are bulky and necrotic and often protrude through the cervical os. There may be deep myometrial involvement, and metastasis is common. The prognosis is very poor.

*References 22, 27, 58, 59, 64, 67, 73, 74.

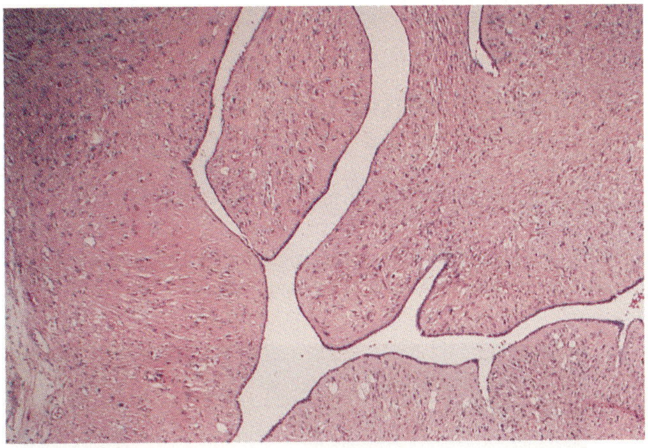

4.77 Low-power view of papillary adenofibroma of the uterus.

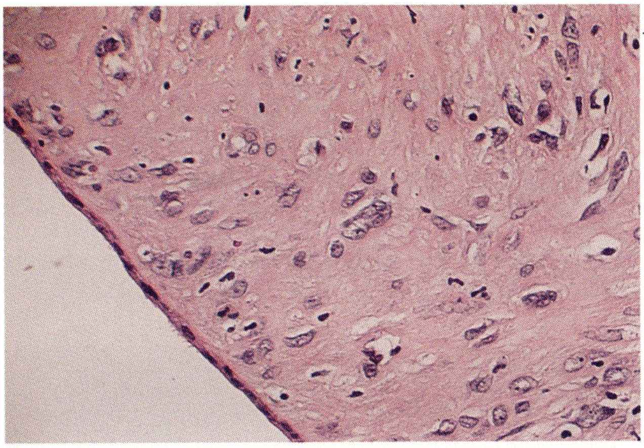

4.78 High-power view of adenofibroma of the uterus demonstrating a bland flattened epithelial lining and a fibroma-like proliferation in the subepithelial area.

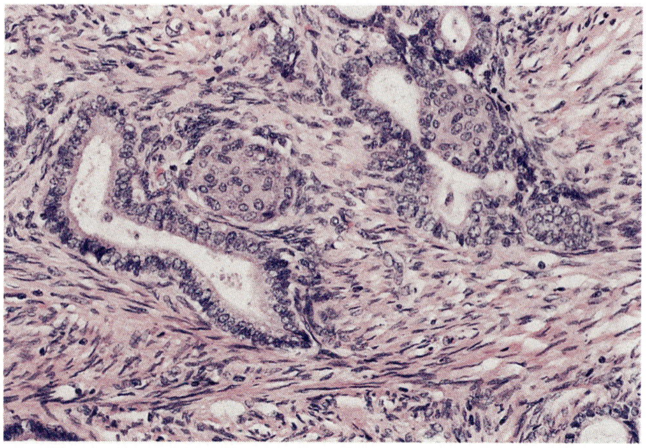

4.79 Atypical polypoid adenomyoma of the uterus with irregular glands showing focal squamous metaplasia embedded in a fibromuscular stroma.

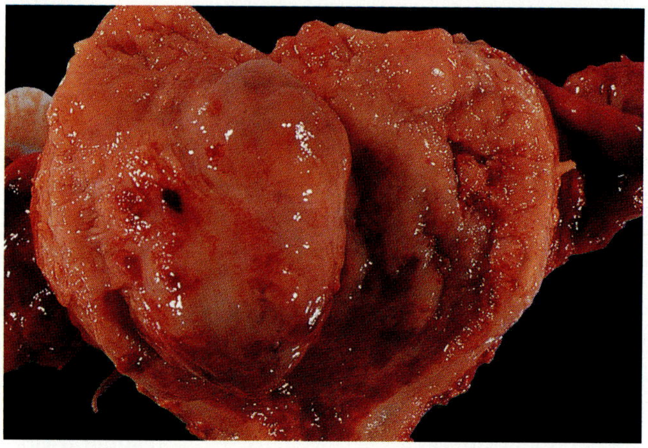

4.80 Gross view of adenosarcoma of the uterus.

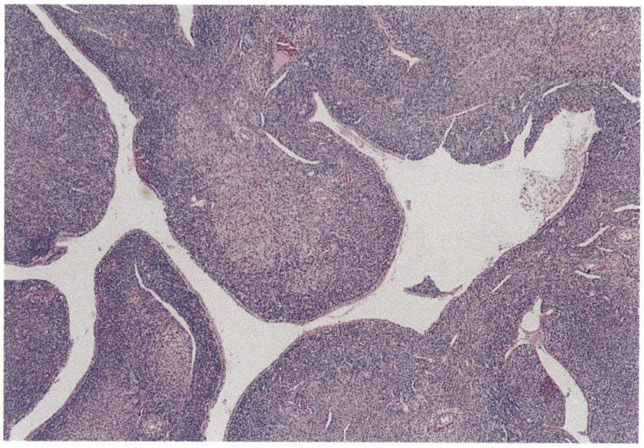

4.81 Adenosarcoma revealing increased cellularity beneath the epithelial layer.

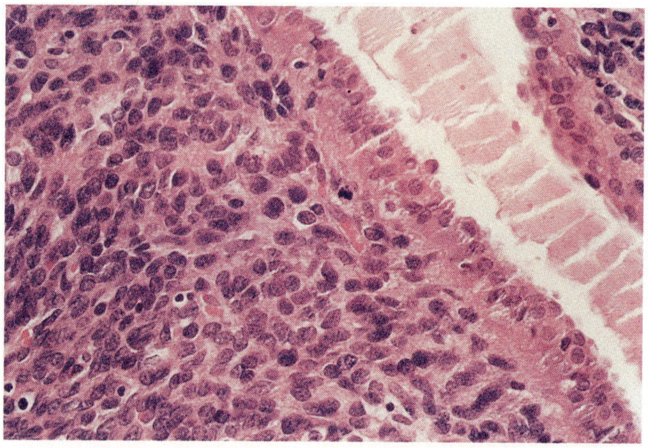

4.82 Adenosarcoma demonstrating the benign glandular lining with underlying endometrial stromal sarcoma.

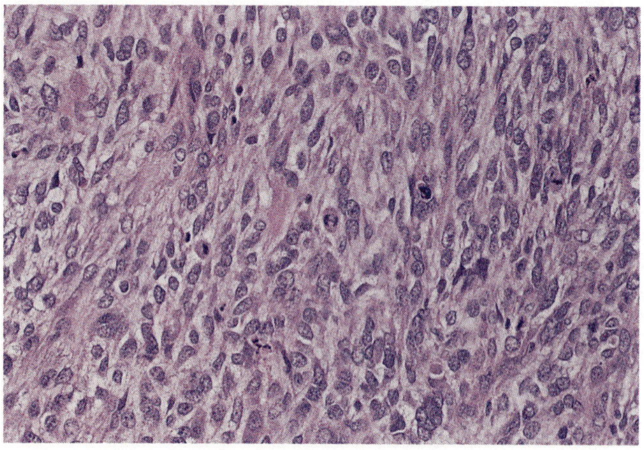

4.83 Adenosarcoma with stromal overgrowth obscuring the benign glandular component.

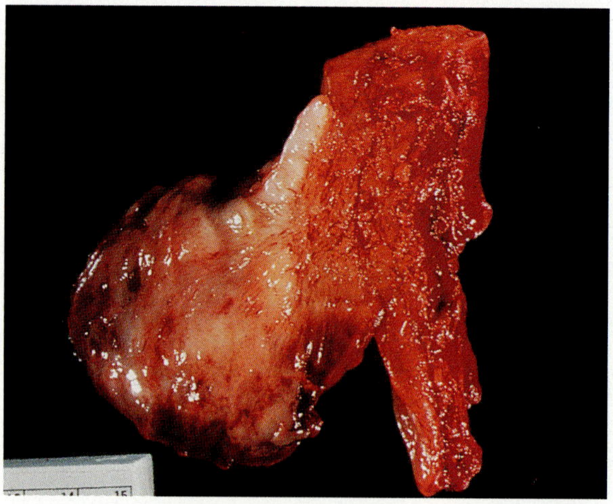

4.84 Gross view of carcinosarcoma of the uterus arising in the endometrium and forming a polypoid mass protruding and extending through the uterine cervix.

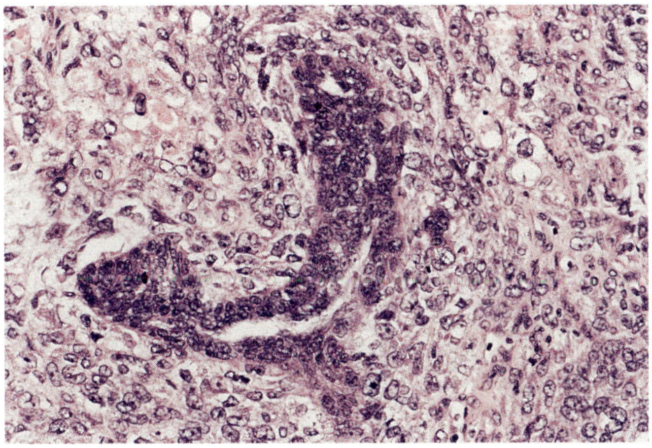

4.85 Carcinosarcoma of the uterus showing a mixed epithelial and mesenchymal component.

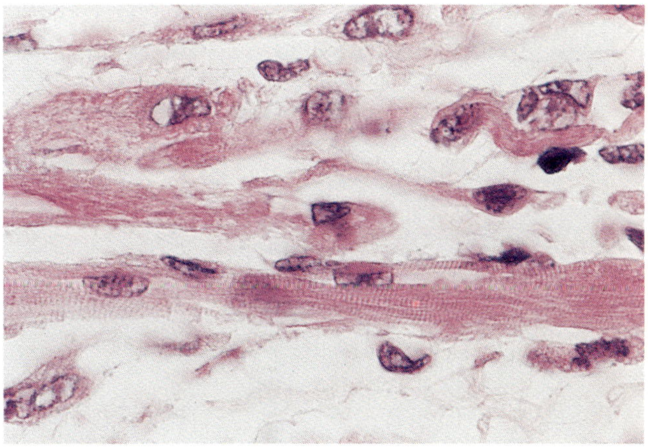

4.86 Carcinosarcoma with rhabdomyoblastic (heterologous) differentiation.

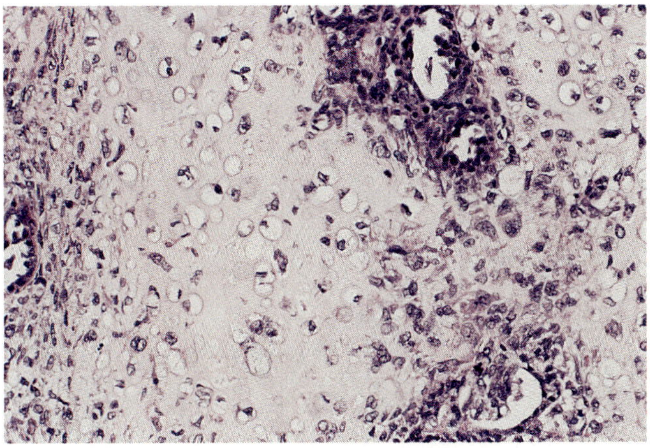

4.87 Carcinosarcoma with chondroid differentiation.

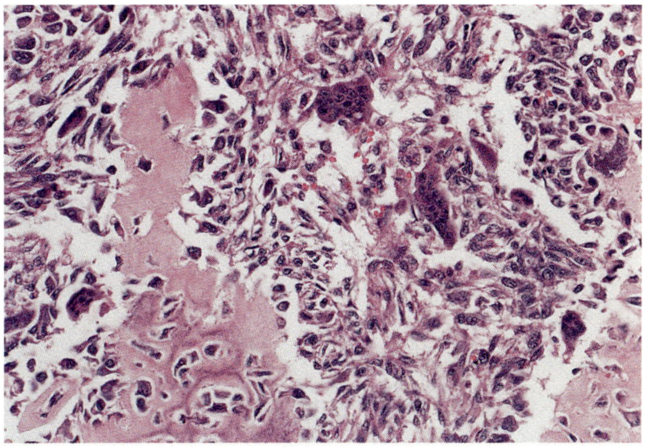

4.88 Carcinosarcoma with osteoid differentiation.

World Health Organization (WHO) Histologic Classification of Tumors of the Uterine Corpus[6]

(with associated systematized nomenclature of medicine [SNOMED] codes)

I. Epithelial Tumors and Related Lesions	SNOMED
A. Endometrial hyperplasia	
1. Simple	72000
2. Complex (adenomatous)	
B. Atypical endometrial hyperplasia	72005
1. Simple	
2. Complex (adenomatous with atypia)	
C. Endometrial polyp	76800
D. Endometrial carcinoma	
1. Endometrioid	
a. Adenocarcinoma	83803
(1) Secretory (variant)	
(2) Ciliated cell (variant)	
b. Adenocarcinoma with squamous differentiation (adenoacanthoma, adenosquamous carcinoma)	85703
2. Serous adenocarcinoma	84413
3. Clear cell adenocarcinoma	83103
4. Mucinous adenocarcinoma	84803
5. Squamous cell carcinoma	80703
6. Mixed carcinoma	83233
7. Undifferentiated carcinoma	80203

II. Mesenchymal Tumors and Related Lesions	
A. Endometrial stromal tumors	
1. Endometrial stromal nodule	89300
2. Endometrial stromal sarcoma, low grade (endolymphatic stromal myosis)	89311
3. Endometrial stromal sarcoma, high grade	89303
B. Smooth muscle tumors	
1. Leiomyoma	88900
a. Cellular (variant)	88920
b. Epithelioid (variant)	88910
c. Bizarre (variant)	88930
d. Lipoleiomyoma (variant)	
2. Smooth muscle tumor of uncertain malignant potential	88971
3. Leiomyosarcoma	88903
a. Epithelioid (variant)	88913
b. Myxoid (variant)	88963
4. Other smooth muscle tumors	
a. Metastasizing leiomyoma	
b. Intravenous leiomyomatosis	88901
c. Diffuse leiomyomatosis	
C. Mixed endometrial stromal and smooth muscle tumors	
D. Adenomatoid tumor	90540
E. Other mesenchymal tumors	
1. Homologous	
2. Heterologous	

III. Mixed Epithelial and Mesenchymal Tumors	
A. Benign	
1. Adenofibroma	90130
2. Adenomyoma	89320
a. Atypical polypoid adenomyoma (variant)	
B. Malignant	
1. Adenosarcoma	89333
a. Homologous	
b. Heterologous	
2. Carcinofibroma	
3. Carcinosarcoma (malignant mesodermal mixed tumor; malignant müllerian mixed tumor)	89803
a. Homologous	
b. Heterologous	

IV. Miscellaneous Tumors	
A. Sex cord–like tumor	
B. Tumors of germ cell type	
C. Neuroectodermal tumors	
D. Lymphoma and leukemia	
E. Others	

V. Secondary Tumors

VI. Tumor-Like Lesions	
A. Epithelial metaplastic and related changes	73220
1. Squamous metaplasia, including morule formation	73320
2. Mucinous metaplasia, including intestinal type	
3. Ciliated cell metaplasia	
4. Hobnail cell metaplasia	
5. Clear cell change	
6. Eosinophilic cell change, including oncocytic	73050
7. Surface syncytial change	69420
8. Papillary change	76050
9. Arias-Stella change	79430
B. Stromal metaplastic and related changes	
1. Smooth muscle metaplasia	
2. Osseous metaplasia and retention of fetal bone	73400
3. Cartilaginous metaplasia and retention of fetal cartilage	73600
4. Adipocyte metaplasia	50080
5. Retention of fetal glial tissue	47320
6. Foam cell change	69520
C. Adenomyosis	76510
D. Epithelial cysts of myometrium	33420
E. Chronic endometritis	43000
F. Lymphoma-like lesions	72290
G. Inflammatory pseudotumor	76820
H. Others	

TNM Staging Classification of Endometrial Carcinoma

Primary Tumor (T): see corresponding FIGO stages

Tis	Carcinoma in situ (atypical hyperplasia)
T1(a, b, c)	
T2(a, b)	
T3(a, b, c)	
T4(a, b)	

Nodal Involvement (N)

NX	Minimum requirements to assess the regional nodes cannot be met
N0	No involvement of regional nodes
N1	Evidence of regional node involvement

Distant Metastasis (M)

MX	Minimum requirements to assess the presence of distant metastasis cannot be met
M0	No (known) distant metastasis
M1	Distant metastasis present: specify site

Residual Tumor (R): Postsurgical treatment

R0	No residual tumor
R1	Microscopic residual tumor
R2	Macroscopic residual tumor: specify site

FIGO Staging Classification of Endometrial Carcinoma

Stage I The carcinoma is confined to the corpus uteri
- Stage IA Tumor limited to the endometrium
- Stage IB Invasion to less than one half the myometrium
- Stage IC Invasion to more than one half the myometrium

Stage II The carcinoma has involved the corpus and the cervix
- Stage IIA Endocervical glandular involvement only
- Stage IIB Cervical stromal invasion

Stage III The carcinoma has extended outside the uterus but not outside the true pelvis
- Stage IIIA Tumor invades serosa and/or adnexa, and/or positive peritoneal cytology
- Stage IIIB Vaginal metastases
- Stage IIIC Metastases to pelvic and/or para-aortic lymph nodes

Stage IV The carcinoma has extended outside the true pelvis or has invaded the mucosa of the bladder or rectum; bullous edema alone does not establish Stage IV disease
- Stage IVA Tumor invasion of bladder and/or bowel mucosa
- Stage IVB Distant metastases including intra-abdominal and/or inguinal lymph nodes

Histopathology: degree of differentiation:

Cases of carcinoma of the corpus should be classified (or graded) according to the degree of histologic differentiation, as follows:

G1 5% or less of a nonsquamous or nonmorular solid growth pattern

G2 6% to 50% of a nonsquamous or nonmorular solid growth pattern

G3 More than 50% of a nonsquamous or nonmorular solid growth pattern

Notes on pathologic grading:

1. *Notable nuclear atypia, inappropriate for the architectural grade; raises Grade 1 or Grade 2 tumor by 1.*
2. *In serous adenocarcinomas, clear cell adenocarcinomas, and squamous cell carcinomas, nuclear grading takes precedence.*
3. *Adenocarcinomas with squamous differentiation are graded according to the nuclear grade of the glandular component.*

Rules related to staging:

1. *Because corpus cancer is now staged surgically, procedures previously used for determination of stages are no longer applicable, such as the findings from fractional D&C (dilatation and curettage) to differentiate between Stage I and Stage II.*
2. *It is appreciated that there may be a small number of patients with corpus cancer who will be treated primarily with radiation therapy. If that is the case, the clinical staging adopted by FIGO in 1971 would still apply, but designation of that staging system would be noted.*
3. *Ideally, the width of the myometrium should be measured along with the depth of tumor invasion.*

BIBLIOGRAPHY

General Reading

1. Hendrickson MR, Kempson RL. Pure Mesenchynal Neoplasms of the Uterine Corpus. In: *Obstetrical and Gynaecological Pathological Pathology,* 3rd edition, Fox H (ed.). New York: Chrucholl Livingston, 1987.
2. Hendrickson MR, Kempson RL: *The uterine corpus.* In Sternberg SS, editor: *Diagnostic surgical pathology,* ed 2, New York, 1994, Raven Press.
3. Kempson RL, Hendrickson MR. The Female Reproductive System. In: *Surgical Pathology,* 2nd edition, Coulson WF (ed.). Philadelphia: JB Lippincott, 1988.
4. Kurman RJ, editor: *Blaustein's pathology of the female genital tract,* ed 4, New York, 1994, Springer-Verlag.
5. Silverberg SG, Kurman RJ: *Tumors of the uterine corpus and gestational trophoblastic disease. Atlas of tumor pathology,* 3rd series, fascicle 3, Washington, DC, 1992, Armed Forces Institute of Pathology.
6. Scully RE, Bonfiglio TA, Kurman RJ, Silverberg SG, Wilkinson EJ: *World Health Organization. Histological classification of tumors of the female genital tract,* New York, 1994, Springer-Verlag.

References

7. Ambros RA, Ballouk F, Malfetano JH, Ross JS: Significance of papillary (villoglandular) differentiation in endometrioid carcinoma of the uterus, *Am J Surg Pathol* 18:569-575, 1994.
8. Arias-Stella J, Arias-Velasquez A, Arias-Stella J: Normal and abnormal mitoses in the atypical endometrial change associated with chronic tissue effect, *Am J Surg Pathol* 18:694-701, 1994.
9. Bell SW, Kempson RL, Hendrickson MR: Problematic uterine smooth muscle neoplasms. A Clinicopathologic study of 213 cases, *Am J Surg Pathol* 18:535-558, 1994.
10. Bitterman P, Chun B, Kurman RJ: The significance of epithelial differentiation in mixed mesodermal tumors of the uterus, *Am J Surg Pathol* 14:317-328, 1990.
11. Buscema J, Carpenter SE, Rosenshein NB, Woodruff JD: Epithelioid leiomyosarcoma of the uterus, *Cancer* 57:1192-1196, 1986.
12. Carcangiu ML, Chambers JT: Early pathologic stage clear cell carcinoma and uterine papillary serous carcinoma of the endometrium: comparison of clinicopathologic features and survival, *Int J Gynecol Pathol* 14:30-38, 1995.
13. Carlier MT, Dardick I, Lagace AF, Sreeram V: Brief communication. Adenomatoid tumor of uterus: presentation in endometrial curettings, *Int J Gynecol Pathol* 5:69-74, 1986.
14. Chang KL, Crabtree GS, Lim-Tan SK, Kempson RL, Hendrickson MR: Primary uterine endometrial stromal neoplasms, *Am J Surg Pathol* 14:416-438, 1990.
15. Chen JL, Trost DC, Wilkinson EJ: Endometrial papillary adenocarcinomas: two clinicopathological types, *Int J Gynecol Pathol* 4:279-288, 1985.
16. Clement PB: Müllerian adenosarcomas of the uterus with sarcomatous overgrowth, *Am J Surg Pathol* 13:28-38, 1989.
17. Clement PB, Young RH, Scully RE: Intravenous leiomyomatosis. A clinicopathological analysis of 16 cases with unusual features, *Am J Surg Pathol* 12:932-945, 1988.
18. Clement PB, Scully RE: Müllerian adenosarcoma of the uterus: a clinicopathologic analysis of ten cases of a distinctive type of müllerian mixed tumor, *Cancer* 34:1138-1149, 1974.
19. Clement PB, Scully RE: Uterine tumors resembling ovarian sex cord tumors: a clinicopathologic analysis of 16 cases, *Am J Clin Pathol* 66:512-525, 1976.
20. Crow J, Gardner RL, McSweeney G, Shaw RW: Morphological changes in uterine leiomyomas treated by GnRH agonist goserelin, *Int J Gynecol Pathol* 14:235-242, 1995.
21. Czernobilsky B, Katz Z, Lancet M, Gaton E: Endocervical-type epithelium in endometrial carcinoma. A report of 10 cases with emphasis on histochemical methods for differential diagnosis, *Am J Surg Pathol* 4:481-489, 1980.
22. DeBrito PA, Silverberg SG, Orenstein JM: Carcinosarcoma (malignant mixed müllerian (mesodermal) tumor) of the female genital tract, *Hum Pathol* 24:132-142, 1993.
23. Eifel PJ, Ross J, Hendrickson M, Cox RS, Kempson R, Martinez A: Adenocarcinoma of the endometrium. Analysis of 256 cases with disease limited to the uterine corpus: treatment comparisons, *Cancer* 52:1026-1031, 1983.
24. Evans HL: Endometrial stromal sarcoma and poorly differentiated endometrial sarcoma, *Cancer* 50:2170-2182, 1982.
25. Evans HL, Chawla SP, Simpson C, Finn KP: Smooth muscle neoplasms of the uterus other than ordinary leiomyoma, *Cancer* 62:2239-2247, 1988.
26. Fekete PS, Vellios F: The clinical and histologic spectrum of endometrial stromal neoplasms: a report of 41 cases, *Int J Gynecol Pathol* 3:198-212, 1984.

27. George E, Lillemoe TJ, Twiggs LB, Perrone T: Malignant mixed müllerian tumor versus high-grade endometrial carcinoma and aggressive variants of endometrial carcinoma: a comparative analysis of survival, *Int J Gynecol Pathol* 14:39-44, 1995.
28. Gitsch G, Friedlander ML, Wain GV, Hacker NF: Uterine papillary serous carcinoma, *Cancer* 75:2239-2243, 1995.
29. Greenwood SM, Moran JJ: Chronic endometritis: morphologic and clinical observations, *Obstet Gynecol* 58:176-184, 1981.
30. Hendrickson MR, Kempson RL: Endometrial epithelial metaplasias: proliferations frequently misdiagnosed as adenocarcinoma. Report of 89 cases and proposed classification, *Am J Surg Pathol* 4:525-542, 1980.
31. Hendrickson MR, Kempson RL: Invited review: the differential diagnosis of endometrial adenocarcinoma. Some viewpoints concerning a common diagnostic problem, *Pathology* 12:35-41, 1980.
32. Hendrickson M, Ross J, Eifel P, Martinez A, Kempson R: Uterine papillary serous carcinoma. A highly malignant form of endometrial adenocarcinoma, *Am J Surg Pathol* 6:93-108, 1982.
33. Hendrickson MR, Ross J, Kempson RL: Toward the development of morphologic criteria for well-differentiated adenocarcinoma of the endometrium, *Am J Surg Pathol* 7:819-838, 1983.
34. Hoevcn KH, Hudock JA, Woodruff JM, Suhrland MJ: Small cell neuroendocrine carcinoma of the endometrium, *Int J Gynecol Pathol* 14:21-29, 1995.
35. Huang SJ, Amparo EG, Fu Y: Endometrial hyperplasia: histologic classification and behavior, *Surg Pathol* 1:215-229, 1988.
36. Huettner PC, Gersell DJ: Arias-Stella reaction in nonpregnant women: a clinicopathologic study of nine cases, *Int J Gynecol Pathol* 13:241-247, 1994.
37. Huntsman DG, Clement PB, Gliks CB, Scully RE: Small-cell carcinoma of the endometrium, *Am J Surg Pathol* 18:364-375, 1994.
38. Jeffrey JF, Krepart GV, Lotocki RJ: Papillary serous adenocarcinoma of the endometrium, *Obstet Gynecol* 67:670-674, 1986.
39. Jones MW, Norris HJ: Clinicopathologic study of 28 uterine leiomyosarcomas with metastasis, *Int J Gynecol Pathol* 14:243-249, 1995.
40. Kaminski PF, Tavassoli FA: Plexiform tumorlet: a clinical and pathologic study of 15 cases with ultrastructural observations, *Int J Gynecol Pathol* 3:135-144, 1984.
41. King ME, Dickersin GR, Scully RE: Myxoid leiomyosarcoma of the uterus, *Am J Surg Pathol* 6:589-598, 1982.
42. Korn AP, Bolan G, Padian N, Ohm-Smith M, Schachter J, Landers DV: Plasma cell endometritis in women with symptomatic bacterial vaginosis, *Obstet Gynecol* 85:387-390, 1995.
43. Kurman RJ, Norris HJ: Mesenchymal tumors of the uterus. VI. Epithelioid smooth muscle tumors including leiomyoblastoma and clear cell leiomyoma, *Cancer* 37:1853-1865, 1976.
44. Kurman RJ, Norris HJ: Evaluation of criteria for distinguishing atypical endometrial hyperplasia from well differentiated carcinoma, *Cancer* 49:2547-2559, 1982.
45. Kurman RJ, Kaminski PF, Norris HJ: The behavior of endometrial hyperplasia. A long-term study of "untreated" hyperplasia in 170 patients, *Cancer* 54:403-412, 1985.
46. Kurman RJ, Scully RE: Clear cell carcinoma of the endometrium. An analysis of 21 cases, *Cancer* 37:872-882, 1976.
47. Longacre TA, Chung MH, Jensen DN, Hendrickson MR: Proposed criteria for the diagnosis of well-differentiated endometrial carcinoma, *Am J Surg Pathol* 19:371-406, 1995.
48. Malpica A, Tornos C, Burke TW, Silva EG: Low-stage clear-cell carcinoma of the endometrium, *Am J Surg Pathol* 19:769-774, 1995.
49. Marshall RJ, Braye SG, Jones DB: Leiomyosarcoma of the uterus with giant cells resembling osteoclasts, *Int J Gynecol Pathol* 5:260-268, 1986.
50. Mazur MT: Atypical polypoid adenomyomas of the endometrium, *Am J Surg Pathol* 5:473-482, 1981.
51. Mazur MT, Hendrickson MR, Kempson RL: Optically clear nuclei. An alteration of endometrial epithelium in the presence of trophoblast, *Am J Surg Pathol* 7:415-423, 1983.
52. Mazur MT, Kraus FT: Histogenesis of morphologic variations in tumors of the uterine wall, *Am J Surg Pathol* 4:59-74, 1980.
53. Mentzel T, Calonje E, Fletcher CDM: Leiomyosarcoma with prominent osteoclast-like giant cells, *Am J Surg Pathol* 18:258-265, 1994.
54. Muller-Holzner E, Ruth NR, Abfalter E, Schrocksnadel H, Dapunt O, Martin-Sances L, Nogales FF: IUD-associated pelvic actinomycosis: a report of five cases, *Int J Gynecol Pathol* 14:70-74, 1995.
55. Mulvany NJ, Slavin JL, Ostor AG, Fortune DW: Intravenous leiomyomatosis of the uterus: a clinicopathologic study of 22 cases, *Int J Gynecol Pathol* 13:1-9, 1994.

56. Norris HJ, Tavassoli FA, Kurman RJ: Endometrial hyperplasia and carcinoma: diagnostic considerations, *Am J Surg Pathol* 7:839-847, 1983.
57. Norris HJ, Taylor HB: Clinical and pathologic study of 53 endometrial stromal tumors, *Cancer* 19:755-766, 1966.
58. Norris HJ, Taylor HB: Mesenchymal tumors of the uterus. II. Clinical and pathologic study of 31 mixed mesodermal tumors, *Obstet Gynecol* 28:57-63, 1966.
59. Norris HJ, Taylor HB: Mesenchymal tumors of the uterus. III. A clinical and pathologic study of 31 carcinosarcomas, *Cancer* 19:1459-1465, 1966.
60. O'Connor DM, Norris HJ: Mitotically active leiomyomas of the uterus, *Hum Pathol* 21:223-227, 1990.
61. Oliva E, Young RH, Clement PB, Bhan AK, Scully RE: Cellular benign mesenchymal tumors of the uterus. A comparative morphologic and immunohistochemical analysis of 33 highly cellular leiomyomas and six endometrial stromal nodules, two frequently confused tumors, *Am J Surg Pathol* 19:757-768, 1995.
62. Orenstein HJ, Richart RM, Fenoglio CM: Müllerian adenosarcoma of the uterus: literature review, case report, and ultrastructural observations, *Ultrastruct Pathol* 1:189-200, 1980.
63. Perrone T, Dehner LP: Prognostically favorable "mitotically active" smooth-muscle tumors of the uterus, *Am J Surg Pathol* 12:1-8, 1988.
64. Peters WA III, Kumar NB, Fleming WP, Morley GW: Prognostic features of sarcomas and mixed tumors of the endometrium, *Obstet Gynecol* 63:550-556, 1984.
65. Piver MS, Rutledge FN, Copeland L, Webster K, Blumenson L, Suh O: Uterine endolymphatic stromal myosis: a collaborative study, *Obstet Gynecol* 64:173-178, 1984.
66. Prayson RA, Hart WR: Mitotically active leiomyomas of the uterus, *Am J Clin Pathol* 97:14-20, 1992.
67. Press MF, Scully RE: Endometrial "sarcomas" complicating ovarian thecoma, polycystic ovarian disease and estrogen therapy, *Gynecol Oncol* 21:135-154, 1985.
68. Ross JC, Eifel PJ, Cox RS, Kempson RL, Hendrickson MR: Primary mucinous adenocarcinoma of the endometrium: a clinicopathologic and histochemical study, *Am J Surg Pathol* 7:715-729, 1983.
69. Schlaen IS, Wong P, Bergeron CB, Naves A, Ferenczy A, Bertoli R: Endometrial polyps: a study of 204 cases, *Surg Pathol* 1:375-382, 1988.
70. Scully RE, Kempson RL, Norris HJ: Editorial: mitosis counting, *Hum Pathol* 7:481-482, 1976.
71. Shlaen I, Bergeron C, Ferenczy A, Wong P, Naves A, Bertoli R: Endometrial polyps: a study of 204 cases, *Surg Pathol* 1:375-382, 1988.
72. Sickel JZ, Sant'Agnese PA: Anomalous immunostaining of "optically clear" nuclei in gestational endometrium, *Arch Pathol Lab Med* 118:831-834, 1994.
73. Silverberg SG, Major FJ, Blesing JA, Fetter B, Askin FB, Liao SY, Miller A: Carcinosarcoma (malignant mixed mesodermal tumor) of the uterus, *Int J Gynecol Pathol* 9:1-19, 1990.
74. Sreenan JJ, Hart WR: Carcinosarcomas of the female genital tract, *Am J Surg Pathol* 19:666-674, 1995.
75. Tavassoli F, Kraus FT: Endometrial lesions in uteri resected for atypical endometrial hyperplasia, *Am J Clin Pathol* 70:770-779, 1978.
76. Tavassoli FA, Norris HJ: Peritoneal leiomyomatosis (leiomyomatosis peritonealis disseminata): a clinicopathologic study of 20 cases with ultrastructural observations, *Int J Gynecol Pathol* 1:59-74, 1982.
77. Vellios F, NG ABP, Reagan JW: Papillary adenofibroma of the uterus, *Am J Clin Pathol* 60:543-551, 1973.
78. Yamamoto Y, Izumi K, Otsuka H, Kishi Y, Mimura T, Okitsu O: Primary squamous cell carcinoma of the endometrium: a case report and a suggestion of new histogenesis, *Int J Gynecol Pathol* 14:75-80, 1995.
79. Young RH, Treger T, Scully RE: Atypical polypoid adenomyoma of the uterus. A report of 27 cases, *Am J Clin Pathol* 86:139-145, 1986.
80. Zaino RJ, Kurman R, Herbold D, Gliedman J, Bundy BN, Voet R, Advani H: The significance of squamous differentiation in endometrial carcinoma, *Cancer* 68:2293-2302, 1991.
81. Zaloudek CJ, Norris HJ: Adenofibroma and adenosarcoma of the uterus: a clinicopathologic study of 35 cases, *Cancer* 48:354-366, 1981.

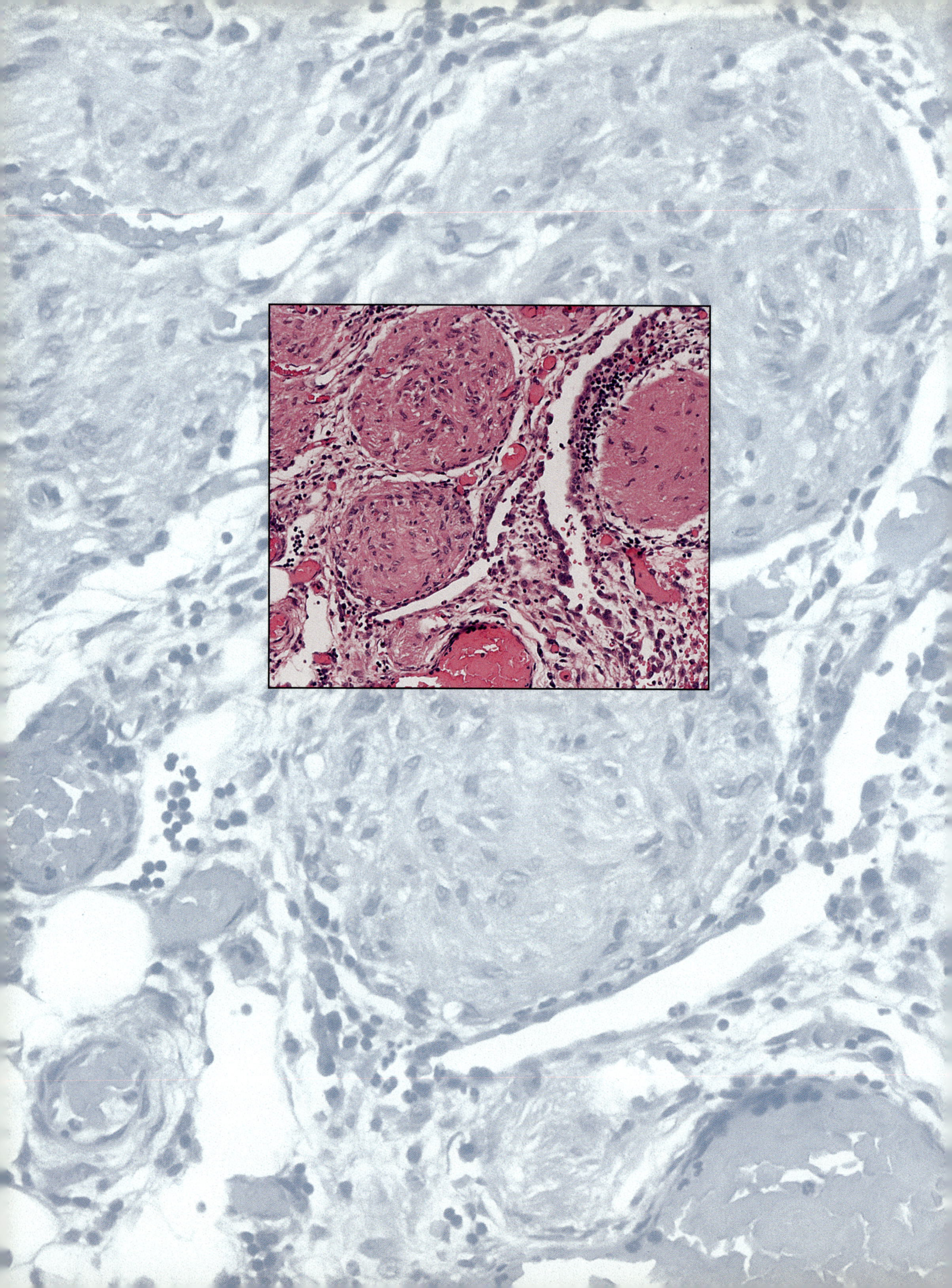

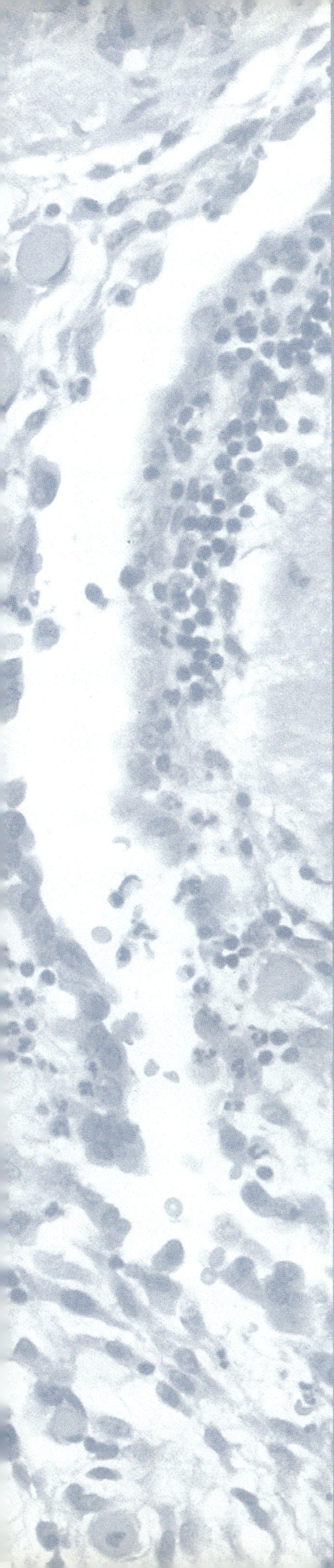

Chapter 5

Pathology of the Fallopian Tube, Broad Ligament and Peritoneum

TUMOR-LIKE LESIONS

The fallopian tube responds in a limited way to hormonal stimuli. The most common functional reaction is decidual reaction in tubal mucosa.[82] The mucosal folds are enlarged and slightly blunted by the decidual reaction (Figures 5-1 and 5-2). This change occurs as the result of pregnancy and is commonly seen in postpartum tubal ligations. The fallopian tube is the most frequent site for an ectopic pregnancy (Figures 5-3 to 5-7).[53] Another benign functional reaction is the metaplastic papillary syncytial tumor.[63] This is an eosinophilic metaplasia of the cytoplasm with bland, round nuclei (Figures 5-8 and 5-9). This unusual reaction has also been reported in postpartum tubal ligations. After tubal ligations, the proximal end of the fallopian tube becomes blunted and slightly dilated (Figure 5-10).[26,70] The epithelium becomes atrophic and the distal portion retains its normal configuration. At the resected edges, there is occasional calcification and psammoma body formation. These psammoma bodies can occasionally be found on a cervical cytologic smear. Transitional cell metaplasia has also been reported in the fallopian tube.[28]

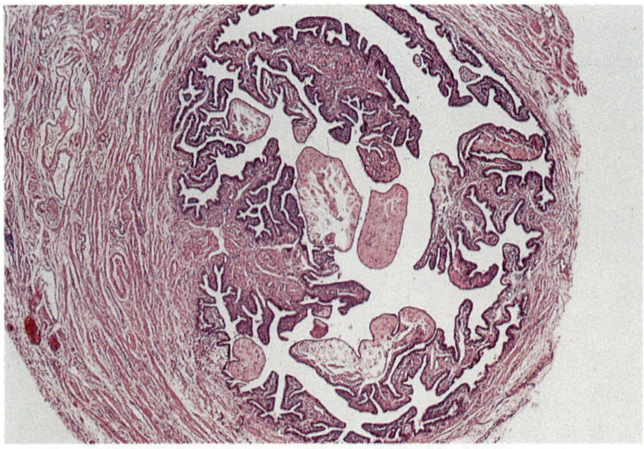

5.1 Fallopian tube showing decidual change.

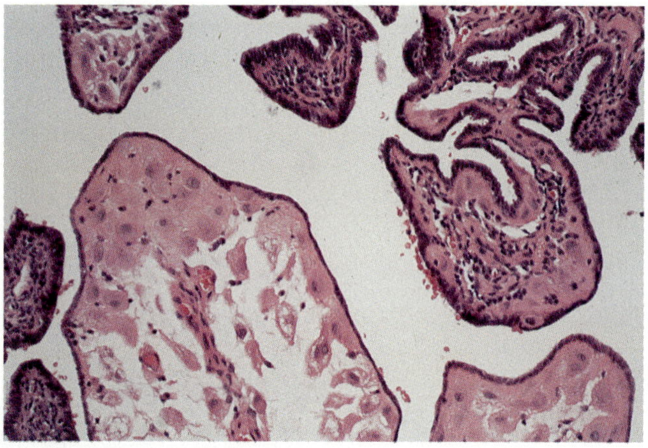

5.2 Decidual change in the stroma of the fallopian tube.

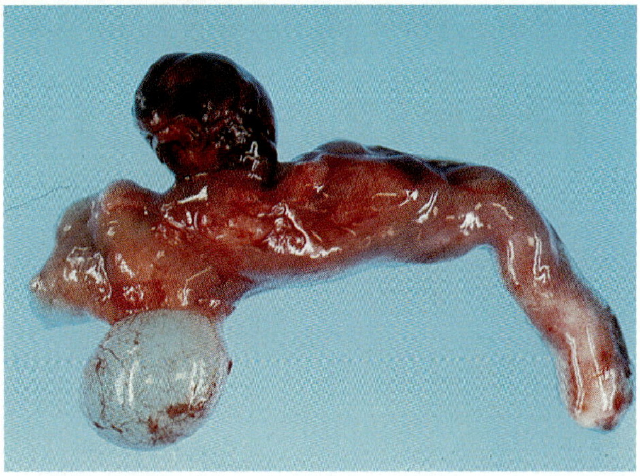

5.3 Fallopian tube with an ectopic pregnancy showing early rupture.

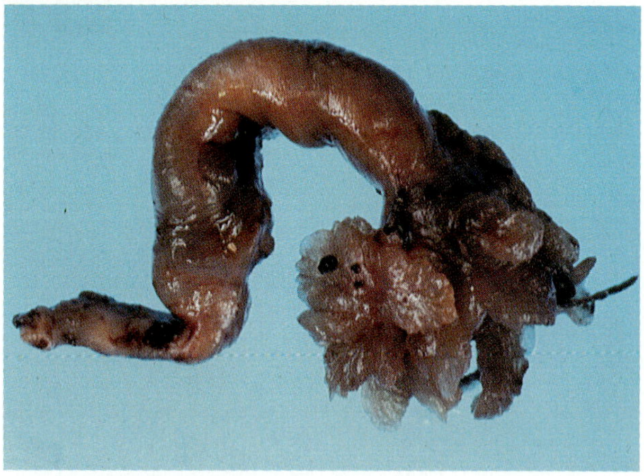

5.4 Edematous fallopian tube in a patient who had an ectopic pregnancy with a tubal abortion.

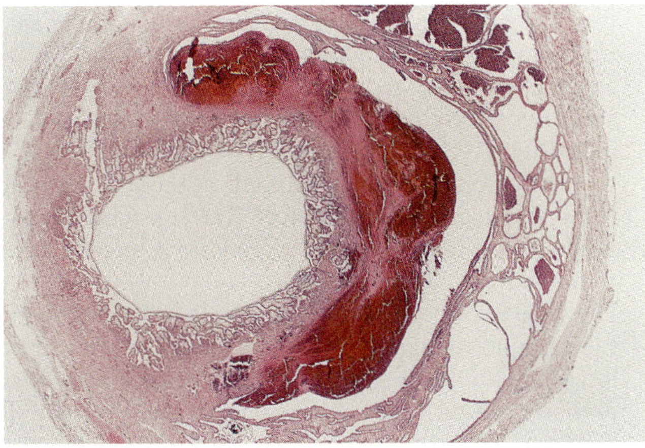

5.5 Fallopian tube containing an ectopic pregnancy showing hemorrhage in the wall of the tube.

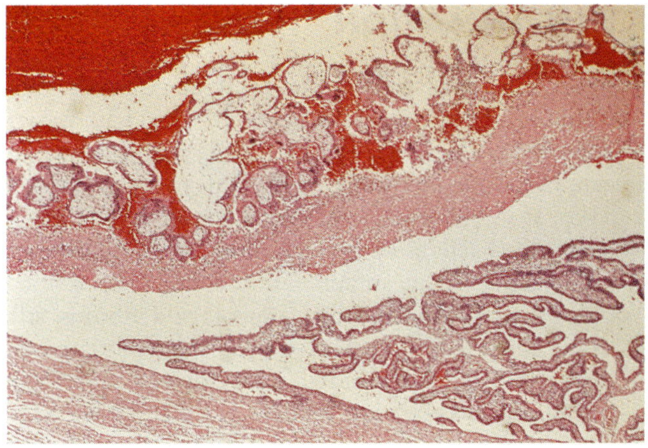

5.6 Ectopic pregnancy in the fallopian tube revealing chorionic villi adjacent to the tubal mucosa.

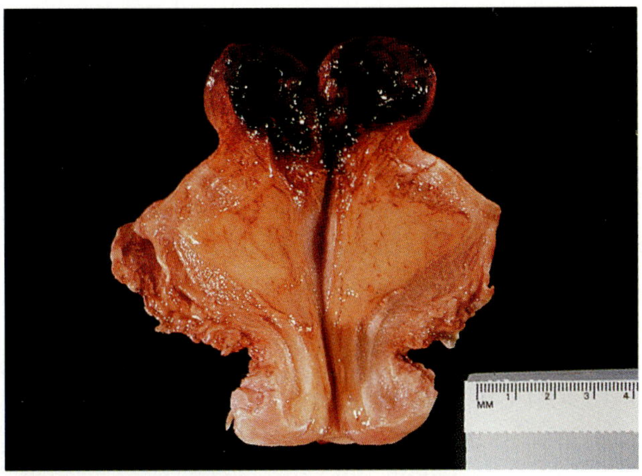

5.7 Hemorrhagic cornual pregnancy.

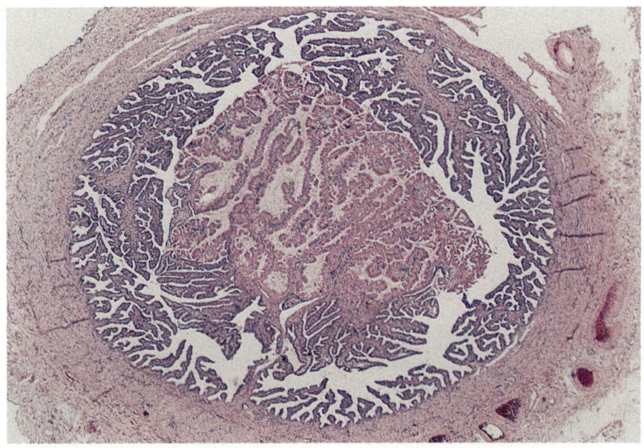

5.8 Metaplastic papillary tumor of the fallopian tube.

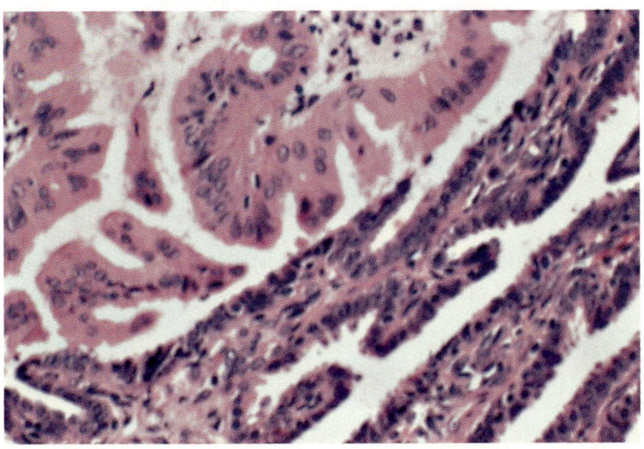

5.9 Metaplastic papillary tumor revealing oncocytic cytoplasm in the metaplastic component.

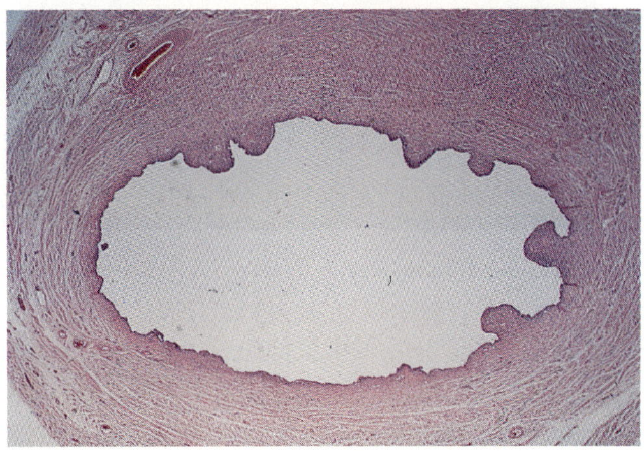

5.10 Proximal dilation of the fallopian tube with blunting and atrophy of the papillary fronds secondary to a previous tubal ligation.

INFLAMMATION

Acute salpingitis is a purulent inflammatory condition secondary to a bacterial infection. Although *Neisseria gonorrhoeae* has been considered the most likely organism, bacteriologic studies reveal that it is rarely cultured from acute infections. More common organisms are anaerobic bacteria as well as some gram-negative aerobic bacteria. Acute inflammation causes destruction of the fallopian tube mucosa, edema, and fibrous adhesions. There can be destruction of the fimbriated end, and if the process continues, it can extend into the ovary, causing a tubo-ovarian abscess (Figure 5-11). As the acute inflammation resolves, the destruction of the tubal mucosa as well as the edema and enlargement may result in a pyosalpinx (Figures 5-12 and 5-13), which eventually gets reabsorbed, leaving a hydrosalpinx (Figure 5-14). If hemorrhage occurs, often as a result of torsion,[9] a hematosalpinx results (Figures 5-15 and 5-16). As the lesion continues to resolve, a subacute inflammation takes place and there is agglutination of the fimbriated end, forming a network-like pattern that has been called salpingitis follicularis (Figures 5-17 and 5-18).

Chronic salpingitis is the result of a smoldering subacute inflammation that continues to cause a lymphoplasmacytic infiltrate with the formation of occasional lymphoid follicles. If the acute process is treated early, the amount of damage can be limited; however, the chronic irritation may continue to form adhesions and strictures in the mucosa, which can eventually lead to infertility.

Tuberculous salpingitis is usually a secondary infection from a systemic presentation.[42] The infection causes a process similar to bacterial salpingitis. Clubbing of the tube can result, as well as edema and purulent inflammation (Figure 5-19). Epithelial hyperplasia is often seen in tuberculous salpingitis (Figure 5-20).[16] Caseating granulomas are formed (Figure 5-21) and acid-fast bacteria are present (Figure 5-22). Actinomycotic infections of the tube may occur in association with intrauterine contraceptive devices (Figures 5-23 and 5-24). Histologically, the "sulfur granules" may be recognized in a purulent exudate. *Chlamydia trachomatis* may also be a cause of acute and chronic salpingitis.

Salpingitis isthmica nodosa[45] presents as outpouchings, or diverticula of the tubular epithelium, usually in the isthmic region (Figures 5-25 and 5-26). It is essentially the tubal counterpart of adenomyosis. The cause is unknown and it has been found in tubes without evidence of inflammation. A similar process occurs as the result of tubal surgery and ectopic pregnancies.

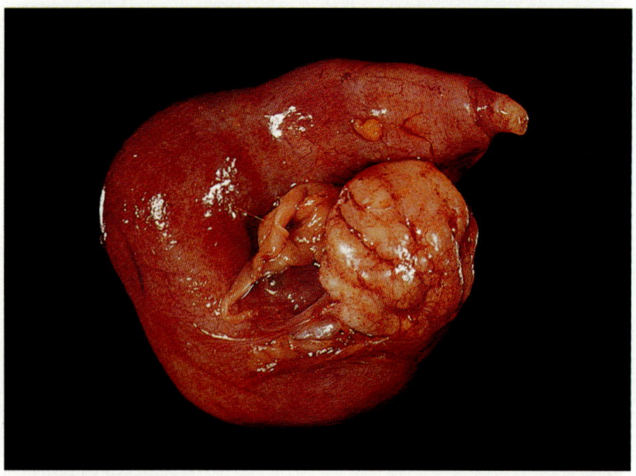

5.11 Tubo-ovarian abscess.

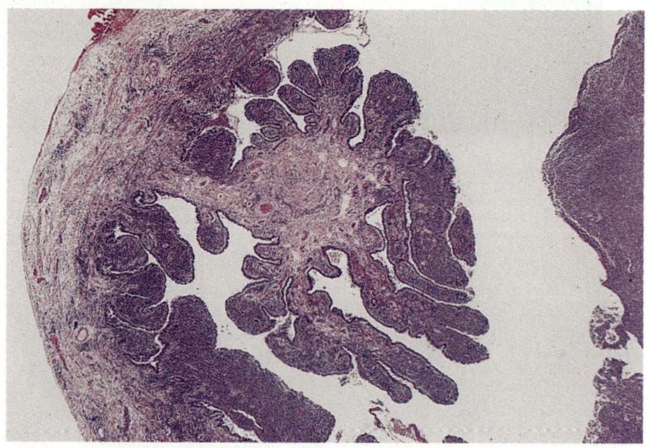

5.12 Acute salpingitis showing dilatation of the fallopian tube and blunting of the papillary fronds.

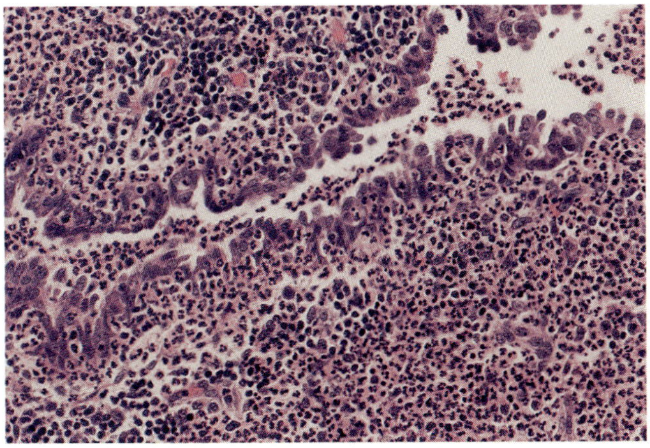

5.13 Acute salpingitis with a mixture of neutrophils, lymphocytes, and plasma cells in the fallopian tube destroying some of the epithelial lining.

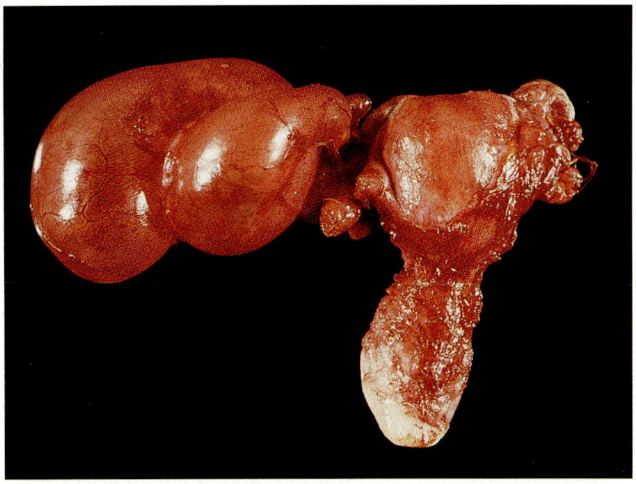

5.14 Hydrosalpinx with marked dilatation of the fallopian tube and blunting of the fimbriated end.

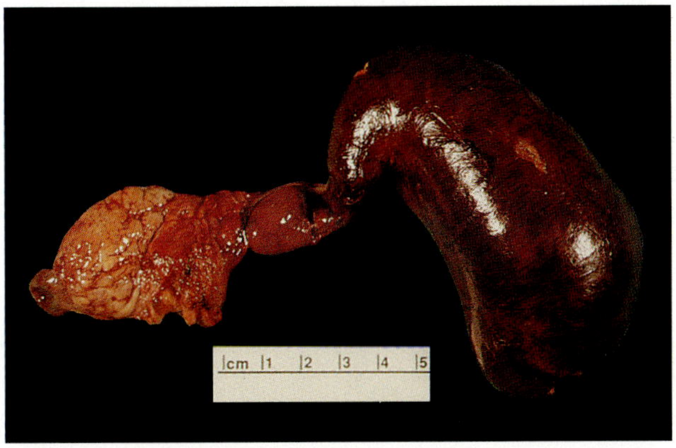

5.15 Hematosalpinx with torsion.

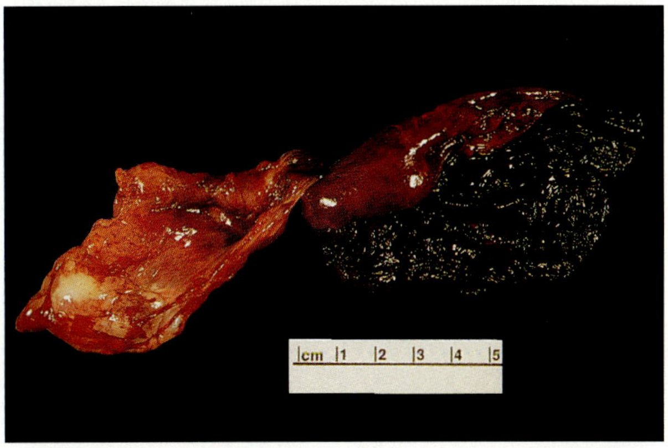

5.16 Hematosalpinx revealing a hemorrhagic mucosa.

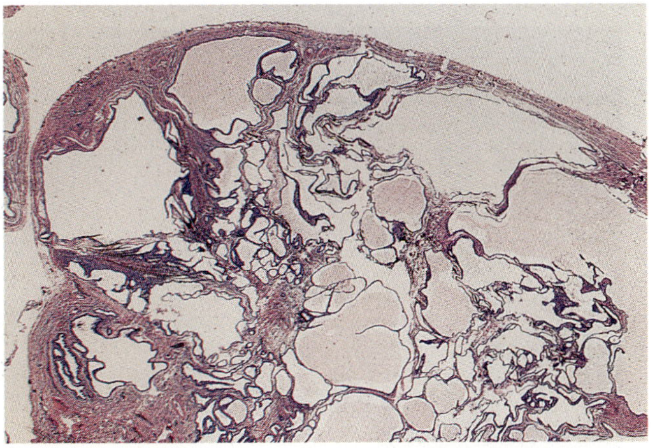

5.17 Salpingitis follicularis revealing irregular anastomosing fibrous areas with dilated, multicystic spaces.

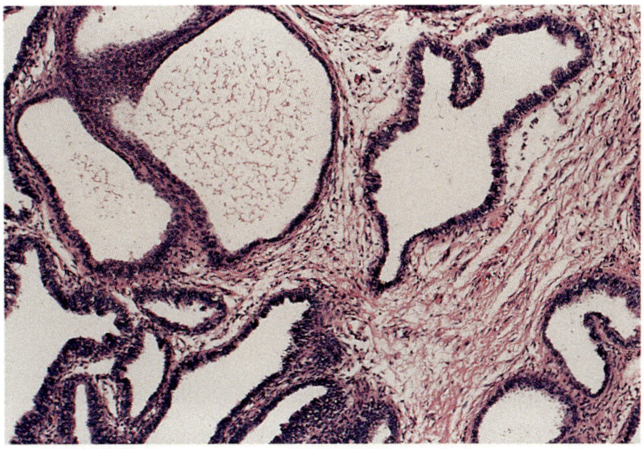

5.18 Salpingitis follicularis showing irregular, cystically dilated, epithelium-lined spaces.

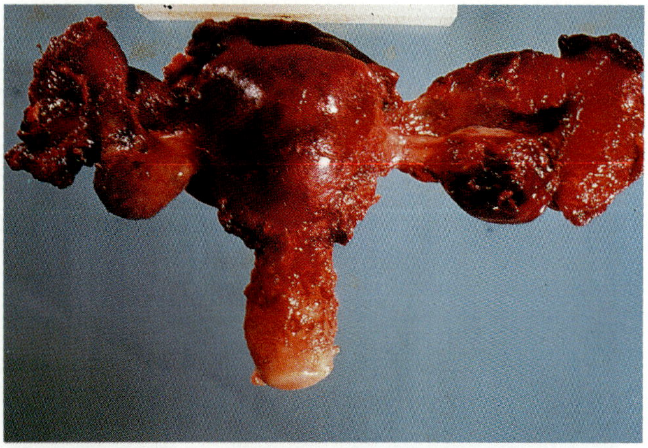

5.19 Tuberculous salpingitis demonstrating dilatation of both fallopian tubes and tubo-ovarian adhesions.

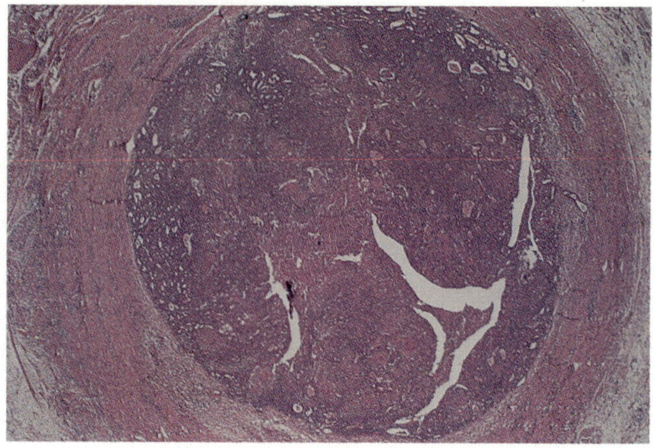

5.20 Tuberculous salpingitis with hyperplasia of the endosalpinx.

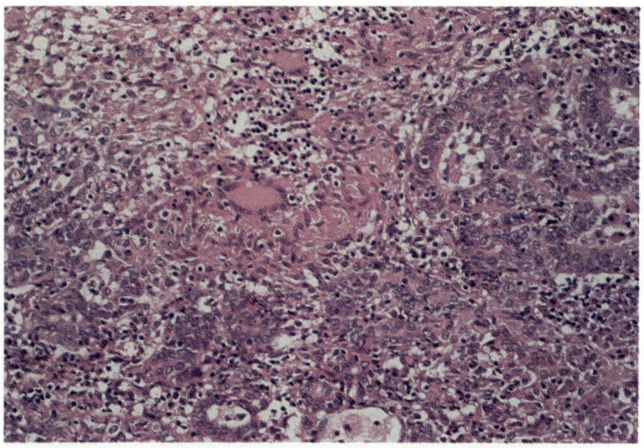

5.21 Tuberculous salpingitis with granulomatous inflammation containing multinucleated giant cells.

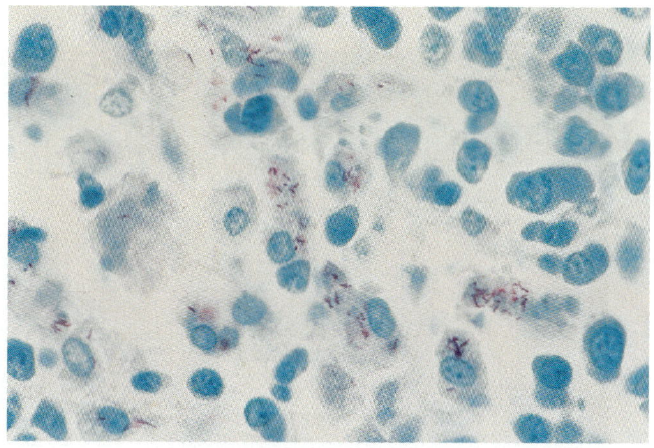

5.22 Acid-fast bacilli.

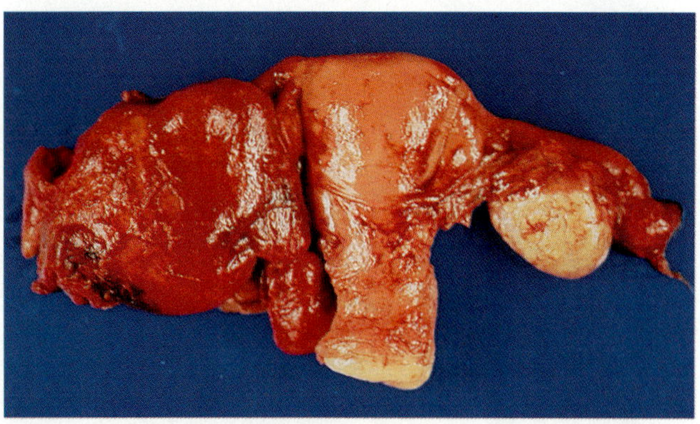

5.23 Unilateral tubo-ovarian abscess in a patient with an intrauterine device and actinomycosis.

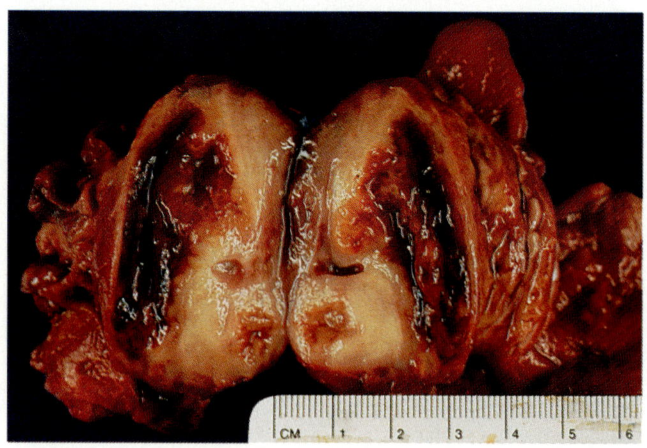

5.24 Unilateral tubo-ovarian abscess due to actinomycosis.

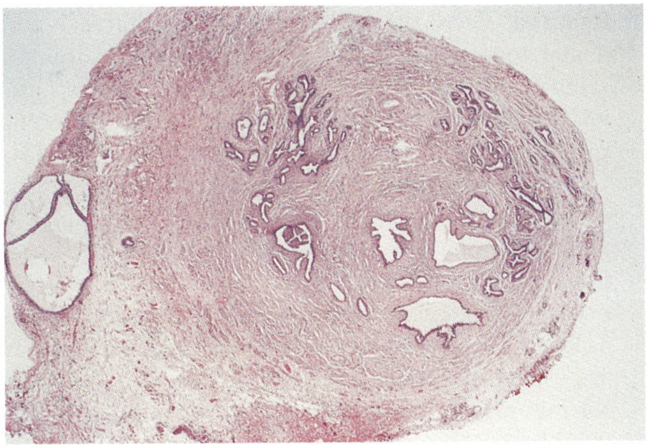

5.25 Salpingitis isthmica nodosa with almost complete obliteration of the lumen and surrounding diverticular extensions of fallopian tube epithelium.

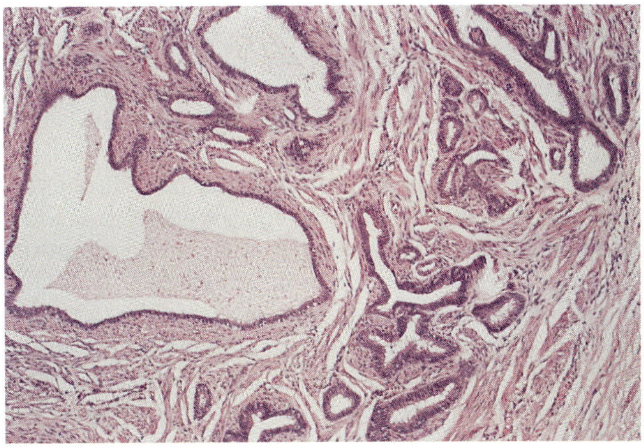

5.26 Salpingitis isthmica nodosa with irregular, partially cystically dilated spaces in the fibromuscular wall of the fallopian tube.

TUMORS

Hyperplasia of the fallopian tube is characterized by a proliferative growth in the endosalpinx with nuclear stratification (Figures 5-27 and 5-28). It can be associated with endometrial hyperplasia and proliferative ovarian lesions.[58,80] The amount of atypia and stratification can be severe enough to warrant the diagnosis of carcinoma in situ or borderline tumor.[50,83]

Primary malignant tumors of the fallopian tube are rare.[30,47,57,60,81] The most common malignant tumor is papillary adenocarcinoma. Since this tumor is similar to ovarian carcinoma, it is likely that there are more cases of primary adenocarcinoma of the tube than have been reported. There are fairly strict criteria (Table 5-1) for a malignancy to qualify as fallopian tube carcinoma (Figures 5-29 to 5-32). Other müllerian types of fallopian tube malignancies have been described (see box on p. 120), including carcinosarcoma (Figure 5-33),[11] Clear cell adenocarcinoma (Figures 5-34 and 5-35),[77] mucinous tumors,[65] transitional cell carcinoma,[43,75] and squamous cell carcinoma.[15] Squamous cell carcinoma in situ of the fallopian tube is usually the result of upward extension from the cervix (Figures 5-36 and 5-37).[78] Trophoblastic tumors of the tube are rare and are usually the result of ectopic gestations. The staging for fallopian tube carcinoma is outlined in the box on p. 121.

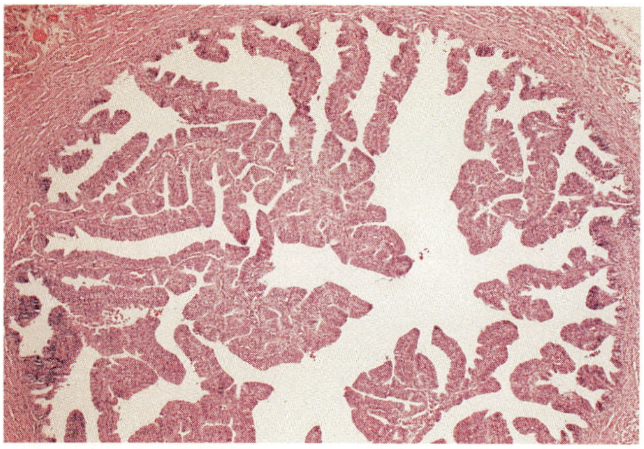

5.27 Epithelial hyperplasia of the fallopian tube mucosa.

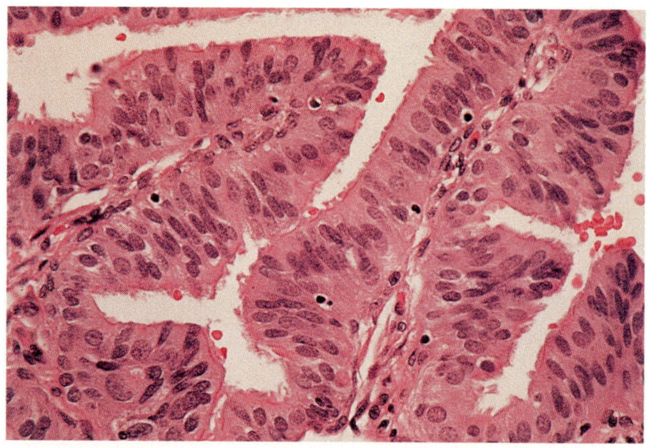

5.28 Hyperplasia with stratified, crowded papillary fronds.

TABLE 5-1 Criteria for a Primary Fallopian Tube Carcinoma

I. GROSS

A. The distal end of the tube is abnormal and the fimbriated end may be occluded, resembling chronic salpingitis
B. There is papillary growth in the endosalpinx
C. The uterus and ovaries are normal or affected by a lesion other than cancer

II. MICROSCOPIC

A. The epithelium of the endosalpinx is replaced in whole or in part by adenocarcinoma
B. The carcinoma is consistent with a tumor arising from tubal epithelium
C. The ovaries and endometrium are normal, or if carcinoma is present, the lesion appears to be metastatic by its size, distribution, and histologic appearance
D. The prime involvement is in the endosalpinx (the perisalpinx and lymphatics of the muscularis and mesosalpinx are rarely involved)
E. Tuberculosis has carefully been excluded

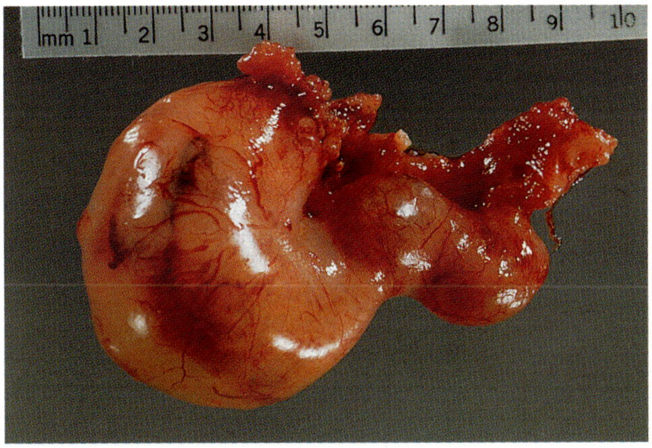

5.29 Adenocarcinoma of the fallopian tube revealing a dilated fallopian tube with an obstructed fimbriated end.

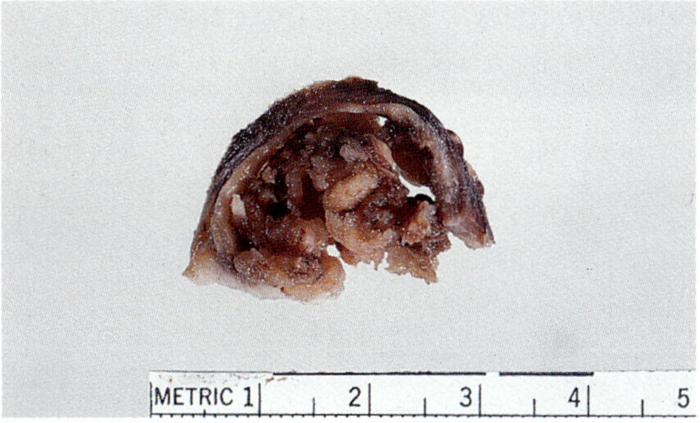

5.30 Cross-section of an adenocarcinoma of the fallopian tube revealing the tumor confined to the endosalpinx.

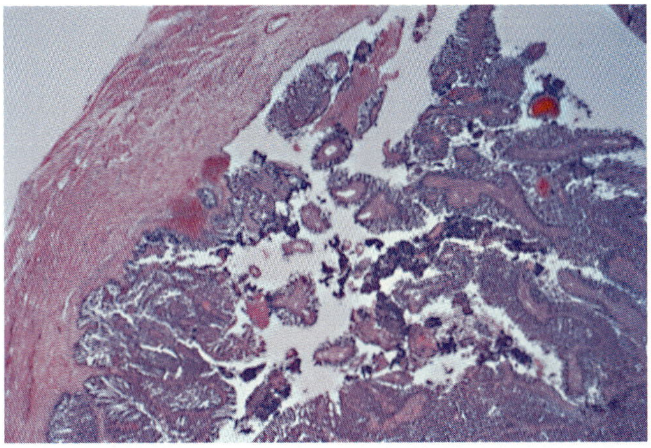

5.31 Adenocarcinoma of the fallopian tube showing the tumor confined to the endosalpinx with minimal invasion into the muscular wall.

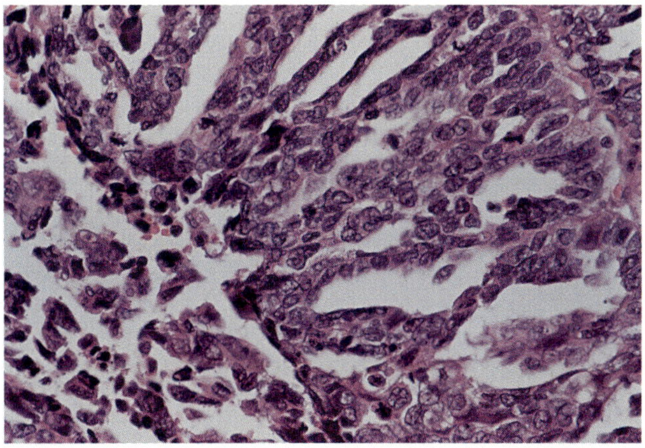

5.32 Moderately differentiated adenocarcinoma of the fallopian tube.

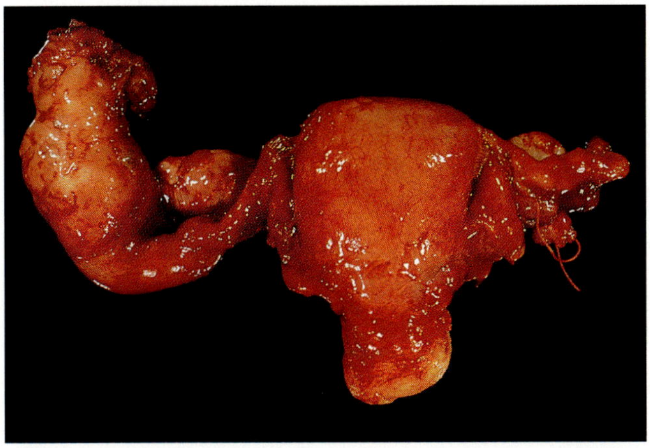

5.33 Carcinosarcoma of the fallopian tube showing gross findings similar to a primary adenocarcinoma.

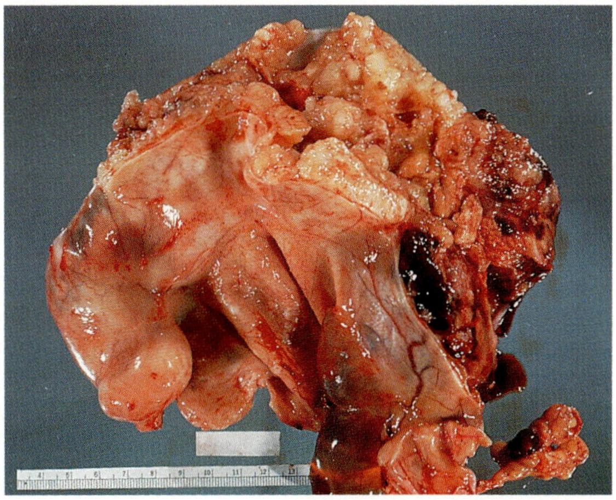

5.34 Primary clear cell carcinoma of the fallopian tube.

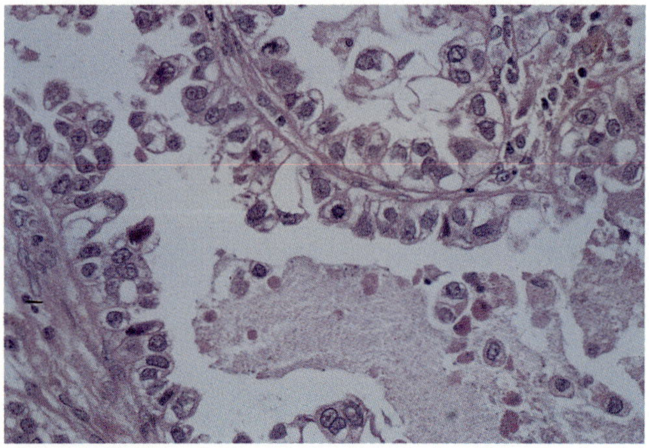

5.35 Clear cell adenocarcinoma of the fallopian tube.

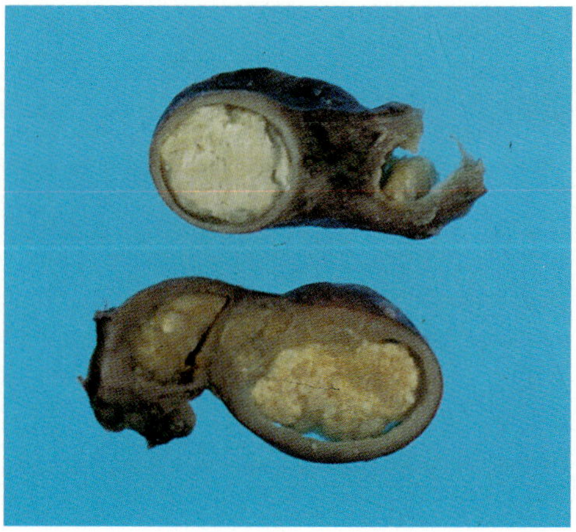

5.36 Dilated fallopian tube containing purulent debris and squamous carcinoma in situ.

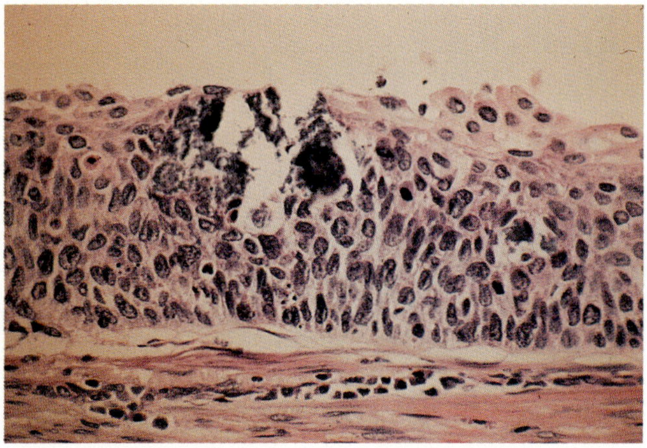

5.37 Squamous carcinoma in situ of the fallopian tube.

PARATUBAL CYSTS AND TUMORS

Paratubal cysts may arise from mesonephric (wolffian) duct remnants (Figure 5-38), paramesonephric (müllerian) duct remnants, or mesothelium.[64] The most common is a müllerian derived serous cyst characterized by the presence of cilia and intracytoplasmic mucin (Figures 5-39 and 5-40).[24] Occasionally, papillary serous cystadenofibromas (Figures 5-41 and 5-42) and borderline tumors[68] occur in the paratubal area, but malignancy is rare.[69] Transitional cell metaplasia (Walthard rests) (Figures 5-43 to 5-45) are commonly present adjacent to the fallopian tube and mesosalpinx.

Tumors in the broad ligament are (see box on p. 121) rare.[6,8,27] Leiomyomas, lipomas (Figure 5-46), and other soft tissue tumors may develop in this area. The female adnexal tumor of probable wolffian origin (Figure 5-47) is an unusual and difficult-to-classify tumor seen in the broad ligament.[23,25,38]

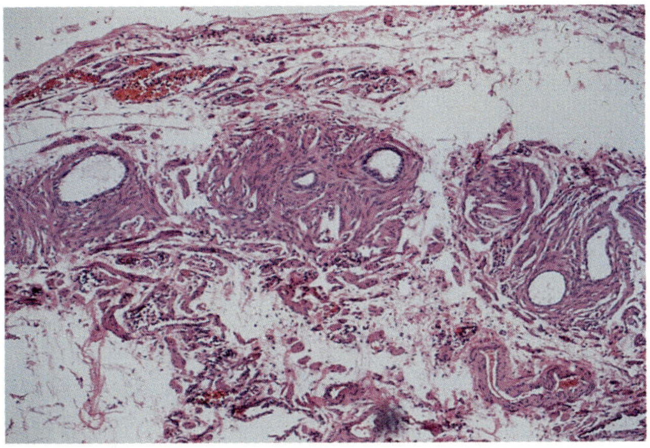

5.38 Mesonephric duct remnants adjacent to the fallopian tube. The remnants contain cuboidal, epithelial-lined spaces surrounded by a proliferation of smooth muscle.

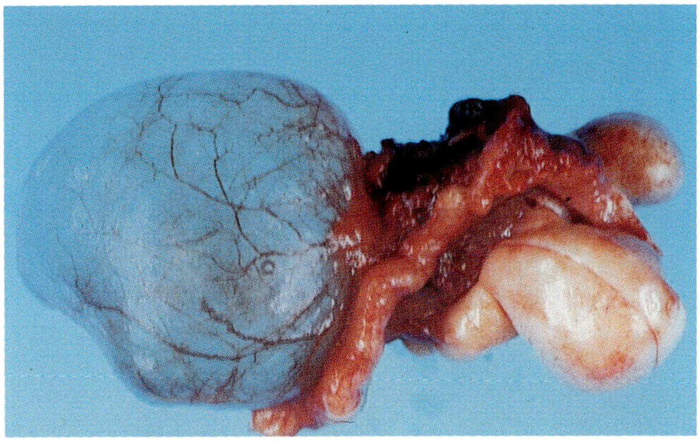

5.39 Thin-walled paratubal cyst.

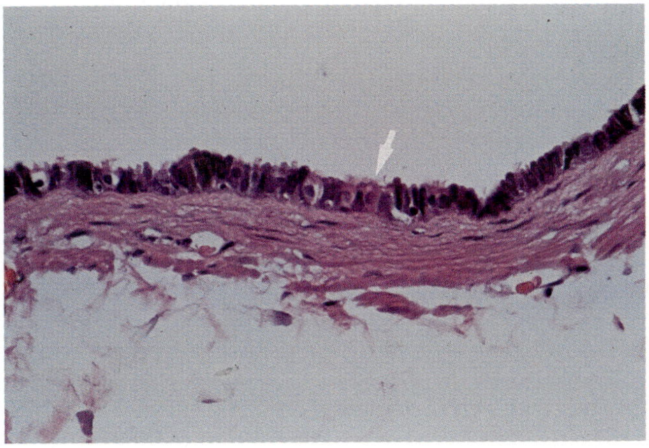

5.40 Paratubal cyst lined with serous ciliated epithelium.

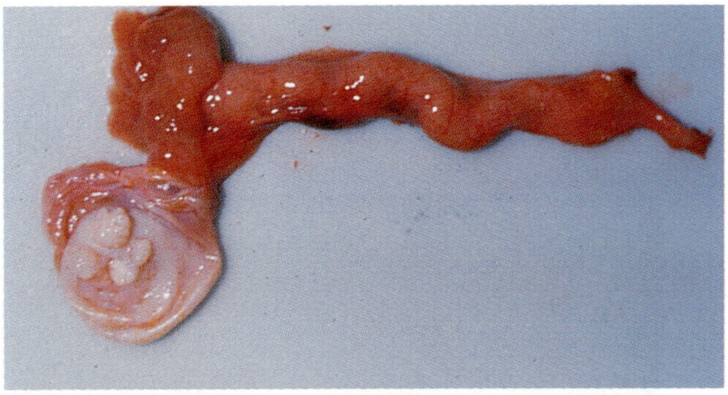

5.41 Paratubal papillary cystadenofibroma showing papillary excrescences on the inner wall of the cyst.

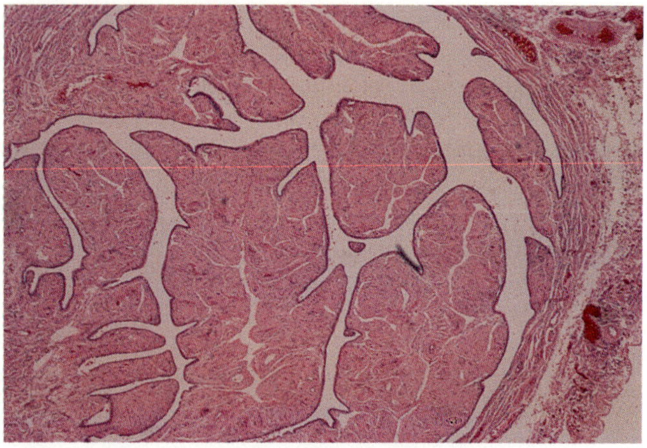

5.42 Adenofibroma showing blunt papillary projections lined with flattened, cuboidal epithelium.

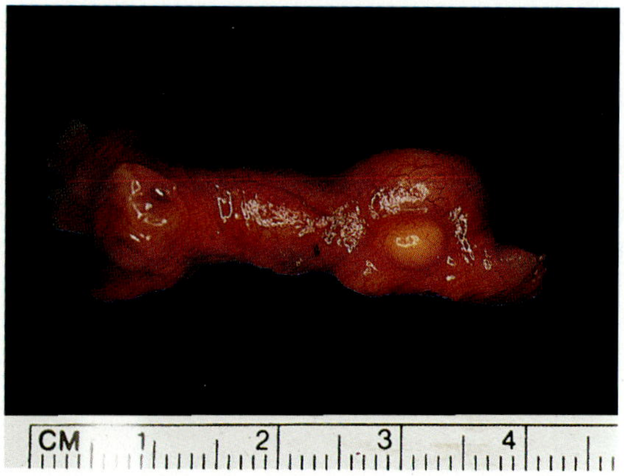

5.43 Walthard rest adjacent to the fallopian tube.

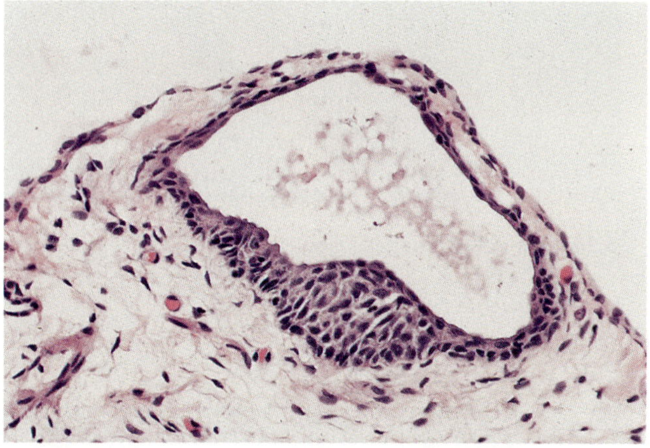

5.44 Walthard rest adjacent to the fallopian tube showing cystic dilatation.

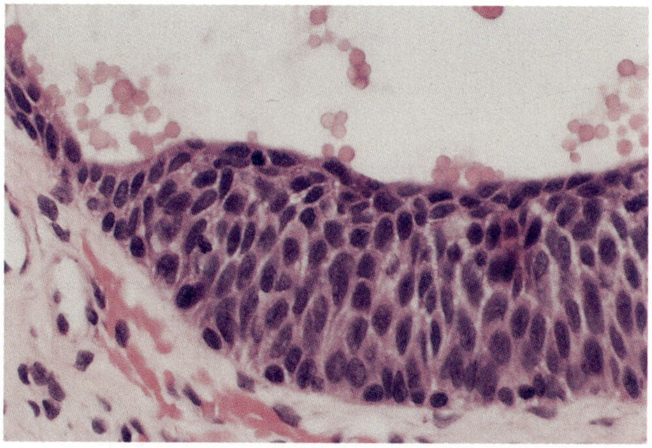

5.45 Walthard rest with transitional epithelium.

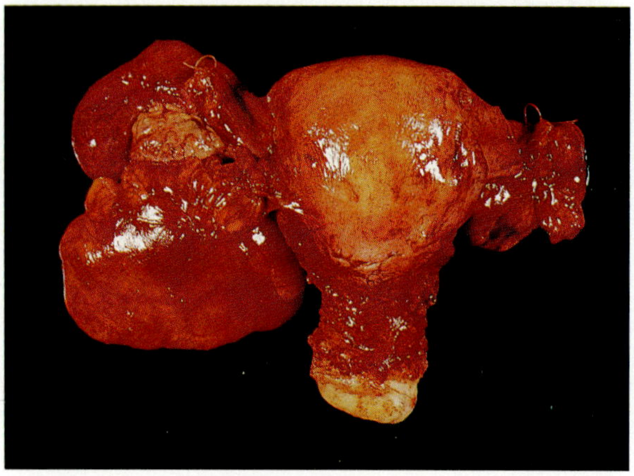

5.46 Lipoma arising in the broad ligament.

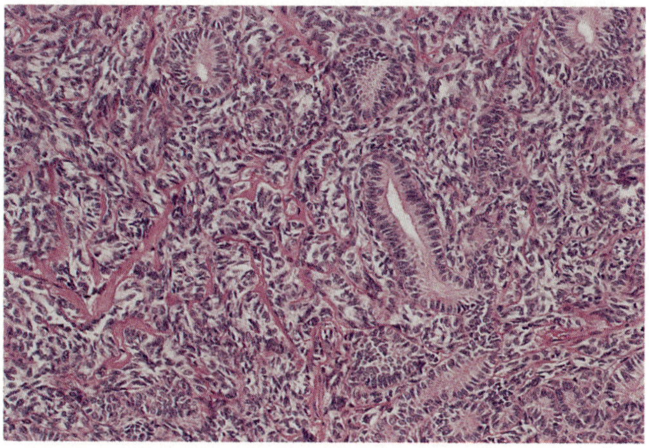

5.47 Female adnexal tumor of probable wolffian origin.

TUMORS AND TUMOR-LIKE LESIONS OF THE PERITONEUM

Mesothelial hyperplasia (Figure 5-48) is often seen in the peritoneum after inflammatory or reactive conditions have occurred. Florid hyperplasia may be confused with a malignant tumor.[18] Multiloculated mesothelial cysts (Figures 5-49 to 5-51), or benign cystic mesotheliomas, are also associated with postinflammatory reactions.* The most common benign tumor of the fallopian tube is the adenomatoid tumor (Figures 5-52 and 5-53).[72] This is a proliferation of the serosal mesothelial lining, giving rise to a firm nodule. The tumor is occasionally large enough to constrict the lumen. Similar lesions have been described in other mesothelium-lined surfaces. Localized papillary mesotheliomas (Figure 5-54) are limited to a localized area of the peritoneum. These are benign tumors that may actually represent localized reactive hyperplasia. It is more important to distinguish them from the more diffuse, well-differentiated papillary mesothelioma (WDPM)(Figures 5-55 and 5-56).[35] Although WDPM usually has an indolent course, it can be unpredictable.[22] Malignant mesotheliomas have more cytologic atypia and are very aggressive tumors. They may be difficult to differentiate from papillary adenocarcinoma. Immunoperoxidase stains may aid in differentiating mesothelial from epithelial tumors of the peritoneum (Figure 5-57).[20,33]

The serosal surfaces of the peritoneum are common sites for endometriosis.[29,31,37,52] The presence of endometrial glands and stroma is required for a definitive histologic diagnosis (Figure 5-58). Areas of hemorrhage with pigmented histocytes are frequently seen. Occasionally, necrotic pseudoxanthomatous nodules may be present.[19,67] Atypia and carcinoma can also develop in endometriosis.[36,66,73] Endosalpingiosis is the serous (tubal) counterpart of endometriosis. Like endometriosis, endosalpingiosis is thought to be a metaplastic change occurring in the mesothelium.[44,74] It can occur on the serosa of the peritoneal cavity, ovary, and omentum[85] and in pelvic lymph nodes.[14,41,48] These areas have ciliated, tube-like epithelium (Figures 5-59 and 5-60). Endosalpingiosis often causes difficulty in its differentiation from implants of a borderline (Figure 5-61) or low-grade malignant ovarian tumor.[54]

Primary papillary serous tumors, borderline and malignant (Figure 5-62), can arise from the peritoneum.[7,10,21,62,84] Diagnostic dilemmas occur when the surface of the ovary is involved over whether the tumor is primary or metastatic to the ovary.[51] Multifocal serous tumors may represent "field effect" on the serosal surfaces or malignant transformation of endosalpingiosis.[55] Other types of müllerian tumors, such as endometrial stromal sarcoma,[13] adenosarcoma,[40] and carcinosarcoma,[32,49] may also arise from the peritoneum.

Peritoneal leiomyomatosis (leiomyomatosis peritonealis disseminata) is a rare metaplastic proliferation of smooth muscle in the subperitoneal tissue.[71] Occasionally, decidua or endometriotic foci can be identified. It is often discovered during a pregnancy or with oral contraceptive use, and presents with multiple nodules that suggest a metastatic tumor (Figures 5-63 to 5-65). Immature teratomas of the ovary are occasionally associated with mature glial implants in the peritoneum, referred to as gliomatosis peritonei (Figure 5-66).[51a] Pseudomyxoma peritonei is characterized by exuberant mucinous material associated with well-differentiated mucinous neoplasm (Figures 5-67 and 5-68). Often both ovaries are involved, but evidence indicates that many of these cases are a result of a primary appendiceal tumor (Figure 5-69).[56,59,79] Poorly differentiated adenocarcinomas involving the peritoneum may occasionally form a mass on the anterior abdominal wall invading the umbilicus (Figures 5-70 to 5-72). This phenomenon is called a "Sister Mary-Joseph nodule" in reference to the nurse at the Mayo Clinic who described it.[45a]

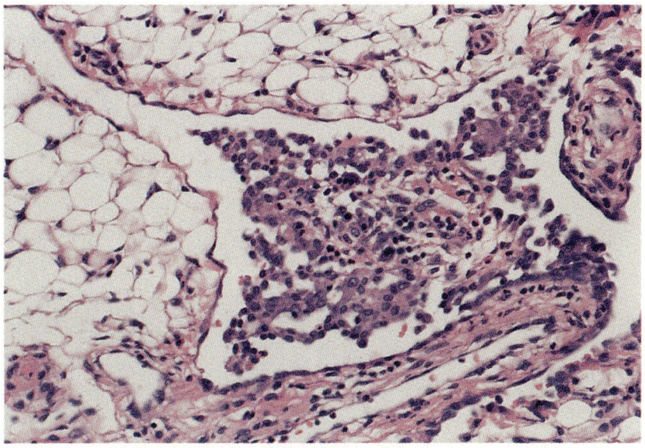

5.48 Mesonephric hyperplasia of the peritoneum lining the omentum.

*References 12, 17, 39, 46, 61, 76.

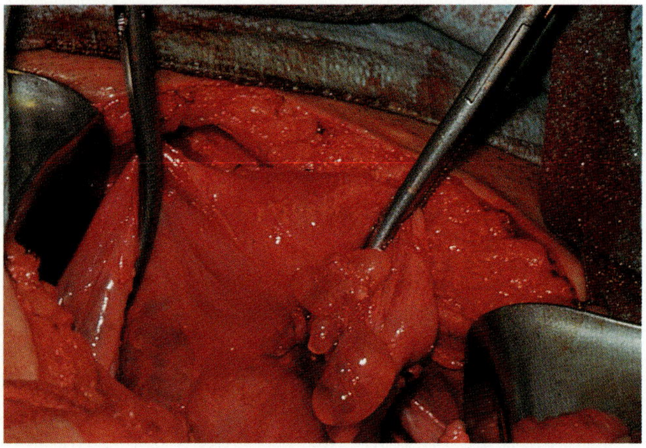

5.49 Intraoperative view of multiloculated cystic mesothelioma.

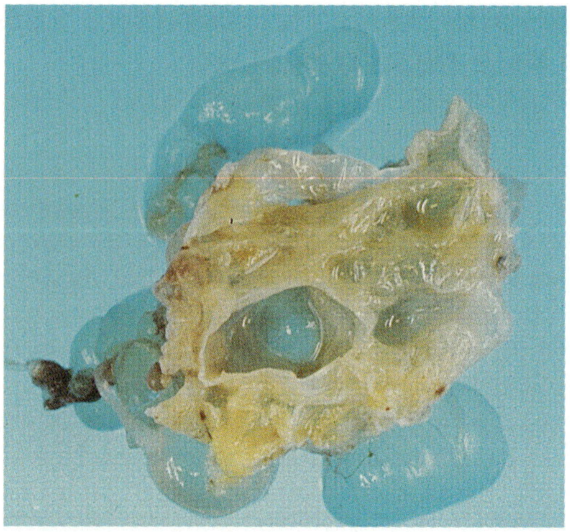

5.50 Multiloculated cystic mesothelioma.

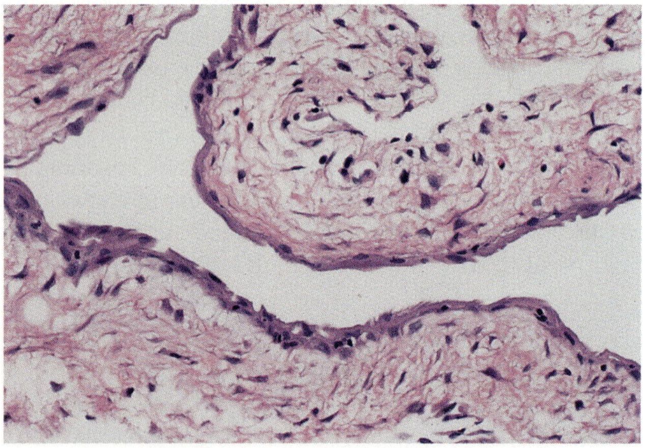

5.51 Cystic mesothelioma lined with flattened mesothelial cells.

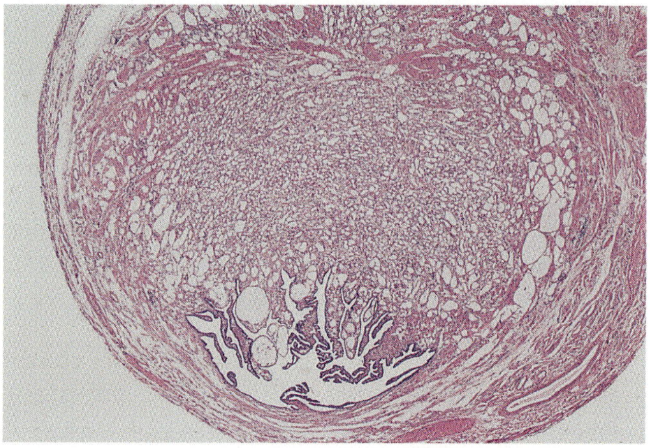

5.52 Adenomatoid tumor arising in the fallopian tube.

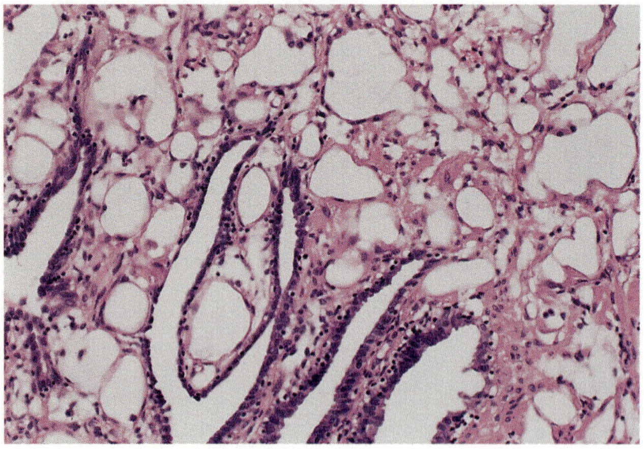

5.53 Adenomatoid tumor showing small cystic spaces lined with flattened mesothelial cells.

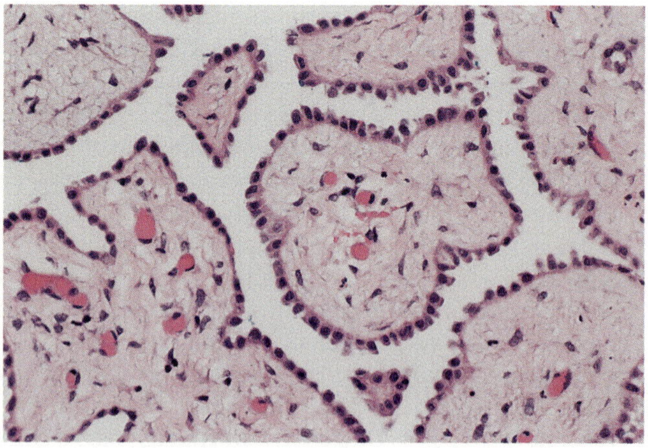

5.54 Localized papillary mesothelioma of the peritoneum with cuboidal, bland mesothelial cells lining papillary fronds with a fibrovascular core.

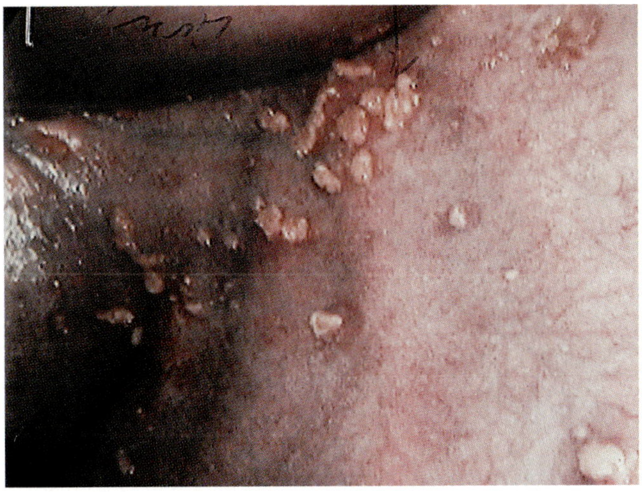

5.55 Intraoperative view of well-differentiated diffuse papillary mesothelioma of the peritoneum. (Courtesy Dr. James Davidson.)

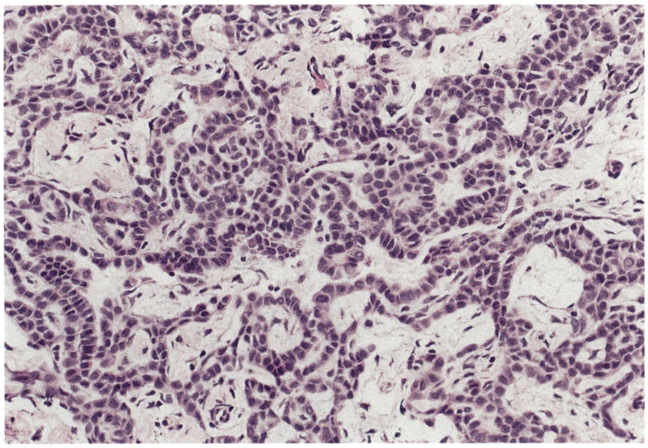

5.56 Well-differentiated diffuse papillary mesothelioma.

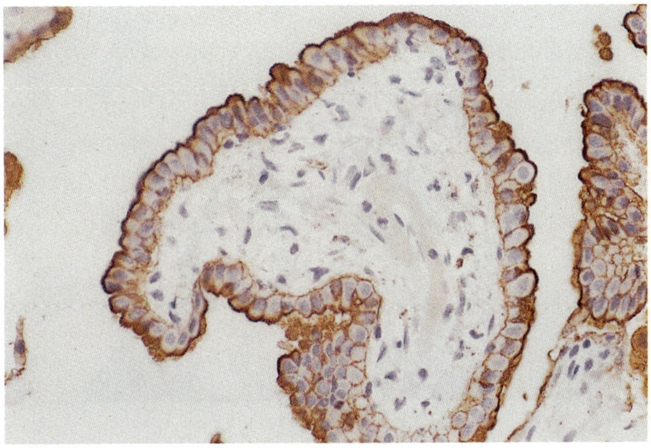

5.57 Well-differentiated diffuse papillary mesothelioma with a positive immunoperoxidase stain for HBME-1.

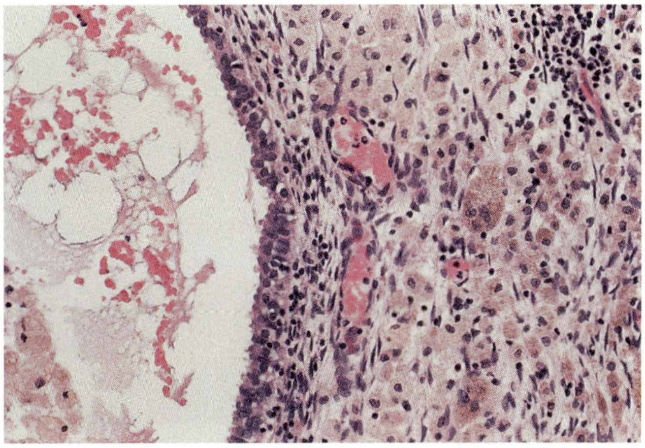

5.58 Endometriosis of the peritoneum with benign endometrial glands, endometrial stromal cells, and pigmented macrophages.

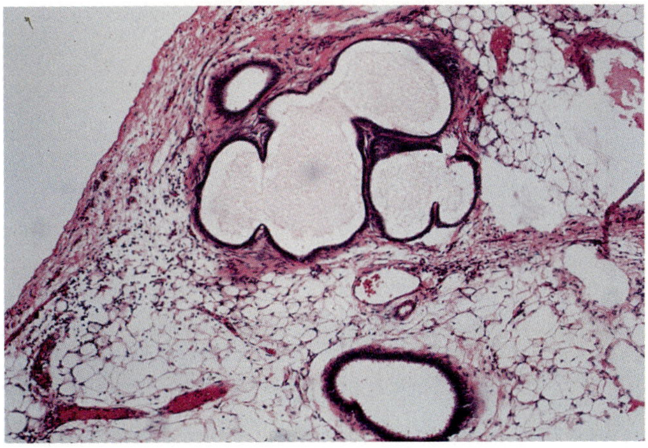

5.59 Endosalpingiosis of the omentum with cystic spaces lined with epithelial cells.

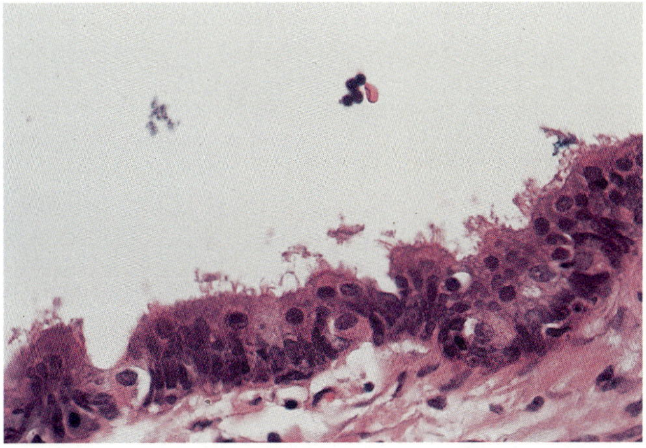

5.60 Endosalpingiosis demonstrating serous glandular epithelium with cilia.

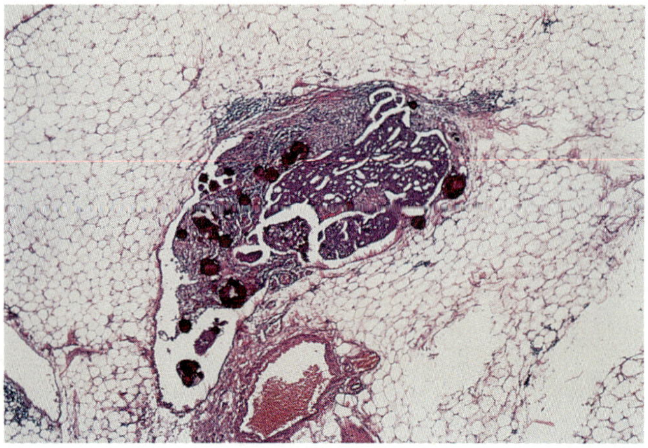

5.61 Implants from a borderline tumor of the ovary occurring in the omentum. The implant is noninvasive and papillary, showing scattered psammoma bodies.

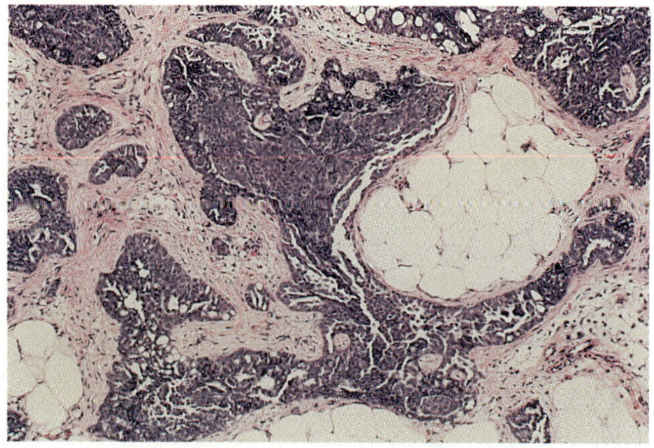

5.62 Primary papillary serous carcinoma arising in the peritoneum.

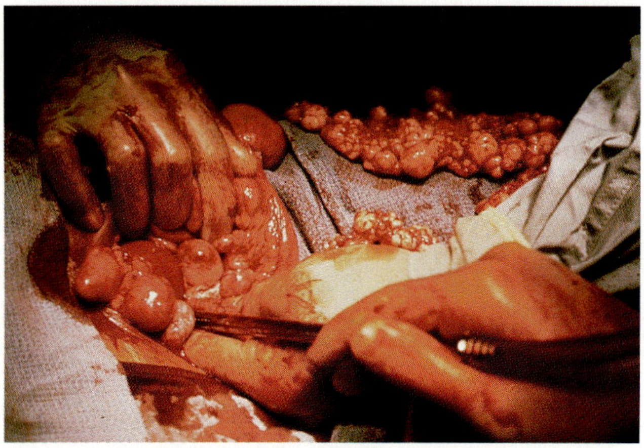

5.63 Intraoperative view of peritoneal leiomyomatosis showing numerous solid nodules. (Courtesy Dr. Herb Buchsbaum.)

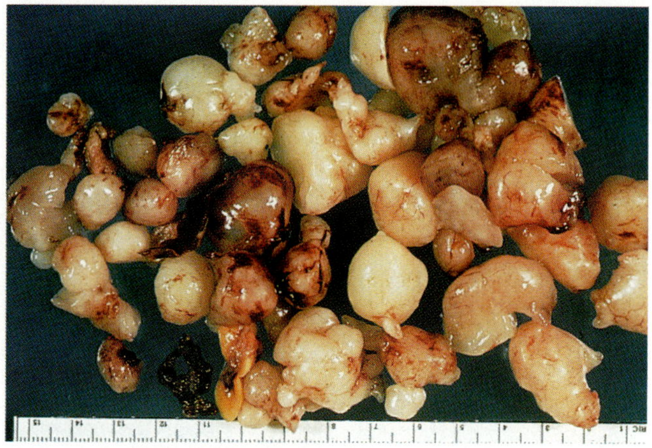

5.64 Gross view of the nodules from disseminated peritoneal leiomyomatosis. (Courtesy Dr. Herb Buchsbaum.)

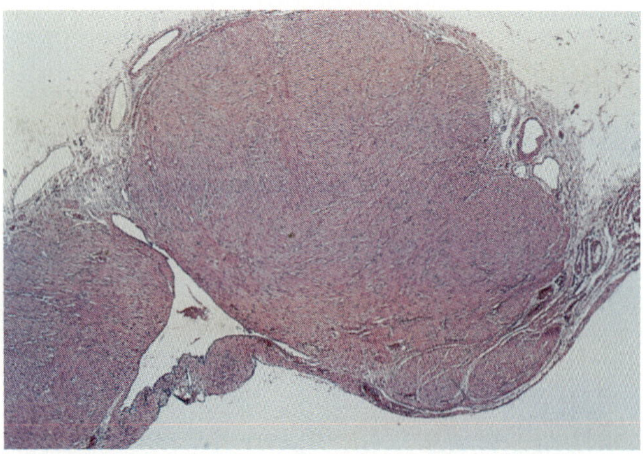

5.65 Peritoneal leiomyomatosis revealing a nodule of bland smooth muscle.

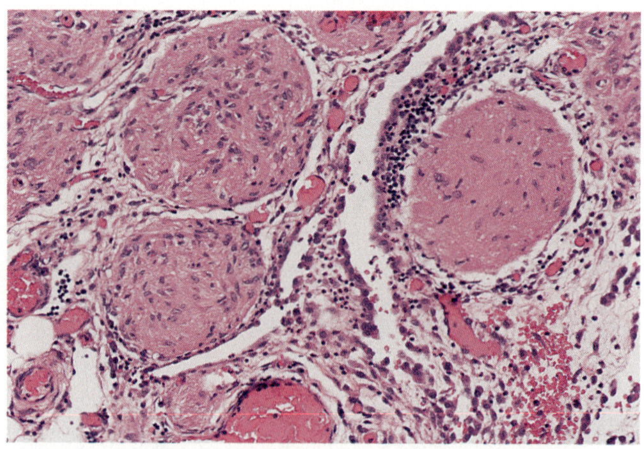

5.66 Gliomatosis peritonei revealing mature glial cells in the omentum.

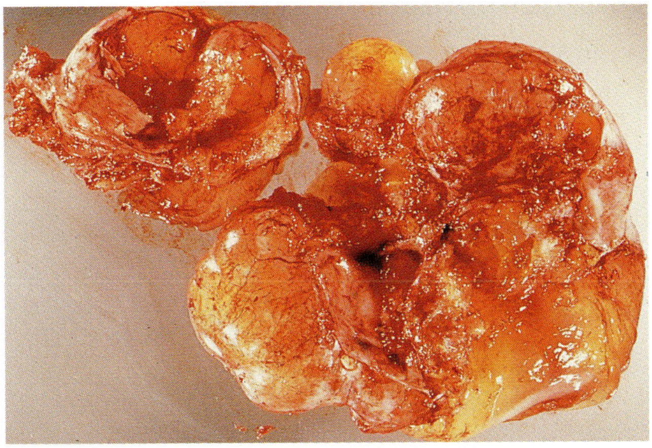

5.67 Pseudomyxoma peritonei demonstrating multiloculated, mucinous material in the omentum.

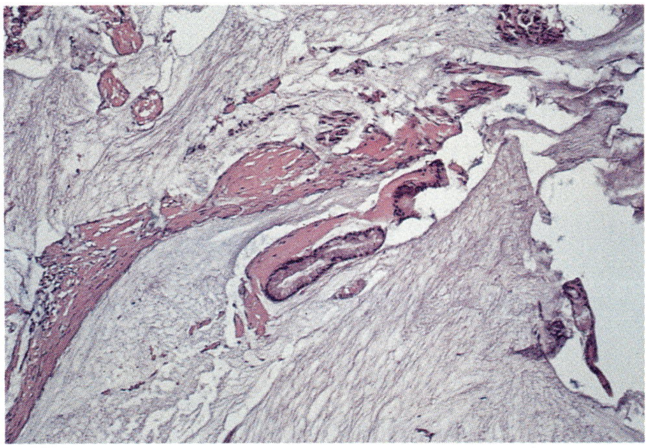

5.68 Pseudomyxoma peritonei containing mucinous epithelium embedded in abundant mucinous material.

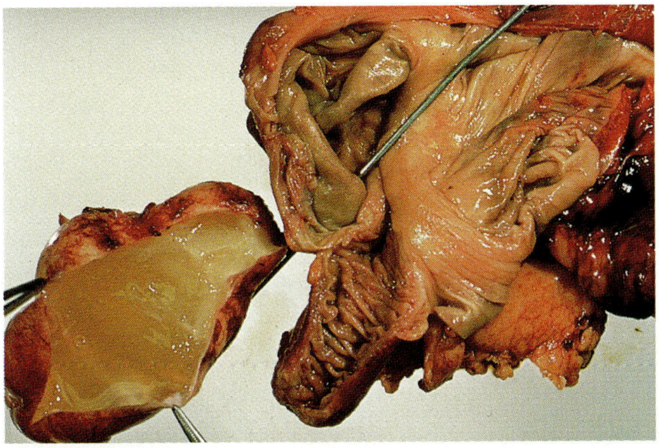

5.69 Primary mucinous tumor of the appendix in a patient with pseudomyxoma peritonei.

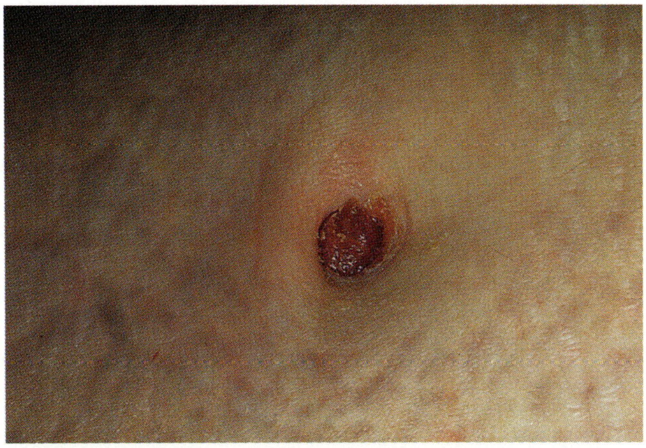

5.70 Clinical view of the umbilicus in a patient with metastatic carcinoma from the ovary (Sister Mary-Joseph nodule).

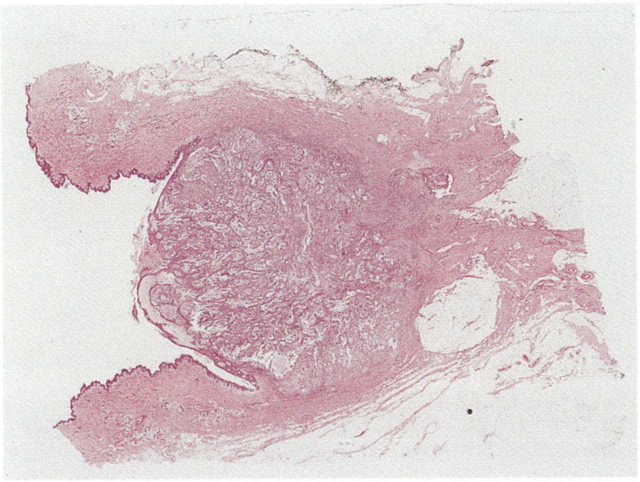

5.71 Histologic section of the umbilicus revealing metastatic adenocarcinoma in a nodular configuration, replacing the umbilicus.

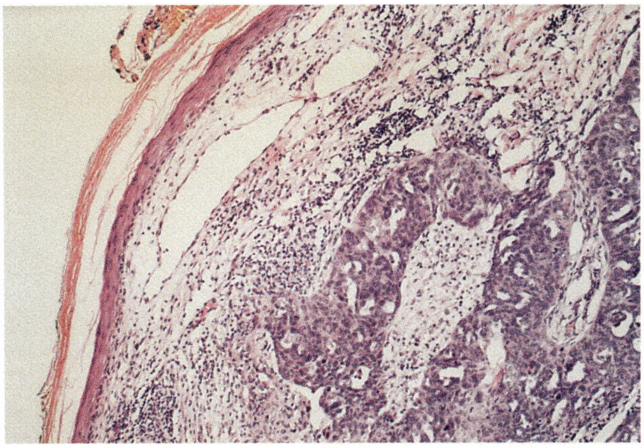

5.72 Intact overlying skin with an underlying poorly differentiated adenocarcinoma in a Sister Mary-Joseph nodule.

Histologic Classification of Tumors and Tumor-Like Lesions of the Fallopian Tube

International Society of Gynecological Pathologists

I. Epithelial tumors
- A. Benign
  1. Adenoma
  2. Papilloma
  3. Endometrioid polyp
  4. Metaplastic papillary tumor
- B. Malignant
  1. Carcinoma in situ
  2. Serous carcinoma
  3. Mucinous carcinoma
  4. Endometrioid carcinoma
  5. Clear cell carcinoma
  6. Transitional cell carcinoma
  7. Squamous cell carcinoma

II. Mixed epithelial-mesenchymal tumors
- A. Benign
  1. Adenofibroma
  2. Adenomyoma
- B. Mesodermal (müllerian) mixed tumor (carcinosarcoma)
  1. Homologous
  2. Heterologous

III. Mesenchymal tumors
- A. Benign
  1. Leiomyoma
  2. Others
- B. Malignant
  1. Leiomyosarcoma
  2. Others

IV. Mesothelial tumors
- A. Adenomatoid tumor
- B. Others

V. Germ cell tumors
- A. Teratoma
  1. Immature
  2. Mature
     - a. Solid
     - b. Cystic
  3. Struma
  4. Carcinoid
- B. Others

VI. Trophoblastic disease
- A. Hydatidiform mole
- B. Placental site trophoblastic tumor
- C. Choriocarcinoma

VII. Lymphomas

VIII. Secondary tumors

IX. Tumor-like lesions
- A. Atypical epithelial hyperplasia
- B. Endometrial colonization and endometriosis
- C. Salpingitis isthmica nodosa
- D. Tuberculous salpingitis with atypical epithelial hyperplasia
- E. Epithelial metaplasia
- F. Heat artifact
- G. Mesothelial hyperplasia
- H. Ectopic pregnancy
- I. Malakoplakia

FIGO Staging for Fallopian Tube Carcinoma

The International Federation of Gynecology and Obstetrics (FIGO)

Stage 0 Carcinoma in situ (limited to tubal mucosa)

Stage I Growth limited to the fallopian tubes
- Stage IA Growth is limited to one tube with extension into the submucosa and/or muscularis but not penetrating the serosal surface; no ascites
- Stage IB Growth limited to both tubes with extension into the submucosa and/or muscularis but not penetrating the serosal surface; no ascites
- Stage IC Tumor either Stage IA or Stage IB but with tumor extension through or onto the tubal serosa; or with ascites present containing malignant cells or with positive peritoneal washings

Stage II Growth involving one or both tubes with pelvic extension
- Stage IIA Extension and/or metastasis to the uterus or ovary
- Stage IIB Extension to other pelvic tissues
- Stage IIC Tumor either Stage IIA or Stage IIB and with ascites present containing malignant cells or with positive peritoneal washings

Stage III Tumor involves one or both fallopian tubes with peritoneal implants outside the pelvis and/or positive retroperitoneal or inguinal nodes. Superficial liver metastasis equals Stage III. Tumor appears limited to the true pelvis but with histologically proven malignant extension to the small bowel or omentum.
- Stage IIIA Tumor is grossly limited to the true pelvis with negative nodes but with histologically confirmed microscopic seeding of abdominal peritoneal surfaces
- Stage IIIB Tumor involving one or both tubes with histologically confirmed implants of abdominal peritoneal surfaces none exceeding 2 cm in diameter; lymph nodes are negative
- Stage IIIC Abdominal implants greater than 2 cm in diameter and/or positive retroperitoneal or inguinal lymph nodes

Stage IV Growth involving one or both tubes with distant metastasis. If pleural effusion is present, there must be positive cytology to be Stage IV. Parenchymal liver metastases equal Stage IV.

Histologic Classification of Tumors and Tumor-Like Lesions of the Broad Ligament

International Society of Gynecological Pathologists

I. Epithelial tumors
- A. Müllerian
  - 1. Serous
    - a. Cystadenoma
    - b. Cystadenoma of borderline malignancy
    - c. Carcinoma
  - 2. Endometrioid
  - 3. Clear cell
  - 4. Mucinous
  - 5. Brenner
- B. Wolffian and probable wolffian
  - 1. Papillary cystadenoma (this tumor may be associated with von Hippel-Lindau syndrome)
  - 2. Adnexal tumor of probable wolffian origin
- C. Ependymoma

II. Mixed epithelial-mesenchymal tumors
- A. Adenomyoma
- B. Others

III. Soft tissue tumors
- A. Benign
  - 1. Leiomyoma
  - 2. Others
- B. Malignant
  - 1. Leiomyosarcoma
  - 2. Others

IV. Germ cell tumors

V. Sex cord–stromal tumors

VI. Steroid cell tumors

VII. Malignant lymphoma

VIII. Secondary tumors

IX. Tumor-like lesions
- A. Cysts
  - 1. Müllerian
  - 2. Wolffian
  - 3. Mesothelial
- B. Endometriosis
- C. Adrenocortical rest hyperplasia
- D. Fibroxanthoma (inflammatory pseudotumor)
- E. Malakoplakia

Histologic Classification of Tumors and Tumor-Like Lesions of the Female Peritoneum and Retroperitoneum

International Society of Gynecological Pathologists

I. Mesothelial tumors
- A. Benign
  1. Localized papillary mesothelioma
  2. Cystic mesothelioma (multilocular peritoneal inclusion cyst)
  3. Adenomatoid tumor
- B. Malignant
  1. Epitheloid type
  2. Sarcomatoid
  3. Biphasic
  4. Undifferentiated

II. Submesothelial tumors
- A. Benign
  1. Fibrous tumor (localized fibrous mesothelioma)
  2. Lymphangioma
  3. Others
- B. Malignant
  1. Fibrous tumor (localized fibrous mesothelioma)
  2. Others

III. Epithelial tumors
- A. Serous
  1. Cystadenoma, retroperitoneal
  2. Cystadenocarcinoma, retroperitoneal
- B. Endometrioid carcinoma
- C. Clear cell carcinoma

IV. Mixed epithelial-mesenchymal tumors
- A. Adenosarcoma
- B. Carcinosarcoma (mesodermal [müllerian] mixed tumors)

V. Disseminated peritoneal leiomyomatosis

VI. Germ cell tumors

VII. Lymphomas

VIII. Others

IX. Secondary tumors
- A. Epithelial
  1. Ovarian serous
     - a. Borderline
     - b. Carcinoma
  2. Ovarian mucinous
     - a. Borderline
     - b. Carcinoma
  3. Other carcinomas
- B. Nonepithelial
  1. Ovarian teratoma
     - a. Mature glial
     - b. Others
  2. Struma (strumosis)
  3. Others

X. Tumor-like lesions
- A. Reactive mesothelial hyperplasia
- B. Endosalpingiosis
- C. Endometriosis
  1. Pseudoxanthomatous necrotic nodules
  2. Other forms
- D. Decidual change
- E. Other metaplasias
  1. Mucinous (endocervicosis)
  2. Transitional (Walthard nests)
  3. Squamous
- F. Fibromatosis
- G. Inflammatory and sclerosing pseudotumors (xanthogranuloma, retractile mesenteritis, panniculitis, sclerosing mesenteritis, retroperitoneal fibrosis)
- H. Retroperitoneal cysts
  1. Mesothelial
  2. Lymphatic
  3. Infectious
  4. Others
- I. Splenosis
- J. Foreign body granulomatous reaction
  1. Secondary to rupture of dermoid cyst (mature cystic tumor)
  2. Secondary to rupture of mucinous ovarian tumor
  3. Keratin granulomas secondary to adenocarcinomas with squamous differentiation
  4. Others
- K. Lymph node lesions
  1. Müllerian inclusion glands and cysts
  2. Decidua
  3. Smooth muscle
- L. Postoperative necrotic nodules
- M. Melanosis peritonei and other pigmented peritoneal lesions
- N. Enlarged pacinian corpuscles

BIBLIOGRAPHY

General Reading

1. Battifora H, McCaughey WTE: *Tumors of the serosal membranes. Atlas of tumor pathology,* 3rd series, fascicle 15, Washington, DC, 1995, Armed Forces Institute of Pathology.
2. Clement PB, Young RH, Scully RE: *Peritoneum.* In Sternberg SS, editor: *Diagnostic surgical pathology,* ed 2, New York, 1994, Raven Press.
3. Kurman RJ, editor: *Blaustein's pathology of the female genital tract,* ed 4, New York, 1994, Springer-Verlag.
4. Thor AD, Young RH, Clement PB: Pathology of the fallopian tube, broad ligament, peritoneum, and pelvic soft tissues, *Hum Pathol* 22:856-867, 1991.
5. Young RH, Clement PB, Scully RE: *The fallopian tube and broad ligament.* In Sternberg SS, editor: *Diagnostic surgical pathology,* ed 2, New York, 1994, Raven Press.

References

6. Aslani M, Scully RE: Primary carcinoma of the broad ligament, *Cancer* 7:1540-1545, 1989.
7. Bell DA, Scully RE: Serous borderline tumors of the peritoneum, *Am J Surg Pathol* 14:230-239, 1990.
8. Bell DA, Woodruff JM, Scully RE: Ependymoma of the broad ligament, *Am J Surg Pathol* 8:203-209, 1984.
9. Bernardus RE, Van Der Slikke JW, Roex AJM, Dijkhuizen GH, Stolk JG: Torsion of the fallopian tube: some considerations on its etiology, *Obstet Gynecol* 64:675-678, 1984.
10. Biscotti VC, Hart WR: Peritoneal serous micropapillomatosis of low malignant potential (serous borderline tumors of the peritoneum). A clinicopathologic study of 17 cases, *Am J Surg Pathol* 16:467-475, 1992.
11. Carlson JA, Ackerman BL, Wheeler JE: Malignant mixed müllerian tumor of the fallopian tube, *Cancer* 71:187-192, 1993.
12. Carpenter HA, Lancaster JR, Lee RA: Multilocular cysts of the peritoneum, *Mayo Clin Proc* 57:634-638, 1982.
13. Chang KL, Crabtree GS, Lim-Tan SK, Kempson RL, Hendrickson MR: Primary extrauterine endometrial stromal neoplasms: a clinicopathologic study of 20 cases and a review of the literature, *Int J Gynecol Pathol* 12:282-296, 1993.
14. Chen KTK: Benign glandular inclusions of the peritoneum and periaortic lymph nodes, *Diagn Gynecol Obstet* 3:265-268, 1981.
15. Cheung ANY, So KF, Ngan HYS, Wong LC: Primary squamous cell carcinoma of fallopian tube, *Int J Gynecol Pathol* 13:92-95, 1994.
16. Cheung ANY, Young RH, Scully RE: Pseudocarcinomatous hyperplasia of the fallopian tube associated with salpingitis, *Am J Surg Pathol* 8:1125-1130, 1994.
17. Clement PB: Reactive tumor-like lesions of the peritoneum, *Am J Clin Pathol* 103:673-676, 1995.
18. Clement PB, Young RH: Florid mesothelial hyperplasia associated with ovarian tumors: a potential source of error in tumor diagnosis and staging, *Int J Gynecol Pathol* 12:51-58, 1993.
19. Clement PB, Young RH, Scully RE: Necrotic pseudoxanthomatous nodules of ovary and peritoneum in endometriosis, *Am J Surg Pathol* 12:390-397, 1988.
20. Coffin CM, Dehner LP: Mesothelial and related neoplasms in children and adolescents: a clinicopathologic and immunohistochemical analysis of eight cases, *Pediatr Pathol* 12:333-347, 1992.
21. Dalrymple JC, Bannatyne P, Russell P, Solomon HJ, Tattersall HN, Atkinson K, Carter J, Duval P, Elliott P, Friedlander M, Murry J, Coppleson M: Extraovarian peritoneal serous papillary carcinoma. A clinicopathologic study of 31 cases, *Cancer* 64:110-115, 1989.
22. Daya D, McCaughey WTE: Well-differentiated papillary mesothelioma of the peritoneum. A clinicopathologic study of 22 cases, *Cancer* 65:292-296, 1990.
23. Daya D, Young RH, Scully RE: Endometrioid carcinoma of the fallopian tube resembling an adnexal tumor of probable wolffian origin: a report of six cases, *Int J Gynecol Pathol* 11:122-130, 1992.
24. De Peralta MN, Delahoussaye PM, Tornos CS, Silva EG: Benign retroperitoneal cysts of müllerian type: a clinicopathologic study of three cases and review of the literature, *Int J Gynecol Pathol* 13:273-278, 1994.
25. Demopoulos RI, Sitelman A, Flotte T, Bigelow B: Ultrastructural study of a female adnexal tumor of probable wolffian origin, *Cancer* 46:2273-2282, 1980.
26. Donnez J, Casanas-Roux F, Ferin J, Thomas K: Tubal polyps, epithelial inclusions, and endometriosis after tubal sterilization, *Fertil Steril* 41:564-568, 1984.

27. D'Ablaing G, Klatt EC, DiRocco G, Hibbard LT: Broad ligament serous tumor of low malignant potential, *Int J Gynecol Pathol* 2:93-99, 1983.
28. Egan AJ, Russell P: Transitional (urothelial) cell metaplasia of the fallopian tube mucosa: morphological assessment of three cases, *Int J Gynecol Pathol* 1:72-76, 1996.
29. Fedele L, Bianchi S, DiNola G, Franchi D, Candiani GB: Endometriosis and nonobstructive müllerian anomalies, *Obstet Gynecol* 79:515-517, 1992.
30. Finn WF, Javert CT: Primary and metastatic cancer of the fallopian tube, *Cancer* 2:803-814, 1949.
31. Fox H, Buckley CH: Current concepts of endometriosis, *Clin Obstet Gynecol* 11:279-287, 1984.
32. Garamvoelgyi E, Guillou L, Gebhard S, Salmeron M, Seematter RJ, Hadji MH: Primary malignant mixed müllerian tumor (metaplastic carcinoma) of the female peritoneum, *Cancer* 74:854-863, 1994.
33. Geary WA, Mills SE, Frierson HF, Pope TL: Malignant peritoneal mesothelioma in childhood with long-term survival, *Am J Clin Pathol* 95:493-498, 1991.
34. George E, Leyser S, Zimmer HL, Simonowitz DA, Agress RL, Nordin DD: Vernix caseosa peritonitis. An infrequent complication of cesarean section with distinctive histopathologic features, *Am J Clin Pathol* 103:681-684, 1995.
35. Goldblum J, Hart WR: Localized and diffuse mesotheliomas of the genital tract and peritoneum in women, *Am J Surg Pathol* 19:1124-1137, 1995.
36. Heaps JM, Nieberg RK, Berek JS: Malignant neoplasms arising in endometriosis, *Obstet Gynecol* 75:1023-1028, 1990.
37. Jenkins S, Olive DL, Haney AF: Endometriosis: pathogenetic implications of the anatomic distribution, *Obstet Gynecol* 67:335-338, 1986.
38. Kariminejad MH, Scully RE: Female adnexal tumor of probable wolffian origin. A distinctive pathologic entity, *Cancer* 31:671-677, 1973.
39. Katsube Y, Mukai K, Silverberg SG: Cystic mesothelioma of the peritoneum, *Cancer* 50:1615-1622, 1982.
40. Kerner H, Lichtig C, Beck D: Extrauterine müllerian adenosarcoma of the peritoneal mesothelium: a clinicopathologic and electron microscopic study, *Obstet Gynecol* 73:510-513, 1989.
41. Kheir SM, Mann WJ, Wilkerson JA: Glandular inclusions in lymph nodes. The problem of extensive involvement and relationship to salpingitis, *Am J Surg Pathol* 5:353-359, 1981.
42. Klein TA, Richmond JA, Mishell DR Jr: Pelvic tuberculosis, *Obstet Gynecol* 48:99-104, 1976.
43. Koshiyama M, Konishi I, Yoshida M, Wang D, Mandai M, Mori T, Fujii S: Transitional cell carcinoma of the fallopian tube: a light and electron microscopic study, *Int J Gynecol Pathol* 13:175-180, 1994.
44. Lauchlan SC: The secondary müllerian system revisited, *Int J Gynecol Pathol* 13:73-78, 1994.
45. Majmudar B, Henderson PH III, Semple E: Salpingitis isthmica nodosa: a high-risk factor for tubal pregnancy, *Obstet Gynecol* 62:73-78, 1983.
45a. Majmudar B, Wiskind AK, Croft BN, Dudley AG: The Sister (Mary) Joseph nodule: its significance in gynecology. *Gynecol Oncol* 40:152-159, 1991.
46. McFadden DE, Clement PB: Peritoneal inclusion cysts with mural mesothelial proliferation, *Am J Surg Pathol* 10:844-854, 1986.
47. McMurray EH, Jacobs AJ, Perez CA, Camel HM, Kao M-S, Galakatos A: Carcinoma of the fallopian tube, *Cancer* 58:2070-2075, 1986.
48. Mills SE: Decidua and squamous metaplasia in abdominopelvic lymph nodes, *Int J Gynecol Pathol* 2:209-215, 1983.
49. Mira JL, Fenoglio-Preiser CM, Husseinzadeh N: Malignant mixed müllerian tumor of the extraovarian secondary müllerian system. Report of two cases and review of the English literature, *Arch Pathol Lab Med* 119:1044-1049, 1995.
50. Moore SW, Enterline HT: Significance of proliferative epithelial lesions of the uterine tube, *Obstet Gynecol* 45:385-390, 1975.
51. Mulhollan TJ, Silva EG, Tornos C, Guerrieri C, Fromm G, Gershenson D: Ovarian involvement by serous surface papillary carcinoma, *Int J Gynecol Pathol* 13:120-126, 1994.
51a. Nielsen SNJ, Scheithauer BW, Gaffey TA. Gliomatosis peritonei. *Cancer* 56:2499-2503, 1985.
52. Olive DL, Henderson DY: Endometriosis and müllerian anomalies, *Obstet Gynecol* 69:411-415, 1987.
53. Pauerstein CJ, Croxatto HB, Eddy CA, Ramzy I, Walters MD: Anatomy and pathology of tubal pregnancy, *Obstet Gynecol* 67:301-308, 1986.
54. Pickartz H: Differential diagnosis of peritoneal lesions of müllerian type and similar epithelial tumors of the peritoneum, *Int J Gynecol Pathol* 12:116-119, 1993.
55. Prade M, Spatz A, Bentley R, Duvillard P, Bognel C, Robboy SJ: Borderline and malignant serous tumor arising in pelvic lymph nodes: evidence of origin in benign glandular inclusions, *Int J Gynecol Pathol* 14:87-91, 1995.

56. Prayson RA, Hart WR, Petras RE: Pseudomyxoma peritonei. A clinicopathologic study of 19 cases with emphasis on site of origin and nature of associated ovarian tumors, *Am J Surg Pathol* 18:591-603, 1994.
57. Roberts JA, Lifshitz S: Primary adenocarcinoma of the fallopian tube, *Gynecol Oncol* 13:301-308, 1982.
58. Robey SS, Silva EG: Epithelial hyperplasia of the fallopian tube: its association with serous borderline tumors of the ovary, *Int J Gynecol Pathol* 8:214-220, 1989.
59. Ronnett BM, Zahn CM, Kurman RJ, Kass ME, Sugarbaker PH, Shmookler BM: Disseminated peritoneal adenomucinous and peritoneal mucinous carcinomatosis. A clinicopathologic analysis of 109 cases with emphasis on distinguishing pathologic features, site of origin, prognosis, and relationship to "pseudomyxoma peritonei," *Am J Surg Pathol* 19:1390-1408, 1995.
60. Rose PG, Piver MS, Tsukada Y: Fallopian tube cancer; the Roswell Park experience, *Cancer* 66:2661-2667, 1990.
61. Ross MJ, Welch WR, Scully RE: Multilocular peritoneal inclusion cysts (so-called cystic mesotheliomas), *Cancer* 64:1336-1346, 1989.
62. Rothacker D, Mobius G: Varieties of serous surface papillary carcinoma of the peritoneum in Northern Germany: a thirty-year autopsy study, *Int J Gynecol Pathol* 14:310-318, 1995.
63. Saffos RO, Rhatigan RM, Scully RE: Metaplastic pap illary tumor of the fallopian tube—a distinctive lesion of pregnancy, *Am J Clin Pathol* 74:232-236, 1980.
64. Samaha M, Woodruff JD: Paratubal cysts: frequency, histogenesis, and associated clinical features, *Obstet Gynecol* 65:691-694, 1985.
65. Seidman JD: Mucinous lesions of the fallopian tube, *Am J Surg Pathol* 18:1205-1212, 1994.
66. Seidman JD: Prognosic importance of hyperplasia and atypia in endometrosis, *Int J Gynecol Pathol* 15:1-9, 1996.
67. Seidman JD, Oberer S, Bitterman P, Aisner SC: Pathogenesis of pseudoxanthomatous salpingiosis, *Mod Pathol* 6:53-55, 1993.
68. Seltzer VL, Molho L, Fougner A, Hong P, Kereszti B, Gero M, Spitzer M: Parovarian cystadenocarcinoma of low-malignant potential, *Gynecol Oncol* 30:216-221, 1988.
69. Stein AL, Koonings PP, Schlaerth JB, Grimes DA, D'Ablaing G: Relative frequency of malignant parovarian tumors: should parovarian tumors be aspirated?, *Obstet Gynecol* 75:1029-1031, 1990.
70. Stock RJ: Histopathologic changes in fallopian tubes subsequent to sterilization procedures, *Int J Gynecol Pathol* 2:13-27, 1983.
71. Tavassoli FA, Norris HJ: Peritoneal leiomyomatosis (leiomyomatosis peritonealis disseminata): a clinicopathologic study of 20 cases with ultrastructural observations, *Int J Gynecol Pathol* 1:59-74, 1982.
72. Taxy JB, Battifora H, Oyasu R: Adenomatoid tumors: light microscopic, histochemical, and ultrastructural study, *Cancer* 34:306-316, 1974.
73. Toki T, Horiuchi A, Shuan-fang L, Nakayama K, Silverberg SG, Fujii S: Proliferative activity of postmenopausal endometriosis: a histopathologic and immunocytochemical study, *Int J Gynecol Pathol* 15:45-53, 1996.
74. Tatschka BG, Lauchlan SC: Endosalpingiosis, *Obstet Gynecol* 55 (suppl):57S-60S, 1980.
75. Uehira K, Hashimoto H, Tsuneyoshi M, Enjoji M: Transitional cell carcinoma pattern in primary carcinoma of the fallopian tube, *Cancer* 72:2447-2456, 1993.
76. Villaschi S, Autelitano F, Santeusanio G, Balistreri P: Cystic mesothelioma of the peritoneum, *Am J Clin Pathol* 94:758-761, 1990.
77. Voet RL, Lifshitz S: Primary clear cell adenocarcinoma of the fallopian tube: light microscopic and ultrastructural findings, *Int J Gynecol Pathol* 1:292-298, 1982.
78. Voet RL, Waisman J, Ballon SC: Intraepithelial epidermoid carcinoma of the cervix, endometrium, and a fallopian tube, *Gynecol Oncol* 8:349-352, 1979.
79. Wertheim I, Fleischhacker D, McLachlin CM, Rice LW, Berkowitz RS, Goff BA: Pseudomyxoma peritonei, *Obstet Gynecol* 84:17-21, 1994.
80. Yanai-Inbar I, Siriaunkgul S, Silverberg SG: Mucosal epithelial proliferation of the fallopian tube: a particular association with ovarian serous tumor of low malignant potential?, *Int J Gynecol Pathol* 14:107-113, 1995.
81. Yoonessi M: Carcinoma of the fallopian tube, *Obstet Gynecol Surv* 34:257-270, 1979.
82. Zaytsev P, Taxy JB: Pregnancy-associated ectopic decidua, *Am J Surg Pathol* 11:526-530, 1987.
83. Zheng W, Wolf S, Kramer EE, Cox KA, Hoda SA: Borderline papillary serous tumor of the fallopian tube, *Am J Surg Pathol* 20:30-35, 1996.
84. Zhou J, Iwasa Y, Konishi I, Kan N, Kannagi R, Kobashi Y, Kim Y, Yamabe H: Papillary serous carcinoma of the peritoneum in women. A clinicopathologic and immunohistochemical study, *Cancer* 76:429-436, 1995.
85. Zinsser KR, Wheeler JE: Endosalpingiosis in the omentum. A study of autopsy and surgical material, *Am J Surg Pathol* 6:109-117, 1982.

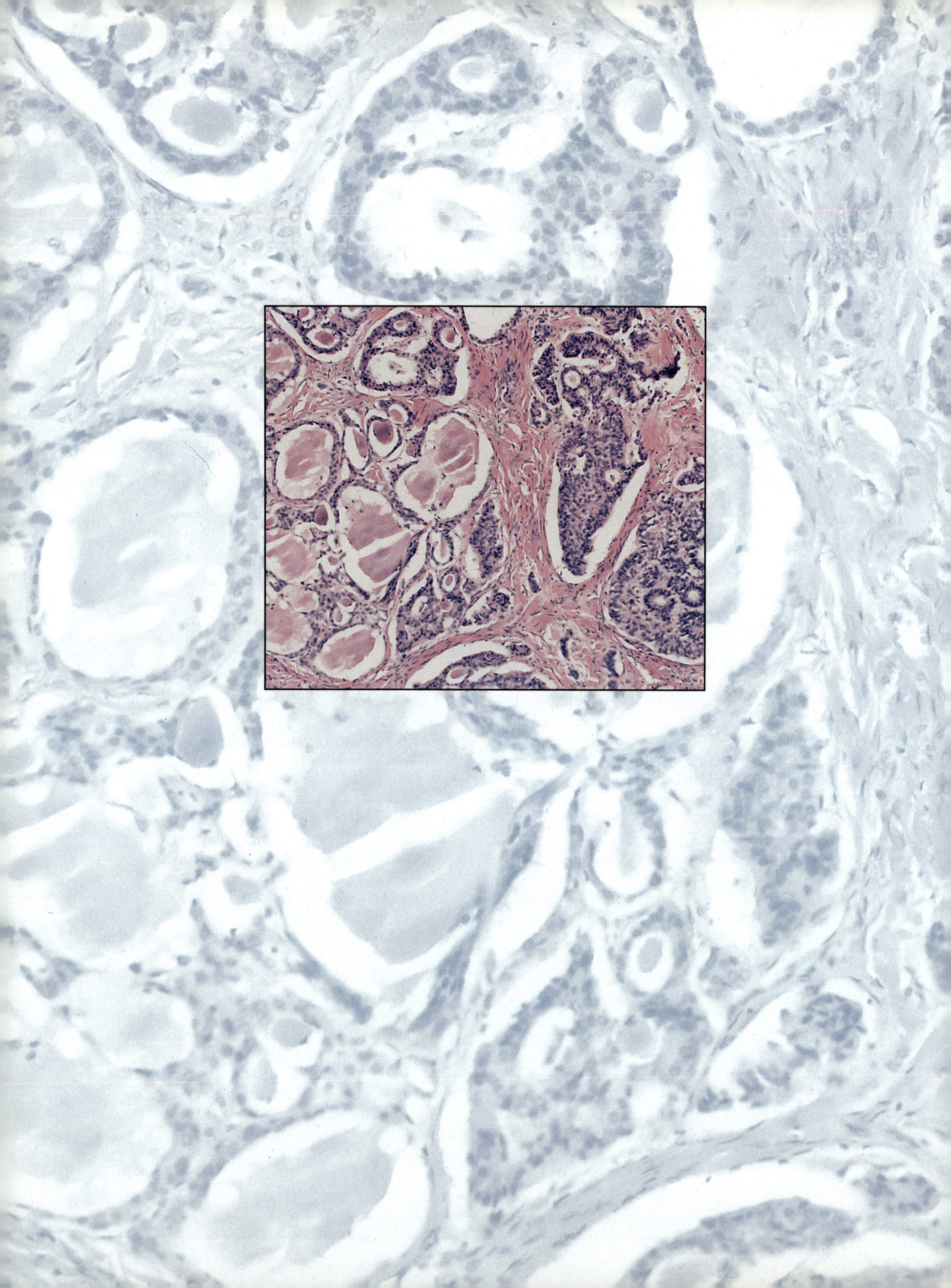

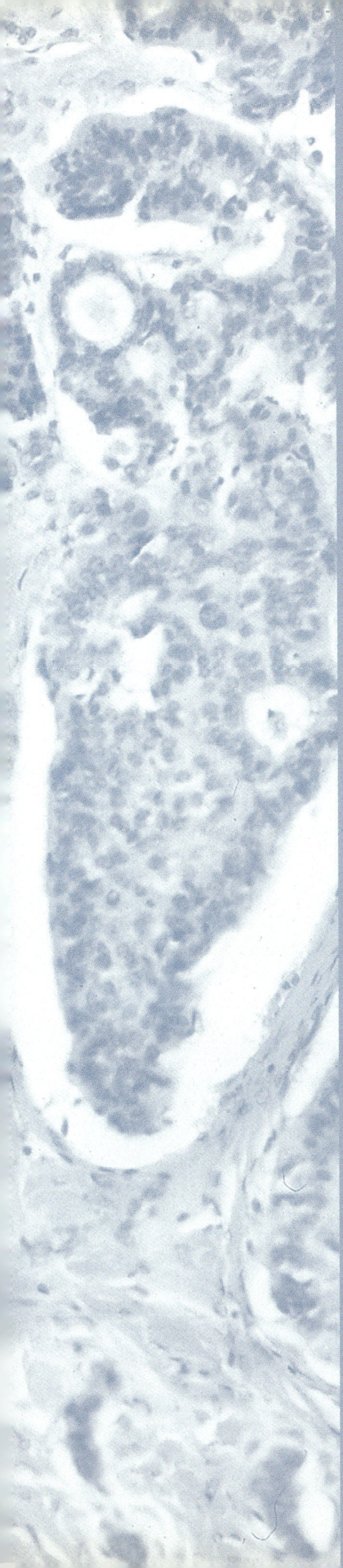

Chapter 6

Pathology of the Ovary

NONNEOPLASTIC LESIONS

Cysts of the developing ovarian follicle (Figure 6-1) are common and vary in size. If the lesion is greater than 2 cm in diameter, it is generally considered to be a follicular cyst. If it is less than 2 cm, it is considered a cystic follicle. They both have the same histologic finding: a granulosa cell layer and a fairly prominent theca interna and externa (Figure 6-2). These lesions can be hemorrhagic and the lining may be denuded. The more generic term hemorrhagic cyst or simple cyst is used if the precise lining cannot be identified. Follicles become cystic in response to gonadotropic hormones. If ovulation does not occur, the follicle usually becomes atretic. In cases of persistent anovulation, there may be numerous cystic follicles.

Polycystic ovaries are usually bilateral and show a mixture of follicular cysts and cystic follicles without evidence of ovulation (Figure 6-3). If there is persistent anovulation, the surface can become fibrotic. In addition to the cystic follicles, there is both follicular and stromal hyperthecosis. Follicular hyperthecosis refers to the luteinization of the theca interna of the cystic follicles. Stromal hyperthecosis refers to isolated islands and nests of luteinized theca cells within the stroma of the ovary (Figure 6-4). This process can exist in combination with the polycystic ovarian syndrome, as an isolated finding in postmenopausal patients, or associated with ovarian tumors.[88]

Corpus luteum cysts usually arise as a result of central hemorrhage into a corpus luteum. There is a typical gross appearance: a corrugated, bright yellow border with central hemorrhage or a cavity containing fibrin (Figure 6-5). The hemorrhage may cause rupture of the cyst and a hemoperitoneum. Corpus luteum cysts are lined by a luteinized granulosa and theca layer (Figure 6-6). If pregnancy occurs, the corpus luteum becomes a corpus luteum of pregnancy with continued hormone secretion. Hyaline droplets are usually identified by this stage. If pregnancy does not occur, the corpus luteum regresses and forms a corpus albicans.

Pregnancy luteomas are usually bilateral, multifocal, and nodular coalescing masses of luteinized cells (Figures 6-7 and 6-8).[14,26] There is a typical dull brown appearance on gross views. The exact cause of this condition is unknown. It is thought by some that it may represent an exaggerated luteinization of a preexisting stromal hyperthecosis. Some of these patients are virilized, and stromal hyperthecosis has been demonstrated in some of the surrounding ovarian parenchyma. These are benign tumors that regress after the pregnancy is terminated.

Theca lutein cysts (hyperreactio luteinalis) are dominated by the theca interna. There is marked luteinization of multiple follicles, which is usually the result of increased gonadotropin stimulation, either exogenous or endogenous. Trophoblastic disease can cause massive bilateral theca lutein cysts. Large, solitary luteinized follicle cysts can be seen in pregnancy and puerperium.[15] They contain luteinized cells with focal nuclear atypia embedded in a fibrotic wall (Figure 6-9).

Bilateral streak gonads can be found in two situations: pure gonadal dysgenesis and Turner syndrome. In adults, the streak gonad is composed almost exclusively of ovarian stroma and a few remnants (Figure 6-10). In the fetal streak ovary, it is similar to the normal ovary. There is a more rapid decline in the number of ova, with an almost complete absence by the time of puberty. Mixed gonadal dysgenesis usually has a unilateral streak gonad and a contralateral testis. True hermaphroditism is defined as the presence of both well-formed ovarian and testicular tissue. This can be seen as testicular tissue on one side with ovarian tissue on the other, or a unilateral or bilateral ovotestis (Figure 6-11). In androgen insensitivity syndrome (testicular feminization), there are immature seminiferous tubules lined by Sertoli cells containing undifferentiated germ cells. There is often a prominent Leydig cell component, as is common in cryptorchid testes. Occasionally, nodules of pure Sertoli cells (Sertoli cell hamartomas) are present (Figures 6-12 and 6-13).

Cysts and tumors of the ovary may produce torsion with subsequent edema and hemorrhage (Figure 6-14). The edema sometimes causes massive enlargement of the ovary (Figure 6-15).[122] Inflammation of the ovary is usually a part of pelvic inflammatory disease with tubo-ovarian abscess formation. If the infection is chronic, xanthogranulomatous changes may develop (Figure 6-16 and 6-17).[66] Primary ovarian ectopic pregnancies are rare and usually implant in the corpus luteum (Figure 6-18 and 6-19).[50]

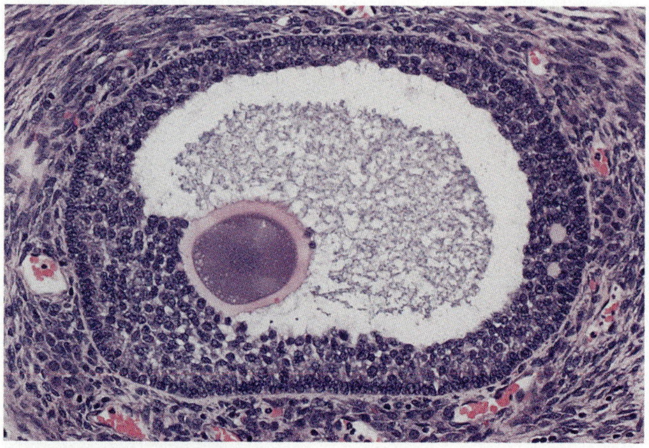

6.1 Early developing follicle containing an oocyte with surrounding granulosa cells.

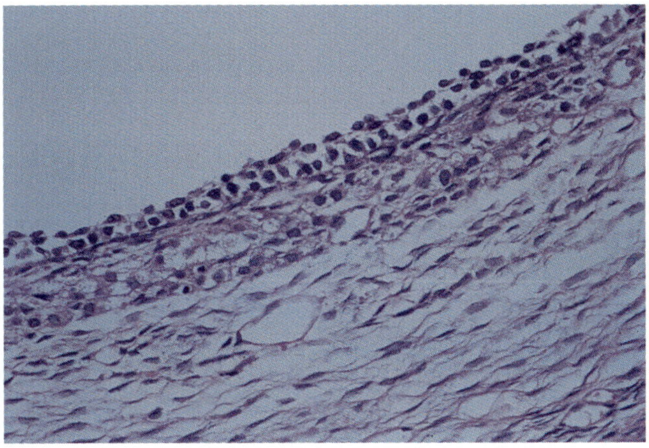

6.2 Follicular cyst lined with granulosa cells and theca cells.

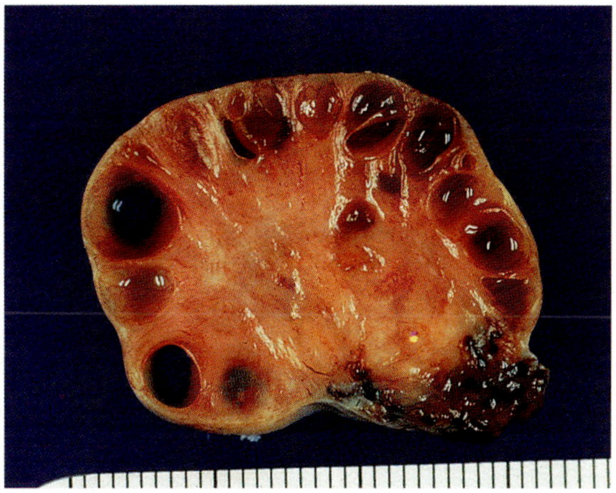

6.3 Polycystic ovary with numerous subcortical cystic follicles and central hyperthecosis characterized by a yellow color.

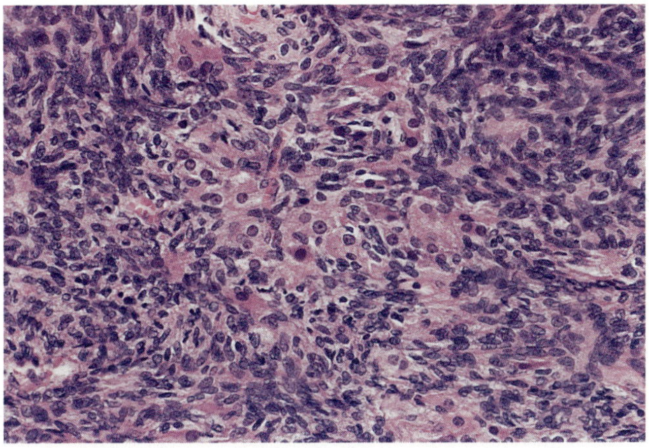

6.4 Hyperthecosis with luteinized stromal cells containing eosinophilic cytoplasm with a round nucleus.

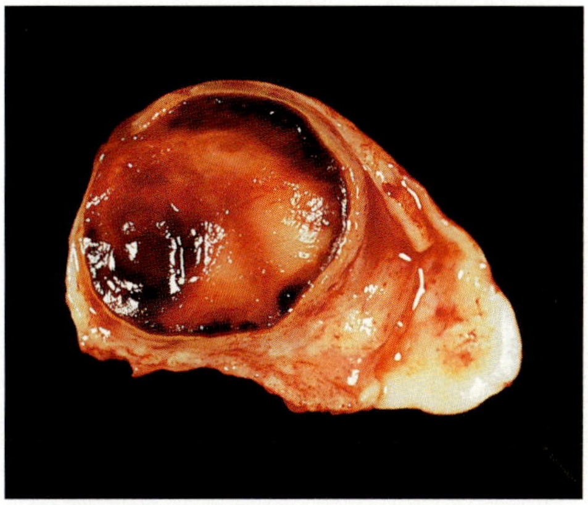

6.5 Hemorrhagic corpus luteum with an outer yellow rim and central hemorrhage.

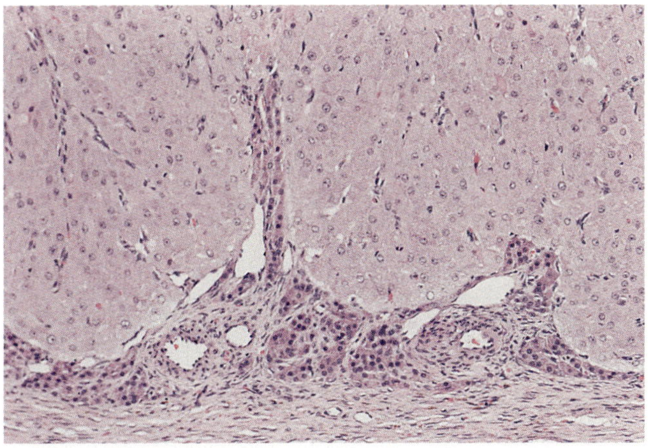

6.6 Corpus luteum with luteinized granulosa cells containing abundant eosinophilic cytoplasm and round nuclei with an outer zone of luteinized theca cells.

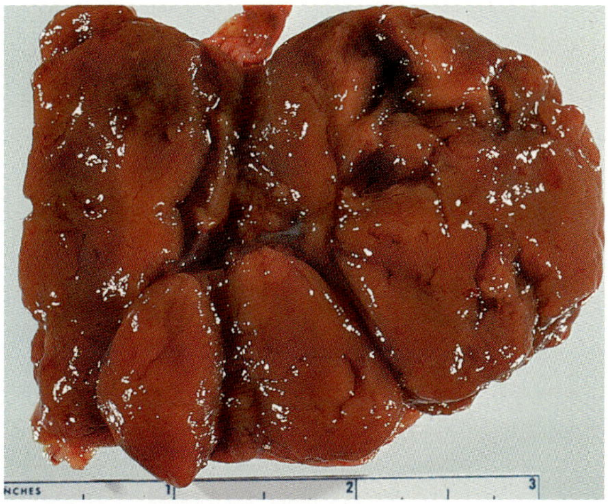

6.7 Luteoma of pregnancy with numerous solid brown nodules.

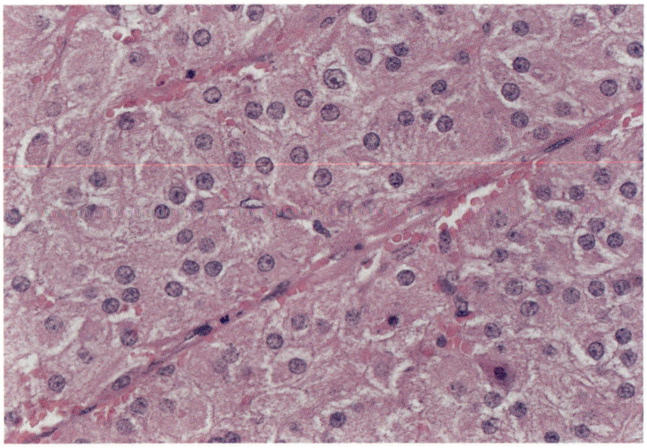

6.8 Luteoma of pregnancy demonstrating a solid proliferation of eosinophilic luteinized cells.

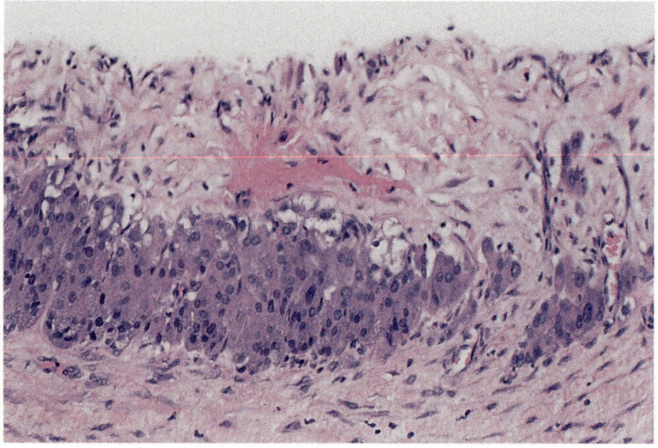

6.9 Solitary luteinized follicle cyst of pregnancy and puerperium containing luteinized cells with focal nuclear atypia embedded in a fibrous wall.

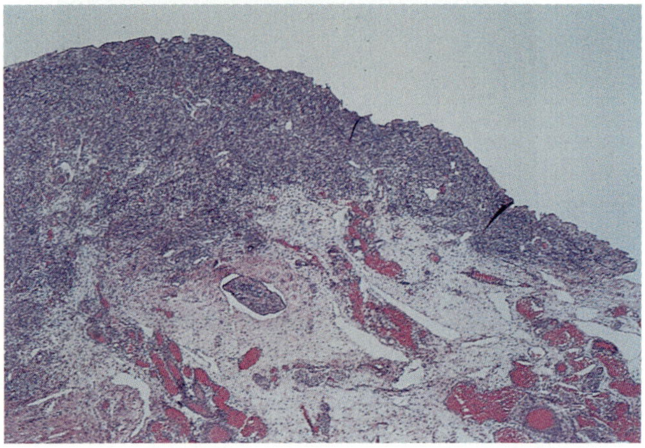

6.10 Streak gonad showing a superficial rim of ovarian tissue.

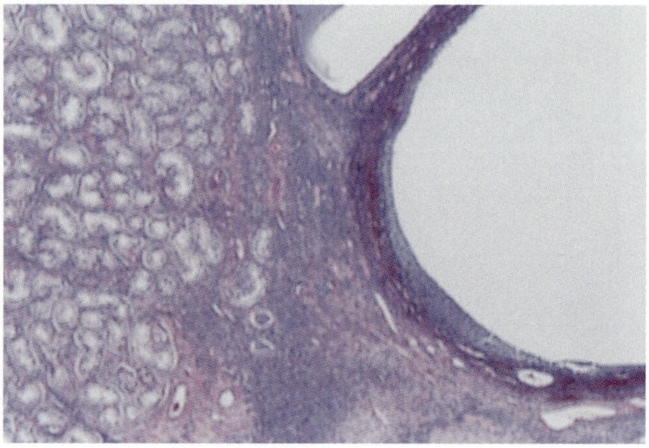

6.11 Ovotestes with a mixture of seminiferous tubules on the left and cystic follicles on the right.

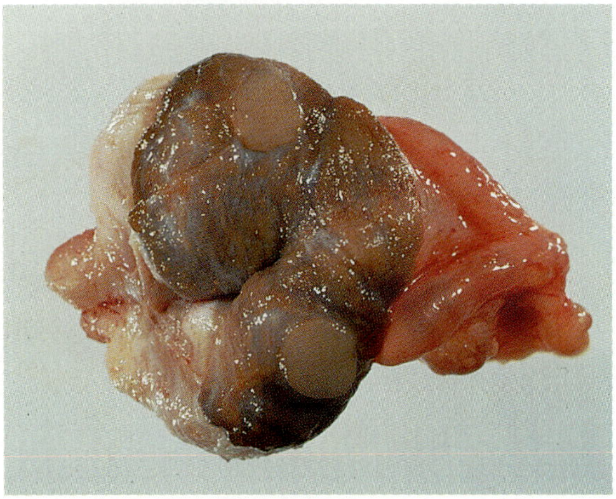

6.12 Testicle from a patient with androgen insensitivity syndrome containing well-circumscribed Sertoli cell nodules.

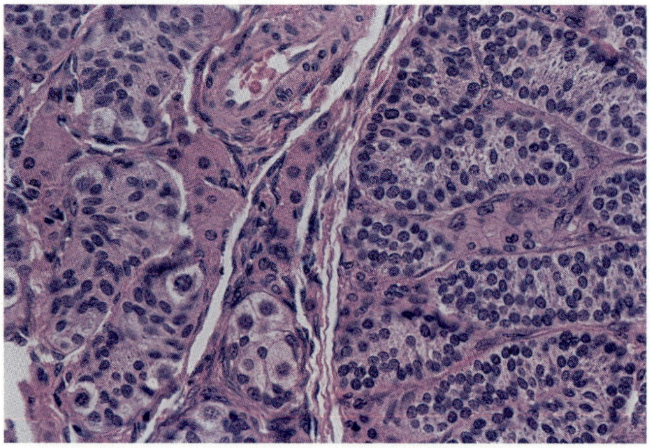

6.13 Sertoli cell nodule on the right, rimming testicular tissue on the left, from a patient with androgen insensitivity syndrome.

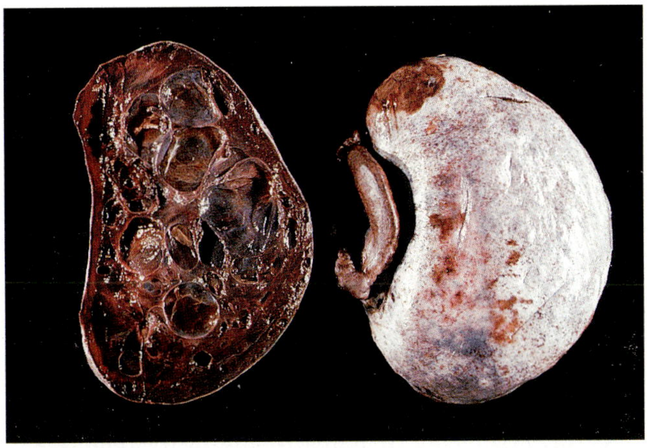

6.14 Massive ovarian edema and hemorrhage from torsion.

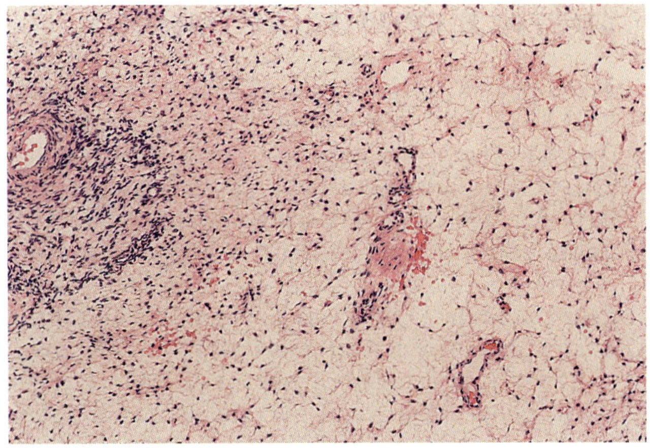

6.15 Massive ovarian edema involving the ovarian stroma.

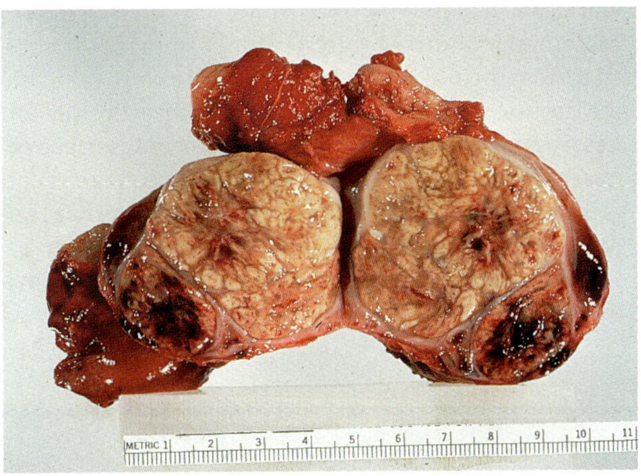

6.16 Xanthogranulomatous oophoritis with a well-circumscribed yellow nodule containing fibrous septa and focal hemorrhage.

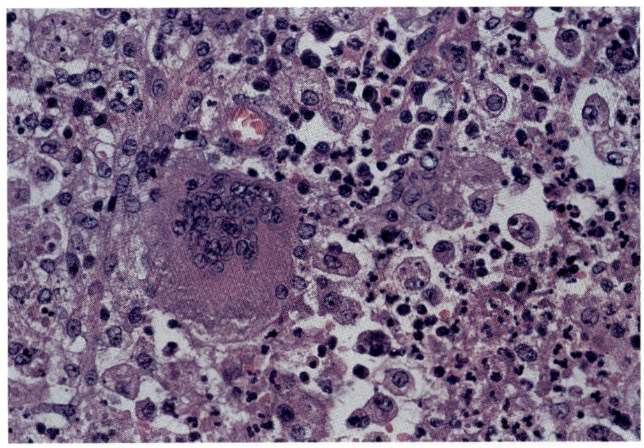

6.17 Xanthogranulomatous oophoritis with multinucleated giant cells, numerous histiocytes, plasma cells, and lymphocytes.

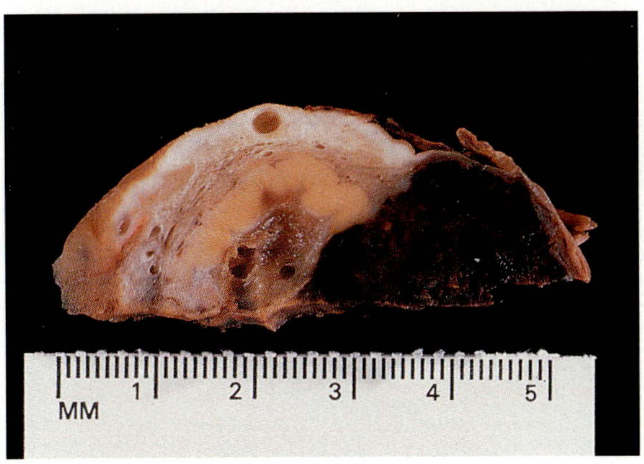

6.18 Ectopic ovarian pregnancy implanting in the corpus luteum.

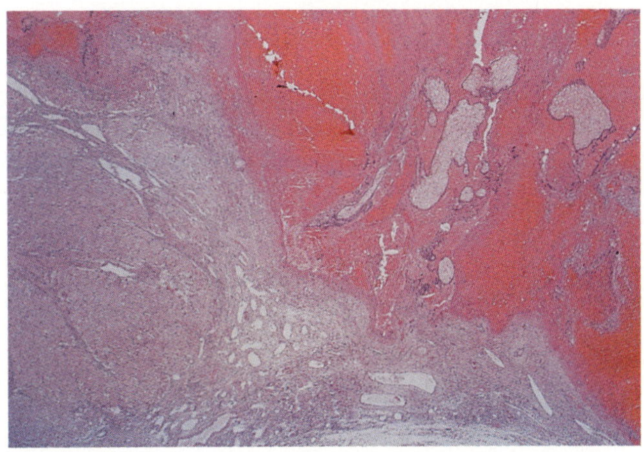

6.19 Ectopic ovarian pregnancy containing degenerating chorionic villi embedded in a blood clot adjacent to the corpus luteum.

SURFACE EPITHELIAL TUMORS

These tumors are presumed to arise from the surface epithelium of the ovary, which is derived from the same coelomic lining that gives rise to the müllerian duct. Therefore, the tumors that arise from the surface epithelium differentiate into cell types similar to those of müllerian origin. Epithelial tumors should be classified according to the best differentiated area and should be graded according to the least differentiated area if a significant pattern is present (more than 5%). The grading of ovarian carcinomas is subjective and takes into account both architectural and cytologic features. These features generally parallel each other, but when there is a discrepancy the cytologic features should be given more weight.

Serous tumors of the ovary are typically unilocular (Figure 6-20) and lined by ciliated epithelium resembling that of the fallopian tube (Figure 6-21); 70% are benign, 10% are of borderline malignancy, and 20% are invasive carcinomas. Occasional internal or external papillary excrescences may be present but are usually minimal. If there is significant papillary formation, the tumor will usually fall into the borderline or low malignant potential category (Figure 6-22).[93] In these tumors, the papillary formations are complex and there is some nuclear pleomorphism and stratification, but there is no stromal invasion (Figures 6-23 and 6-24). Focal early invasion (microinvasion) does not appear to change the good prognosis in serous borderline tumors.[7,31,101] Peritoneal implants may be present and have been divided into noninvasive (Figure 6-25), including desmoplastic (Figure 6-26), and invasive types (Figure 6-27).[9,29,52] Invasive implants are associated with a borderline tumor of worse prognosis. Implants of borderline serous tumors need to be distinguished from endosalpingiosis (see Chapter 5). The concept of borderline ovarian tumors is being challenged, since most patients do well.[47,49] Recent studies indicate that the micropapillary pattern in serous tumors may be a subtype with a worse prognosis. Serous cystadenocarcinoma of the ovary (Figure 6-28) usually pursues a rapidly malignant course with extensive peritoneal implantation and ascites. One of the hallmarks of papillary serous tumors is the formation of psammoma bodies (Figure 6-29). Psammoma bodies are characteristically found in papillary serous tumors, but the tumor may be benign, borderline, or malignant. Occasionally the tumors are limited to the surface of the ovary (Figure 6-30).[8] Benign serous tumors are bilateral in approximately 10% of patients. Borderline serous tumors are bilateral in approximately 25% of cases; serous cystadenocarcinoma is bilateral in approximately two-thirds of all cases.

Grading of Serous Tumors

Gynecologic Oncology Group

Grade 0 Low Malignant Potential (borderline malignancy)
A *noninvasive* serous tumor containing cellular stratification, with several cell layers piled on top of each other; cellular budding or tufting, which refers to small nests of cells projecting from papillary formations and often appearing as detached clusters at the end of papillae; cytologic atypia; and mitotic activity. From a cytologic standpoint, the cells do *not* show unmistakable changes of malignancy.

Grade 1 Well-Differentiated Carcinoma
An *invasive* serous tumor with well-formed papillary processes and glands. There is minimal disorientation of nuclei with only mild stratification. Nuclear pleomorphism and hyperchromatism are minimal.

Grade 2 Moderately Differentiated Carcinoma
This tumor forms more complex papillary and glandular structures with more pronounced nuclear changes. Small areas of solid tumor formation may be seen.

Grade 3 Poorly Differentiated Carcinoma
This tumor is still recognizable as serous but contains large areas of solid cellularity with marked pleomorphism, nuclear hyperchromatism, and giant cell formation. The papillary and glandular formation is minimal.

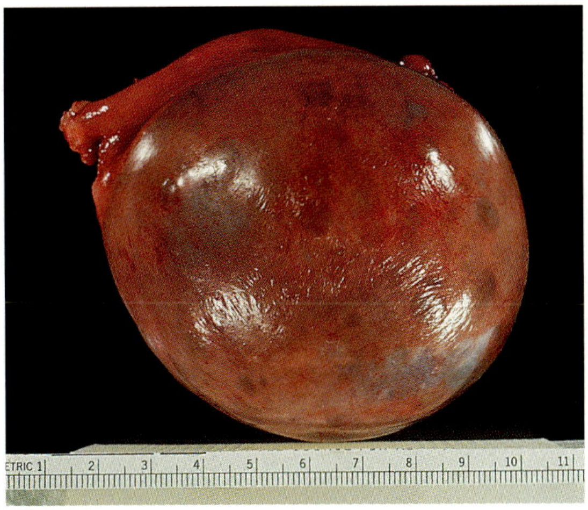

6.20 Serous cystadenoma of the ovary.

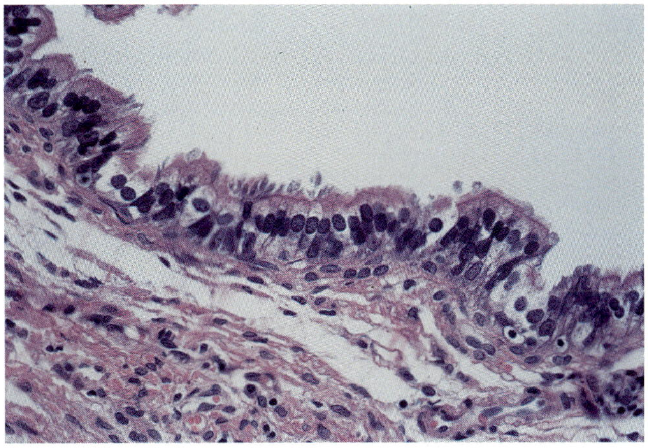

6.21 Serous cystadenoma of the ovary lined with ciliated epithelium.

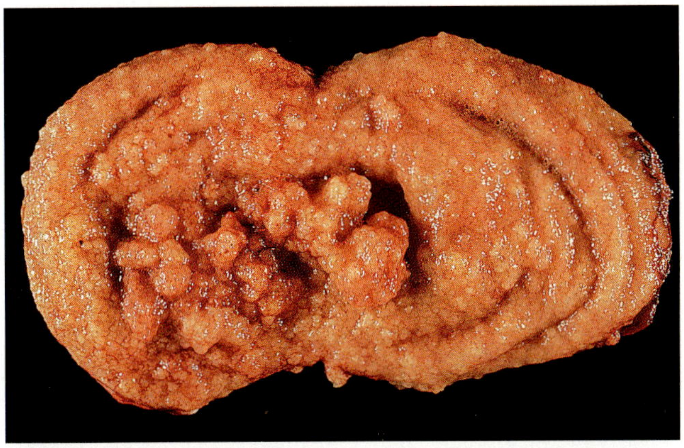

6.22 Papillary serous tumor of low malignant potential containing numerous papillary excrescences on the inner cyst wall.

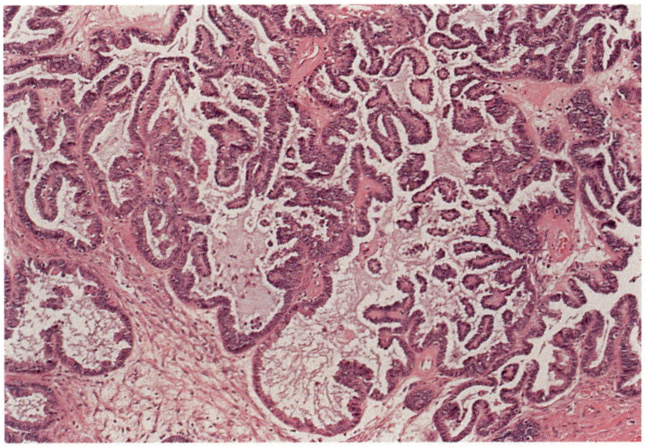

6.23 Serous tumor of low malignant potential demonstrating complex papillary architecture.

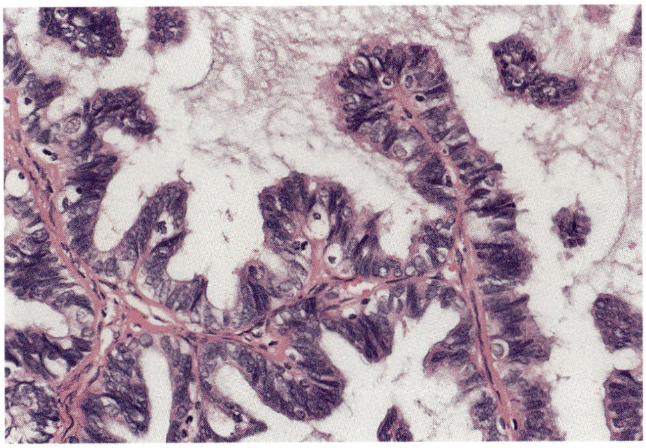

6.24 Serous tumor of low malignant potential with complex papillary fronds lined with serous epithelium.

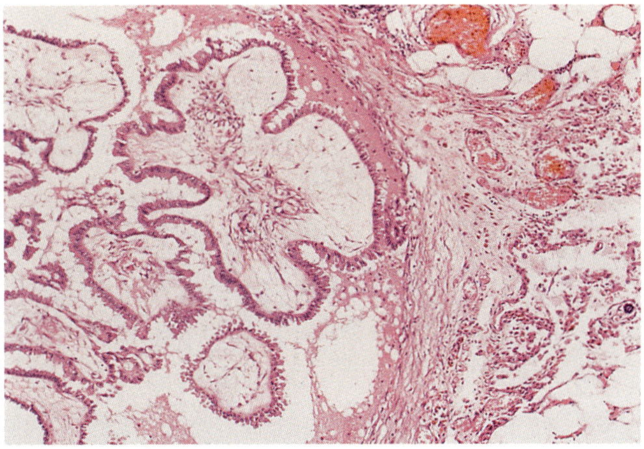

6.25 Noninvasive implant of a papillary serous tumor of low malignant potential on the omentum.

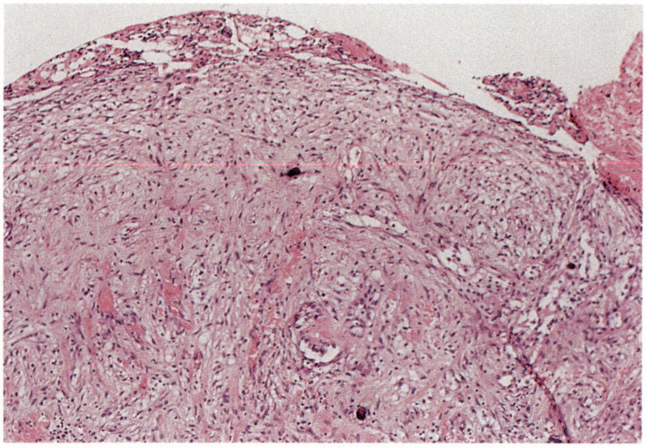

6.26 Noninvasive implant of a papillary serous tumor of low malignant potential desmoplastic on the surface of the peritoneum.

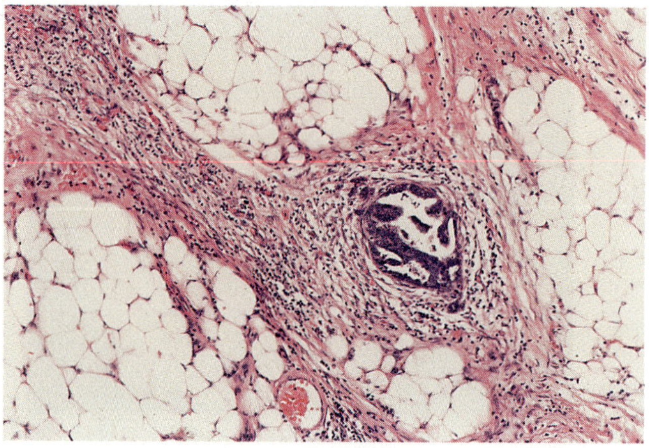

6.27 Invasive implant of a serous ovarian tumor of low malignant potential involving the omentum.

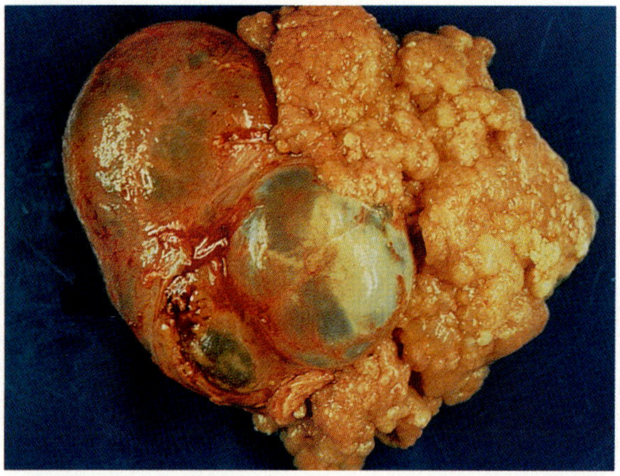

6.28 Papillary serous adenocarcinoma of the ovary with a cystic component and excrescences on the surface.

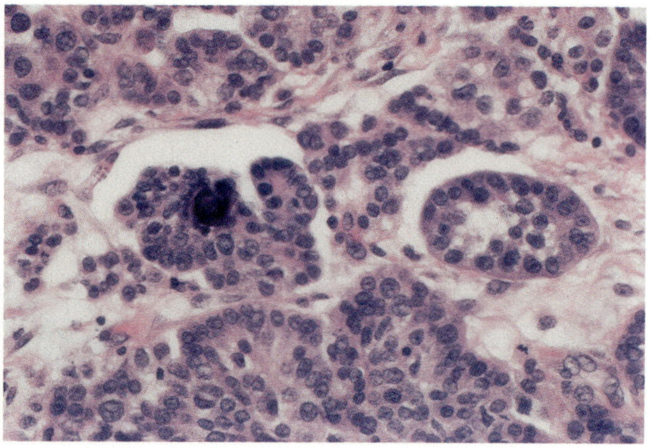

6.29 Papillary serous adenocarcinoma of the ovary with psammoma bodies.

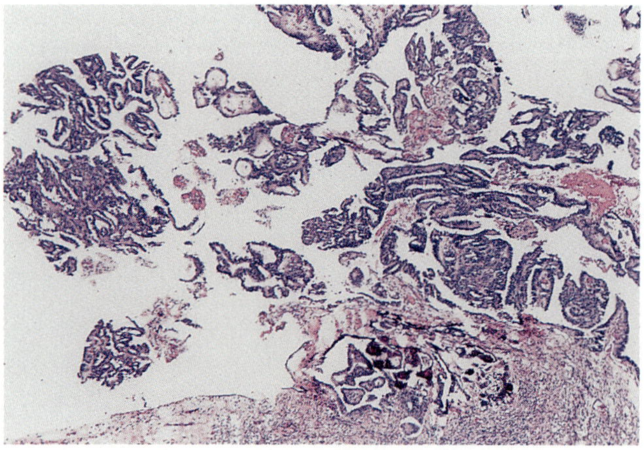

6.30 Serous surface papillary adenocarcinoma of the ovary with a small focus of tumor arising on the surface of the ovary.

Mucinous tumors of the ovary are often multilocular (Figure 6-31) and are usually lined by columnar mucinous epithelium resembling that of the endocervix (Figure 6-32). The epithelial lining may also resemble that of the intestine and may contain goblet cells (Figure 6-33).[58, 86] Although most mucinous neoplasms are considered to be surface epithelial tumors, it is thought that some mucinous tumors may arise from germ cells as part of a teratoma. Mucinous tumors have also been associated with Brenner tumors. Mucinous tumors tend to be some of the largest ovarian tumors reported; some have been up to 30 cm in diameter and up to 4000 g in weight. The largest tumor of record was estimated to be 328 pounds. Benign mucinous tumors are bilateral in less than 5% of cases, whereas borderline and invasive forms are bilateral in approximately 15% of cases. Borderline mucinous tumors are usually complex, multilocular masses with a smooth external surface (Figure 6-34).[91] Histologically, they contain stratification of the nuclei up to, but not exceeding, four cell layers in thickness and a complex architecture.[95] Areas with a transition from benign to atypical are often seen (Figure 6-35). Mixed serous and mucinous epithelium may be present (Figure 6-36).[87,90] Occasionally, solid mural nodules are present in the cyst wall of mucinous tumors (Figure 6-37). The nodules usually contain benign, reactive spindle cells (Figure 6-38) but may have areas of sarcoma.[3,57,69,70] Mucinous carcinomas usually have solid, focally necrotic areas on gross appearance (Figure 6-39). Since mucinous tumors are multiloculated and complex in architecture, invasion is sometimes difficult, if not impossible, to determine with certainty. For this reason, mucinous cystadenocarcinomas can be identified without clear-cut evidence of invasion.[32,33] Mucinous cystadenocarcinomas have stratification of more than four cell layers with nuclear pleomorphism and increased mitoses (Figure 6-40). Mucinous neoplasms of the ovary may be associated with pseudomyxoma peritonei (see Chapter 5).

Grading of Mucinous Tumors

Gynecologic Oncology Group

Grade 0 Low Malignant Potential (borderline malignancy)
A mucinous tumor with complicated glandular pattern showing no stromal invasion. The glands are lined by up to three layers of cells exhibiting mild to moderate atypia. Tumors with marked overgrowth of atypical cells, severely anaplastic nuclei, solid areas, or papillary or cribriform intraglandular proliferations should not be classified as being of low malignant potential.

Grade 1 Well-Differentiated Carcinoma
A glandular tumor with epithelial stratification of four or more cell layers with moderate to marked atypia. The glands are usually well formed, but cribriform or papillary structures without connective tissue cores indicate malignancy. Stromal invasion is usually present but may be difficult to assess. In order to study their biologic behavior, these tumors should be subclassified as follows:

IA: No Stromal invasion
IB: Stromal invasion identified

Grade 2 Moderately Differentiated Carcinoma
This tumor shows usually more complex glands or smaller glands with an increase in the degree of nuclear atypia. Stratification is greater and invasion is more easily seen.

Grade 3 Poorly Differentiated Carcinoma
This tumor is characterized by marked nuclear atypia, pleomorphism, and multinucleated cell formation. The glands are poorly formed, and large sheets of tumor without glands are seen. The mucous secretion may be lost in most of the cells.

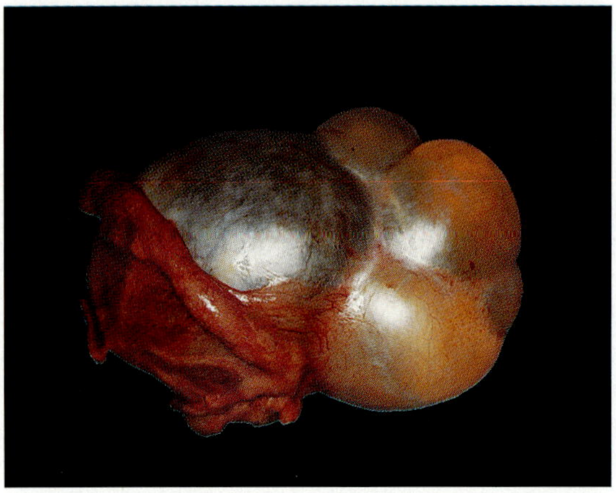

6.31 Multiloculated mucinous cystadenoma of the ovary.

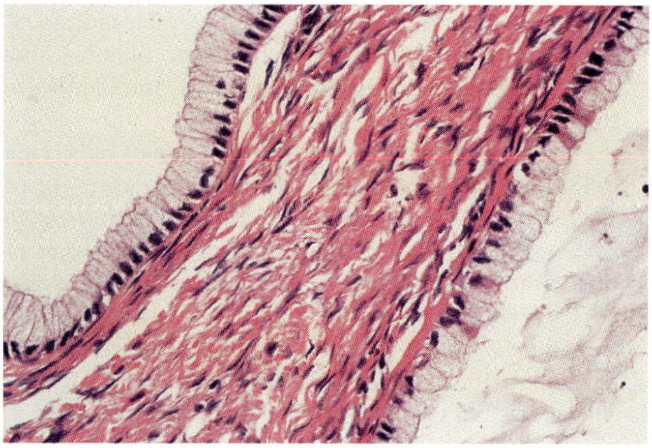

6.32 Mucinous cystadenoma with müllerian (endocervical) differentiation.

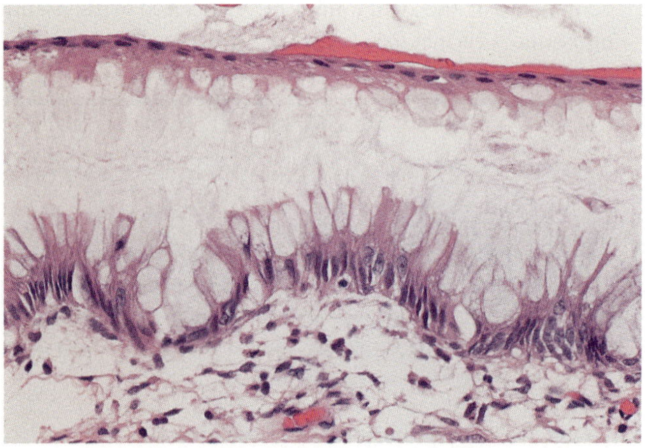

6.33 Mucinous cystadenoma with intestinal differentiation.

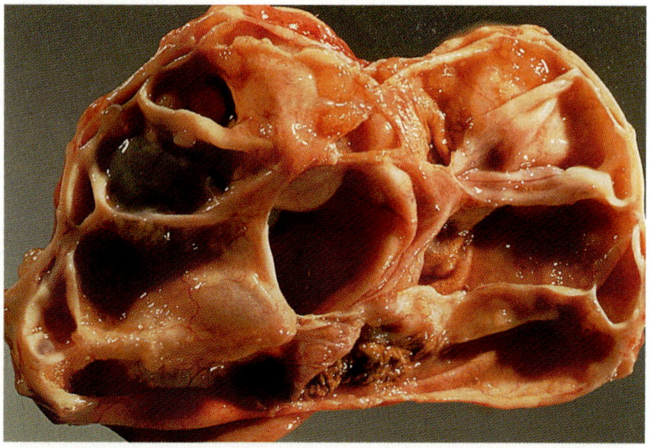

6.34 Multiloculated mucinous tumor of low malignant potential with focal solid areas.

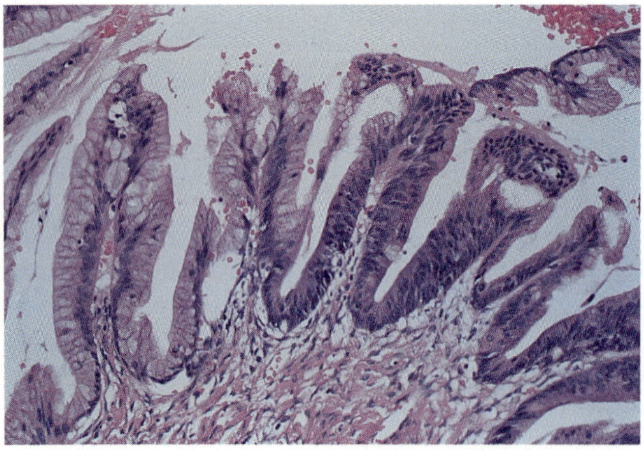

6.35 Mucinous tumor of low malignant potential with villoglandular architecture and transitional areas from benign to atypical epithelium.

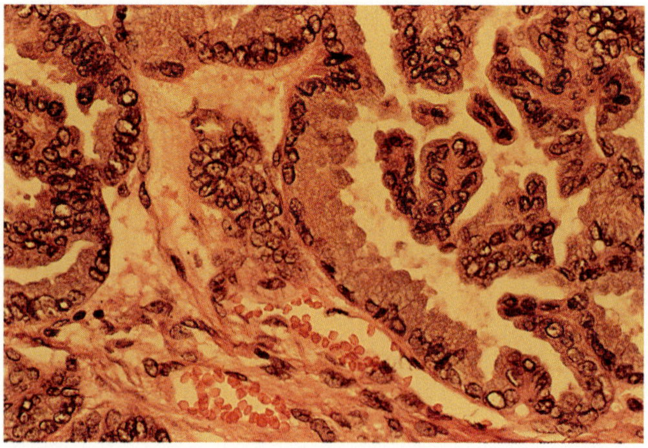

6.36 Mixed epithelial borderline tumor with areas of mucinous and serous differentiation.

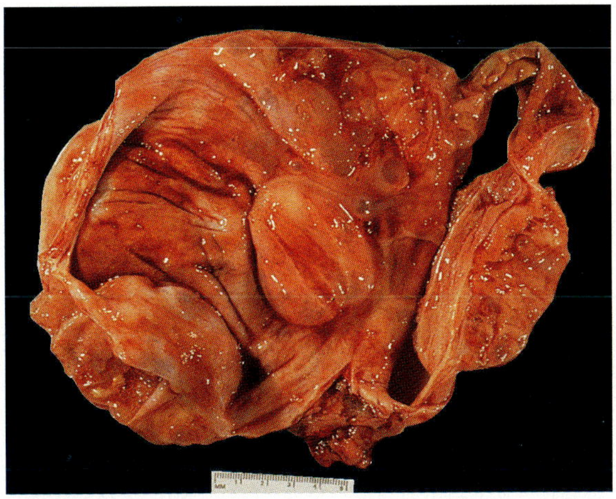

6.37 Mucinous ovarian tumor of low malignant potential with solid mural nodules.

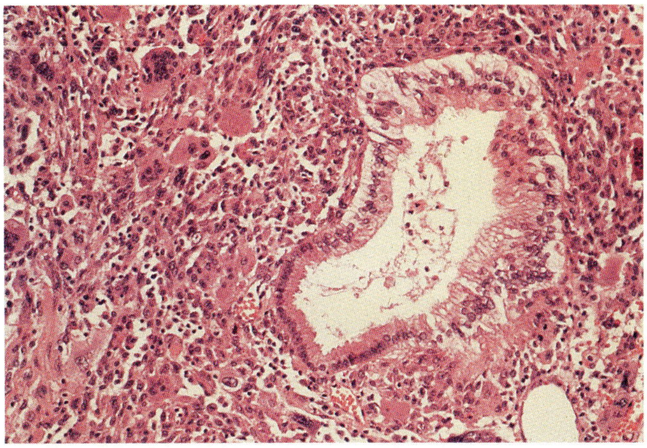

6.38 Mural nodule from a borderline mucinous ovarian tumor with a spindled stroma and numerous multinucleated giant cells.

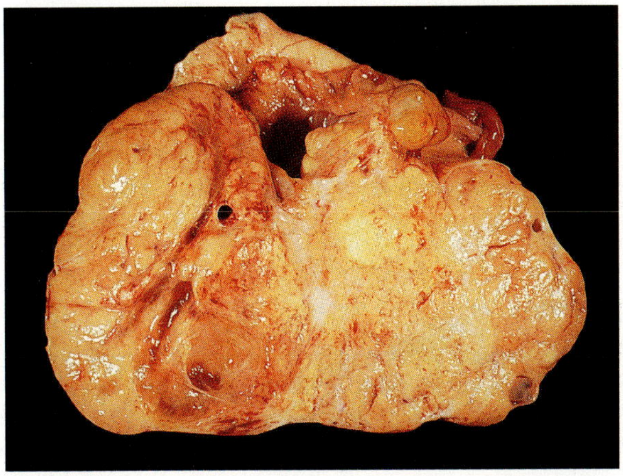

6.39 Mucinous adenocarcinoma of the ovary with a predominant solid pattern replacing the ovary.

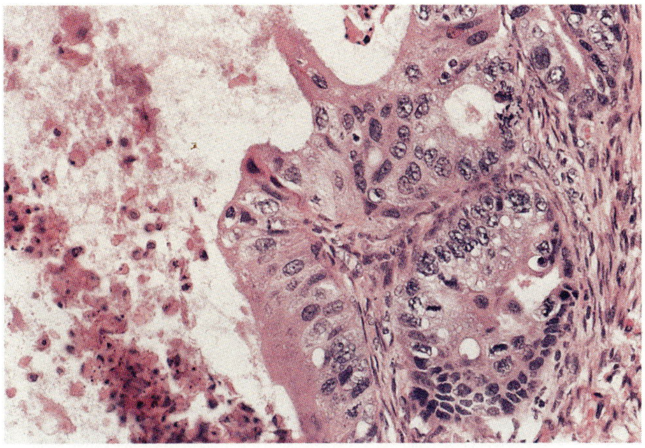

6.40 Mucinous adenocarcinoma of the ovary with areas of necrosis and marked nuclear atypia with numerous mitotic figures.

Endometrioid tumors of the ovary are characterized by epithelial and/or stromal elements that closely resemble those of the endometrium.[20,105] Endometriosis is not considered a neoplasm, but cystic masses are often referred to as endometriomas (Figures 6-41 and 6-42).[37] The borderline category is ill defined and often has an adenofibromatous component[5,63,96] with areas resembling atypical hyperplasia of the endometrium (Figures 6-43 and 6-44). Endometrioid carcinomas are associated with endometriosis in about 10% of cases and may develop in an endometriotic cyst (Figure 6-45). Histologically, the tumors resemble endometrial carcinoma and often contain squamous differentiation (Figure 6-46).

Grading of Endometrioid Tumors

Gynecologic Oncology Group

Grade 0 Low Malignant Potential (borderline malignancy)
A noninvasive tumor that resembles atypical hyperplasia of the endometrium. Squamous differentiation is often present.

Grade 1 Well-Differentiated Carcinoma
This tumor resembles the typical adenocarcinoma of the endometrium. The glands are well formed with the nuclei oriented toward the base of the cell with little nuclear atypia. There is minimal cell stratification and pleomorphism. No solid sheets of tumor are present. Benign-appearing squamous epithelium may be present.

Grade 2 Moderately Differentiated Carcinoma
The glands are more complex with increased stratification and nuclear abnormalities. Occasional small solid nests of tumor are seen but are a minor component. There may be papillary areas. Atypical squamous epithelium may be present.

Grade 3 Poorly Differentiated Carcinoma
This tumor consists of poorly formed glands, nests, and large sheets of pleomorphic cells. Many have squamous differentiation, and there is abundant mitotic activity.

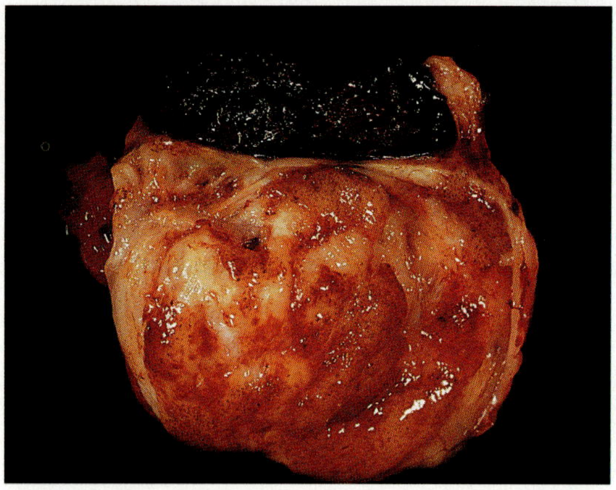

6.41 Endometrioma of the ovary.

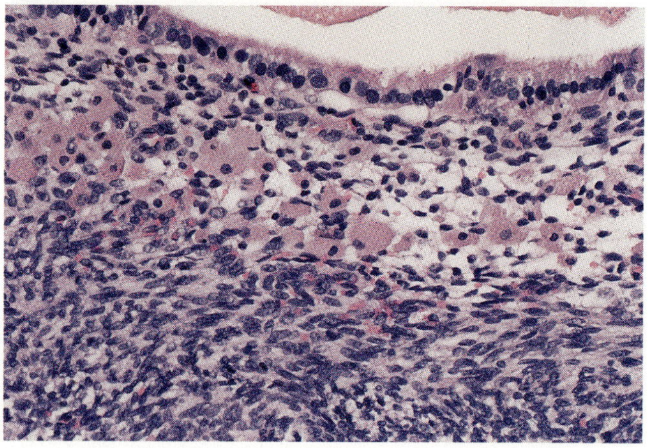

6.42 Endometriosis of the ovary with pigmented macrophages.

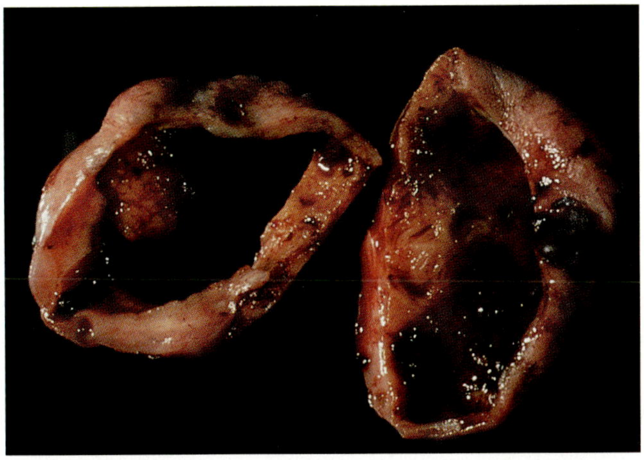

6.43 Atypical endometrioid adenofibroma with a thickened cyst wall.

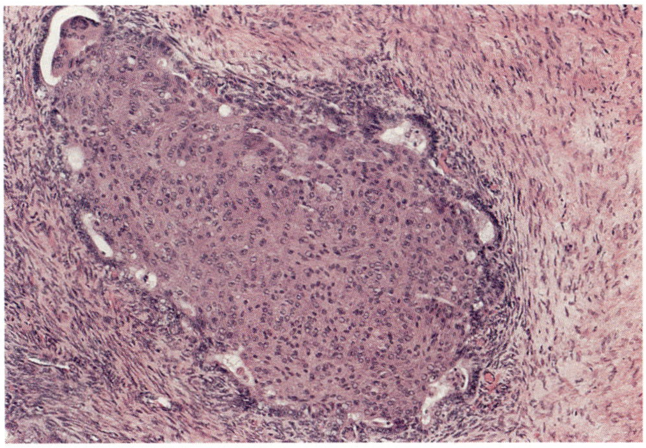

6.44 Atypical endometrioid adenofibroma with endometrioid glands and marked squamous differentiation.

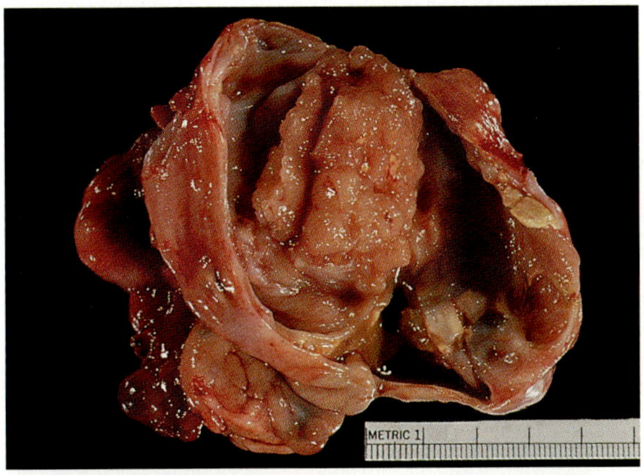

6.45 Endometrioid adenocarcinoma arising in an endometriotic cyst.

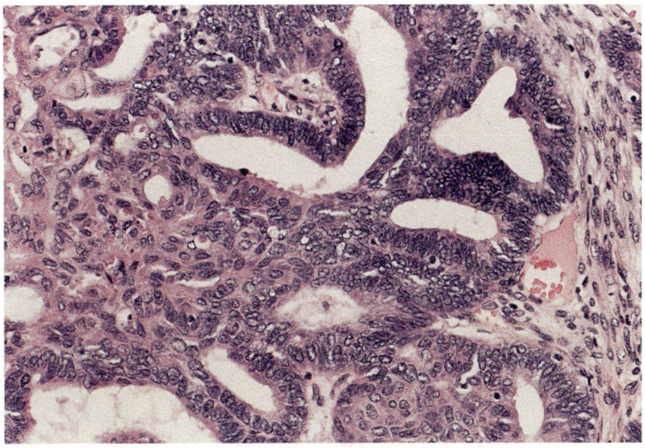

6.46 Endometrioid adenocarcinoma with focal squamous differentiation.

Endometrioid stromal sarcoma (Figure 6-47), adenosarcoma, and carcinosarcoma (malignant mixed mesodermal tumor) (Figures 6-48 and 6-49) are variants of endometrioid tumors of the ovary.[10,22] The same classification for carcinosarcomas of the uterus applies to tumors of the ovary. The sarcomas can be either heterologous or homologous. The most common heterologous element in the ovary is chondrosarcoma, whereas in the uterus it is rhabdomyosarcoma. Benign mixed tumors (adenofibromas) of the ovary may have serous (Figures 6-50 to 6-52), mucinous (Figure 6-53),[4] endometrioid (Figure 6-54)[41] or clear cell (Figure 6-55)[6,83] epithelial differentiation. Clear cell carcinoma of the ovary (Figures 6-56 and 6-57) is considered by some to be a variant of endometrioid carcinoma since it may be seen in association with endometriosis or combined with more typical endometrioid carcinoma.[42,54]

Brenner tumors have the gross appearance of a white, fibrous tumor similar to a fibroma (Figure 6-58). Histologically, they contain nests of transitional epithelium, usually with a central core of mucinous cells, embedded in a fibrous stroma (Figures 6-59 and 6-60). Proliferative (borderline) Brenner tumors have a papillary configuration that resembles low-grade papillary transitional cell carcinoma of the urinary bladder (Figures 6-61 and 6-62).[53,81,84] Malignant Brenner tumors are invasive and must show an association with an otherwise benign or proliferative Brenner tumor (Figure 6-63).[80,94] If no Brenner component is present, the tumor is classified as transitional cell carcinoma (Figure 6-64).[82]

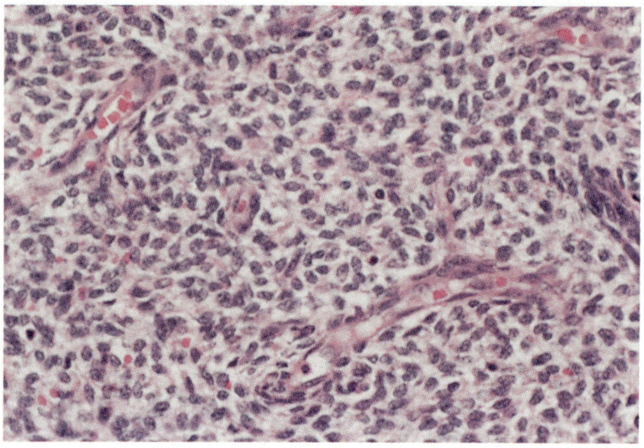

6.47 Endometroid stromal sarcoma, low grade, with vascular channels similar to those seen in the endometrium.

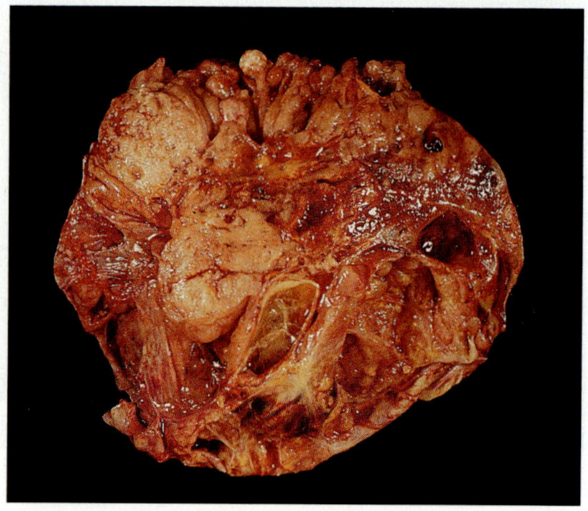

6.48 Carcinosarcoma of the ovary showing a mixture of solid and cystic areas with focal hemorrhage.

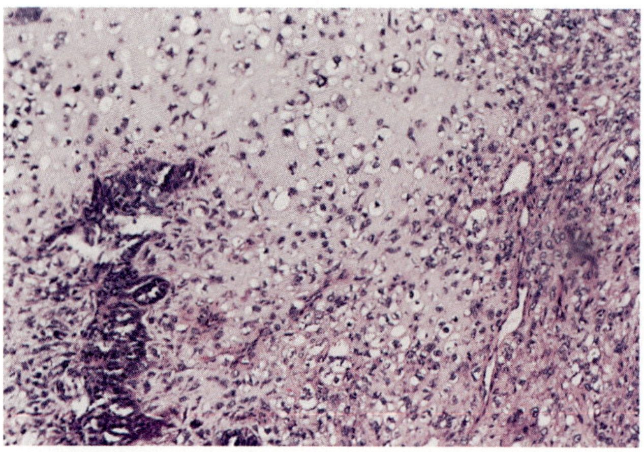

6.49 Carcinosarcoma of the ovary with cartilaginous (heterologous) differentiation.

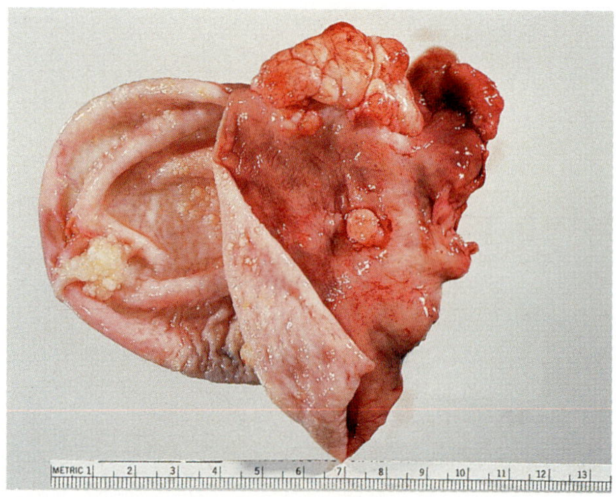

6.50 Papillary adenofibroma of the ovary showing external and internal papillary excrescences.

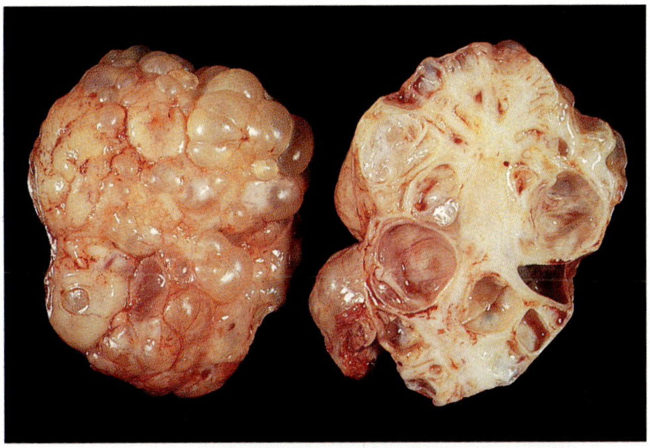

6.51 Solid and cystic adenofibroma of the ovary.

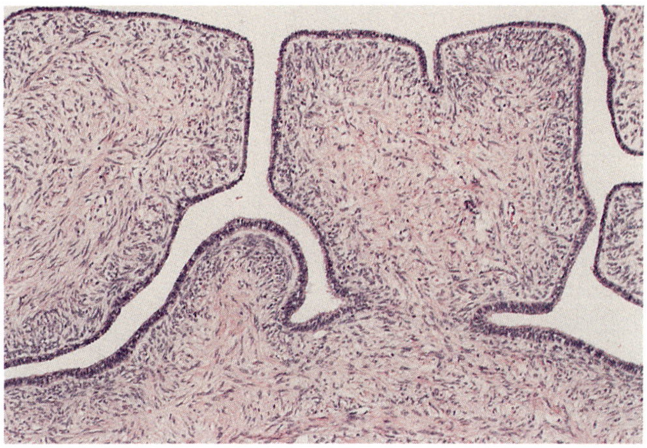

6.52 Papillary serous adenofibroma with bland serous epithelium lining blunt papillary fronds containing dense fibrous tissue.

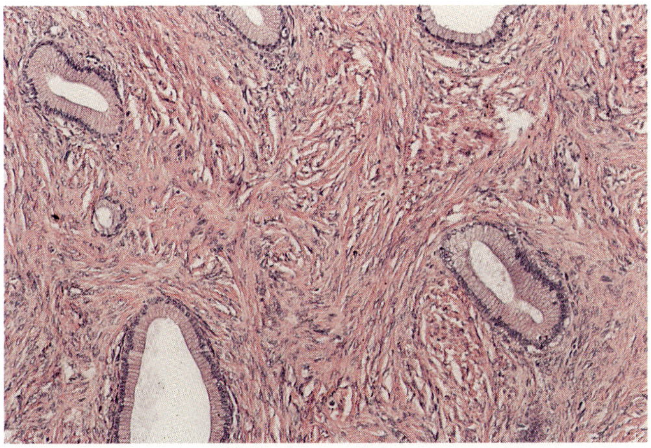

6.53 Mucinous adenofibroma containing benign mucinous glands embedded in a dense fibrous stroma.

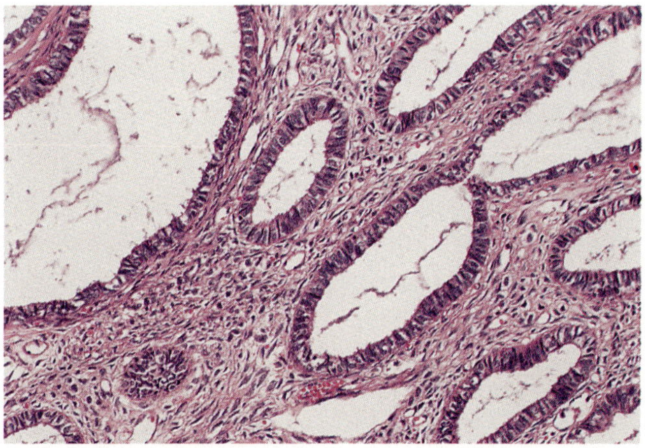

6.54 Endometrioid adenofibroma with endometrioid glands embedded in a fibrous stroma.

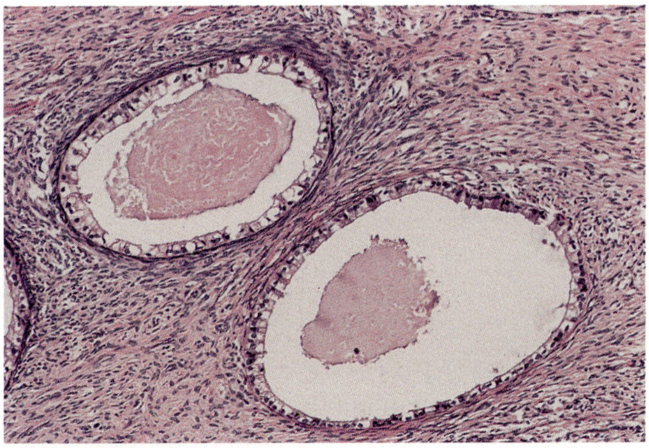

6.55 Clear cell adenofibroma.

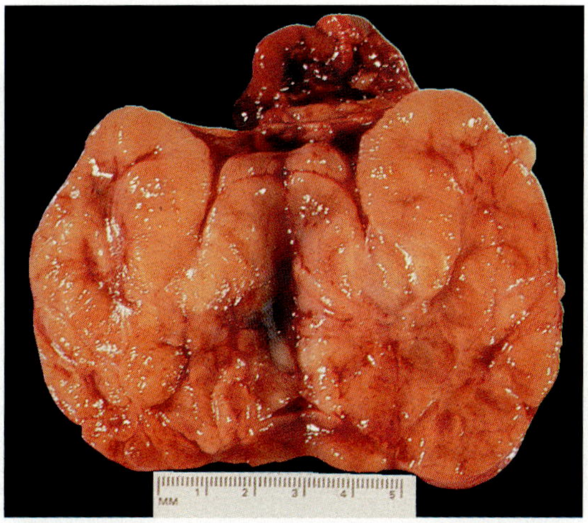

6.56 Clear cell adenocarcinoma of the ovary consisting of a solid lobulated tumor replacing the ovary.

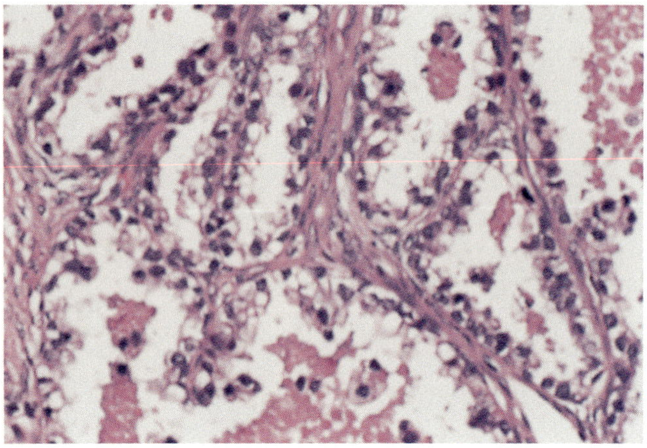

6.57 Clear cell adenocarcinoma of the ovary with a tubulocystic pattern demonstrating hobnail cells.

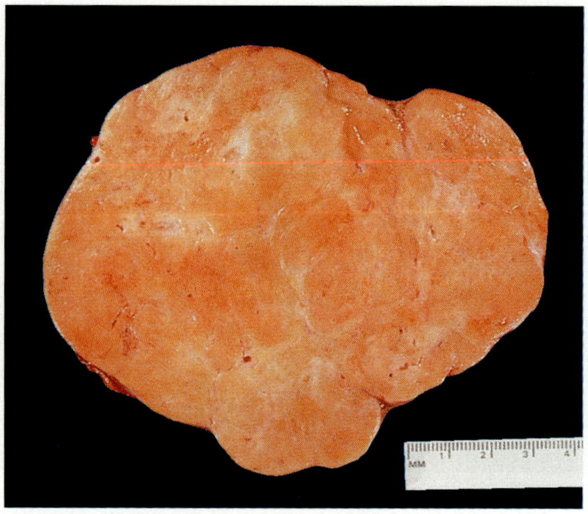

6.58 Brenner tumor of the ovary composed of a solid, fibrous-appearing mass with focal cystic areas.

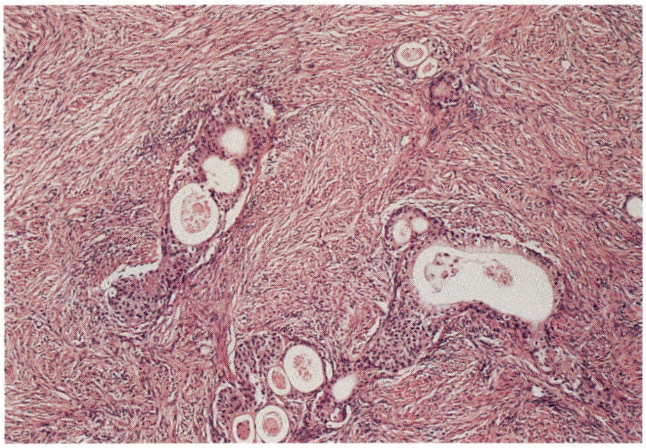

6.59 Brenner tumor of the ovary with nests of transitional epithelium and focal cystic change embedded in a dense fibrous stroma.

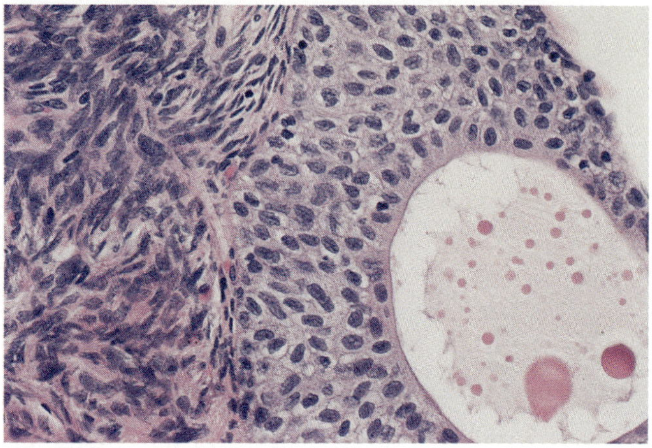

6.60 Brenner tumor of the ovary demonstrating transitional epithelium with nuclear grooves.

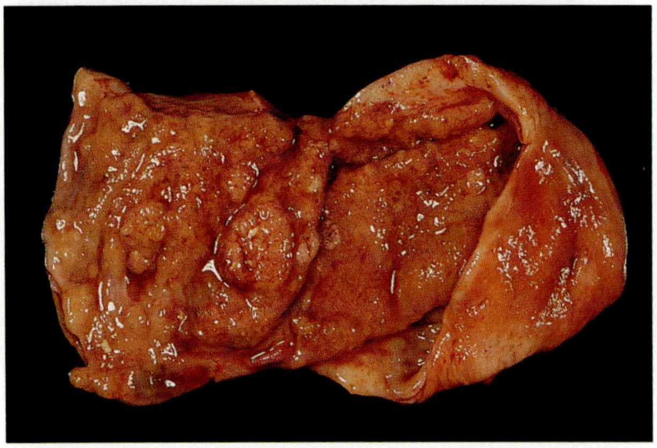

6.61 Proliferative Brenner tumor of the ovary with cystic change and papillary areas in the inner lining of the cyst wall.

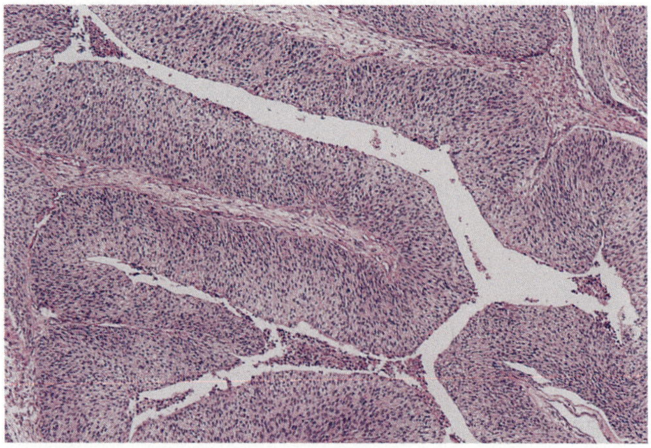

6.62 Proliferative Brenner tumor of the ovary having an appearance similar to a low-grade papillary transitional cell carcinoma of the urinary bladder.

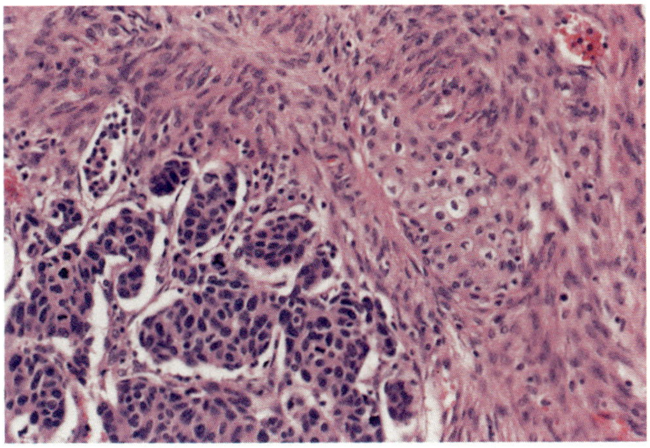

6.63 Malignant Brenner tumor composed of malignant transitional cells arising in a Brenner tumor.

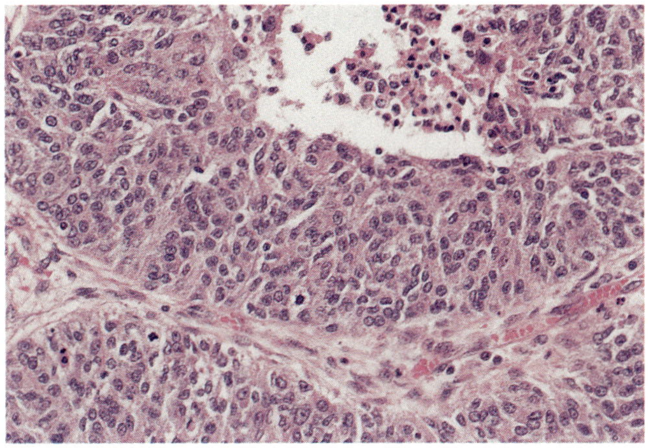

6.64 Transitional cell carcinoma of the ovary with malignant transitional cells and no Brenner component.

GONADAL STROMAL TUMORS OF THE OVARY

Granulosa cell tumors often have a cystic component mixed with solid and hemorrhagic areas (Figure 6-65). The tumors have morphologic features of granulosa cells and form the typical Call-Exner bodies. These are pseudorosettes of granulosa cells that have a central hyalinized area most likely the result of nuclear degeneration (Figure 6-66). One of the characteristic histologic features of granulosa cell tumor is the coffee bean–type nuclear groove (Figure 6-67). Granulosa cell tumors are considered to be of low malignant potential and can persist and recur, often many years after the initial presentation. The tumors are often feminizing and may cause precocious pseudopuberty in children and postmenopausal bleeding with endometrial hyperplasia or carcinoma in postmenopausal patients.[24,98] Granulosa cell tumors have been subdivided according to their manner of growth into several subtypes: macrofollicular (Figure 6-68), microfollicular (Figure 6-66), insular (Figure 6-69), trabecular (Figure 6-70), moiré-silk, and diffuse or sarcomatoid (Figure 6-71). These patterns are commonly mixed in the same neoplasm.[114]

Juvenile granulosa cell tumor (Figure 6-72) is a variant that most often occurs in patients under age 30 years.[111–113,127] These tumors have large, immature granulosa cells forming solid nodules and a lipid-rich cytoplasm (Figure 6-73). Call-Exner bodies and nuclear grooves are uncommon. This variant appears to have a better prognosis and rare recurrences, especially with Stage I tumors.

Grading of Granulosa Cell Tumors

Gynecologic Oncology Group

Grade 1 Well-Differentiated
The follicular form is the best differentiated. The macrofollicular pattern is characterized by the presence of large follicles resembling graafian follicles. The hallmark of the microfollicular pattern is the Call-Exner body.

Grade 2 Intermediate Differentiation
The insular, trabecular, and cylindromatous patterns are characterized by sharply demarcated groups of well-differentiated granulosa cells that are not forming follicles.

Grade 3 Poorly Differentiated
The moiré-silk pattern, in which the granulosa cells are arranged in slender zigzag columns, often merges with the sarcomatoid pattern, in which the tumor cells are growing diffusely and the nuclei are generally rounded and closely packed. Mitotic activity may be prominent in Grade 3 tumors. The nuclei typically lack the pleomorphism and hyperchromatism of adenocarcinomas and undifferentiated carcinomas. The presence of nuclear grooves in granulosa cells is often helpful in the differential diagnosis.

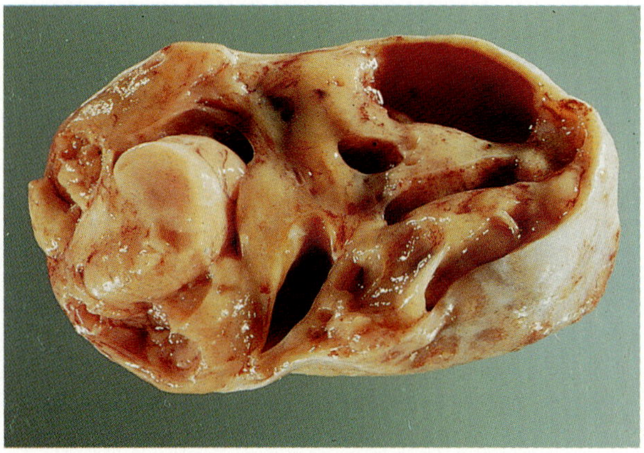

6.65 Granulosa cell tumor of the ovary with solid and cystic areas.

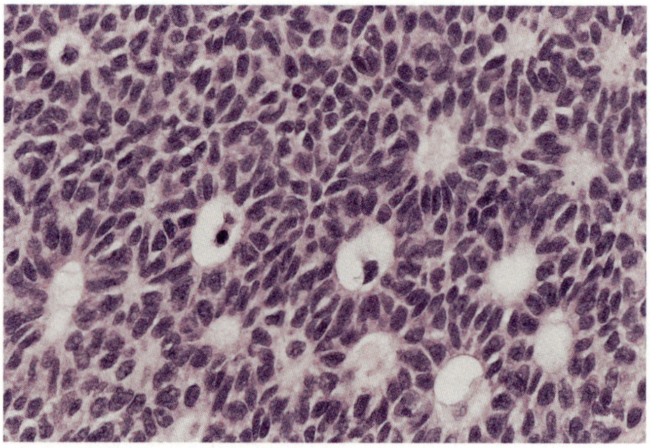

6.66 Microfollicular granulosa cell tumor of the ovary demonstrating the characteristic Call-Exner bodies with granulosa cells rimming a pseudorosette with degenerating nuclei.

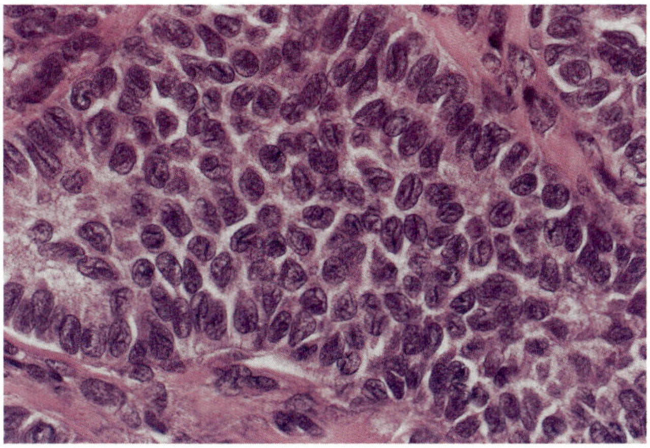

6.67 Granulosa cell tumor of the ovary with characteristic nuclear grooves.

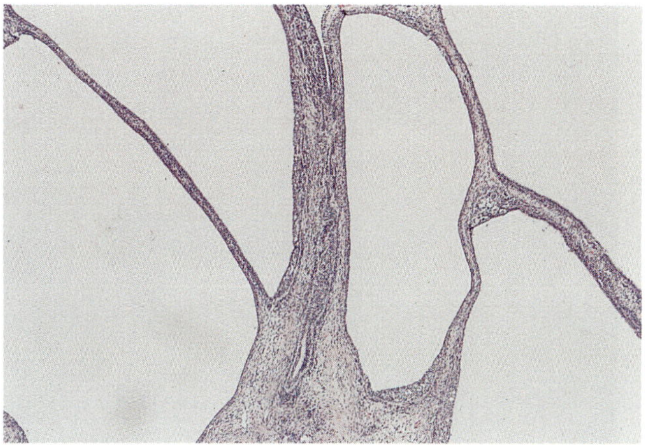

6.68 Granulosa cell tumor of the ovary showing macrofollicular differentiation forming follicle-like structures.

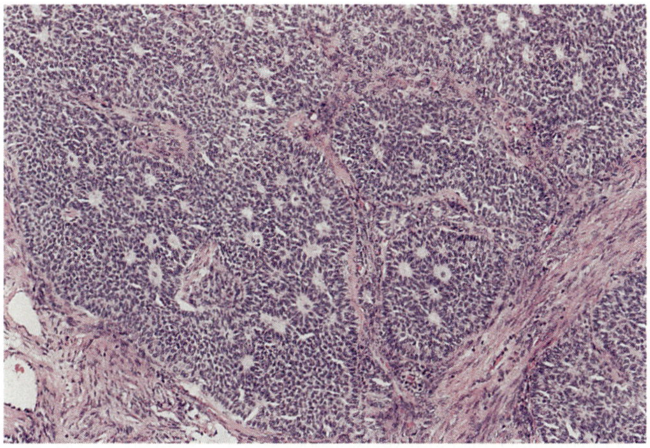

6.69 Granulosa cell tumor of the ovary showing an insular pattern.

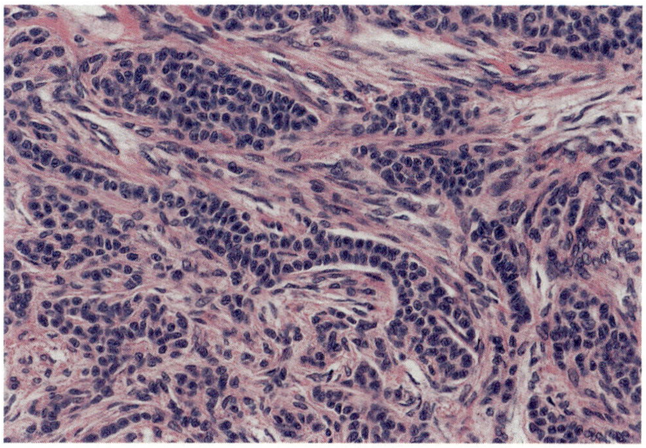

6.70 Granulosa cell tumor of the ovary with a trabecular pattern.

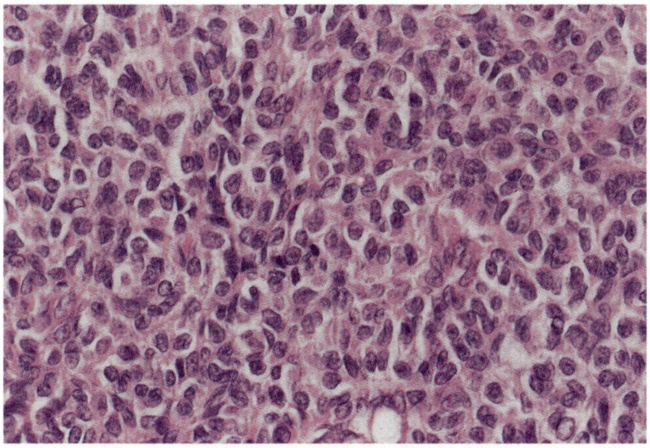

6.71 Granulosa cell tumor of the ovary with a diffuse (sarcomatoid) pattern.

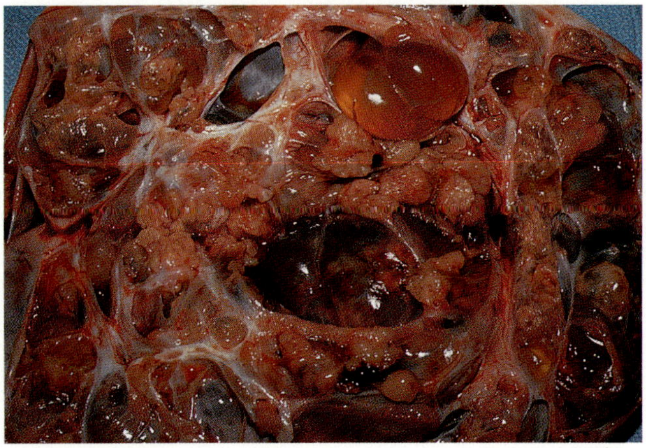

6.72 Juvenile granulosa cell tumor of the ovary with a prominent cystic component.

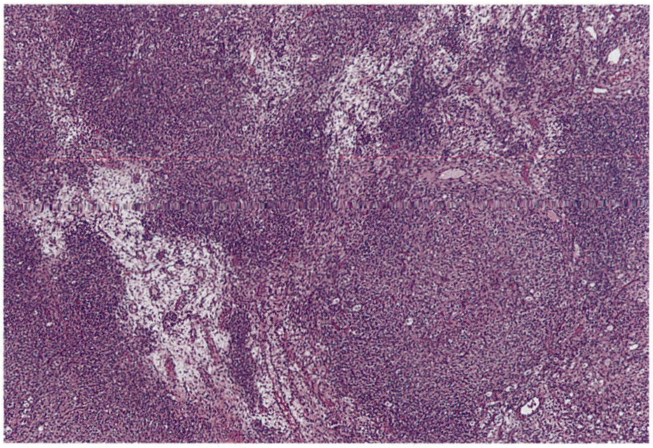

6.73 Juvenile granulosa cell tumor of the ovary with solid nodules separated by fibrous septa.

Fibrothecoma is another category of gonadal stromal tumors that, at one end of the spectrum, is a pure fibroma. Pure fibromas are usually tumors in elderly patients and have a firm, white, whorled appearance (Figure 6-74). Some of these tumors can become large, having cystic degeneration. The fibroma has been described as occasionally causing ascites and right hydrothorax (Meigs syndrome). Histologically, the tumor is seen to be composed of bland, dense fibrous tissue (Figure 6-75). Occasionally, cellular variants (Figure 6-76) and other cell types can be seen.[71,72,75,92] At the opposite end of the spectrum is the thecoma (Figure 6-77).[16] This tumor has lipid-rich luteinized theca cells (Figure 6-78) and is usually estrogenic in function. In reality, most of the tumors in both categories contain a component of the other to a greater or lesser extent. Hence, the term fibrothecoma (Figures 6-79 and 6-80) is applied to many tumors in this category. Sclerosing stromal tumors are a distinctive subtype of stromal tumors that occur in younger patients.[13] They consist of well-circumscribed nodules that often show some cystic change (Figure 6-81). Histologically, they are seen to be composed of nodules with a mixture of dense spindled cells and loose, vacuolated stromal cells (Figure 6-82).

Sertoli-Leydig cell tumors (androblastomas) are tumors that differentiate toward a testicular cell line (Figure 6-83).[79,110,119,125,128] Well-differentiated Sertoli cell tumors are composed of uniform tubules (Figure 6-84).[102,123] Most mixed Sertoli-Leydig cell tumors are androgenic and produce testosterone. The combined Sertoli-Leydig cell tumor can be well (Figure 6-85), intermediately (Figure 6-86), or poorly (Figure 6-87) differentiated, depending on the differentiation of the Sertoli cells. The Leydig cell component in all these tumors is fairly uniform, containing polygonal cells with abundant eosinophilic cytoplasm and occasional Reinke crystals.[85,99]

Grading of Sertoli-Leydig Cell Tumors

Gynecologic Oncology Group

Grade 1 Well-Differentiated
These tumors are composed of either pure Sertoli cell tubules (tubular adenoma), pure Leydig cells (Leydig cell tumor), or mixtures of both (Sertoli-Leydig cell tumor).

Grade 2 Intermediate Differentiation
These tumors have a wide variety of patterns. Typically, they consist of immature Sertoli cells arranged in islands and trabecular cords or ribbons resembling embryonic testicular sex cords. Well-defined tubules may be present and mature Leydig cells are usually identifiable.

Grade 3 Poorly Differentiated
These tumors, also called sarcomatoid, are largely composed of tissue resembling that of the indifferent gonad. They may resemble sarcomas with prominent atypia and mitotic activity. The presence of cords of Sertoli cells, aggregates of Leydig cells, or other elements makes it possible to identify the lesion as a Sertoli-Leydig cell tumor.

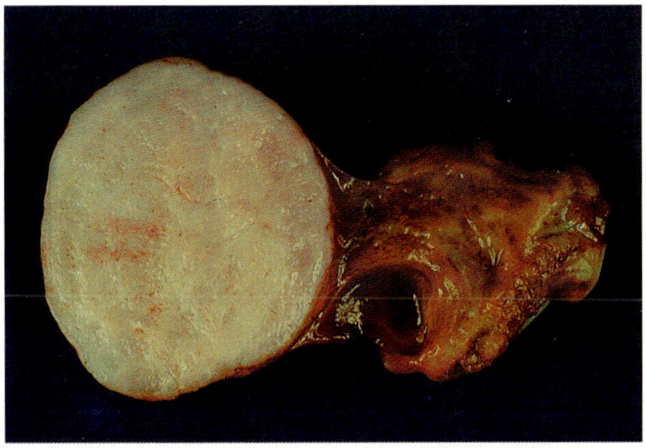

6.74 Fibroma of the ovary with a well-circumscribed, light tan mass.

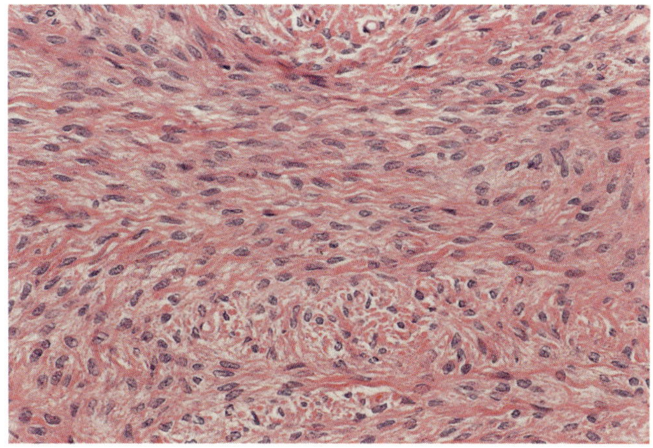

6.75 Fibroma of the ovary demonstrating bland fibrous differentiation.

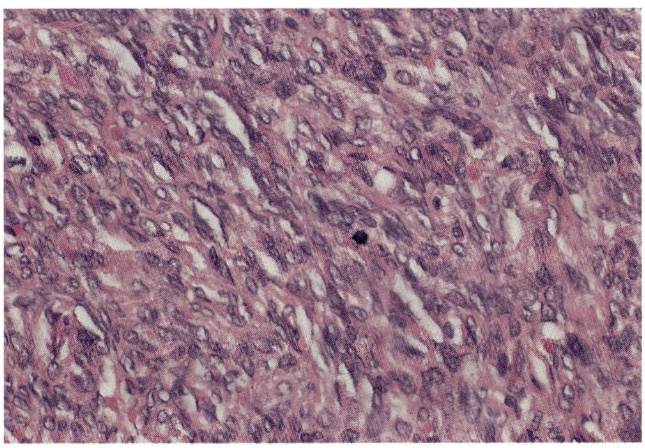

6.76 Cellular fibroma of the ovary with mild nuclear atypia and scattered mitotic figures.

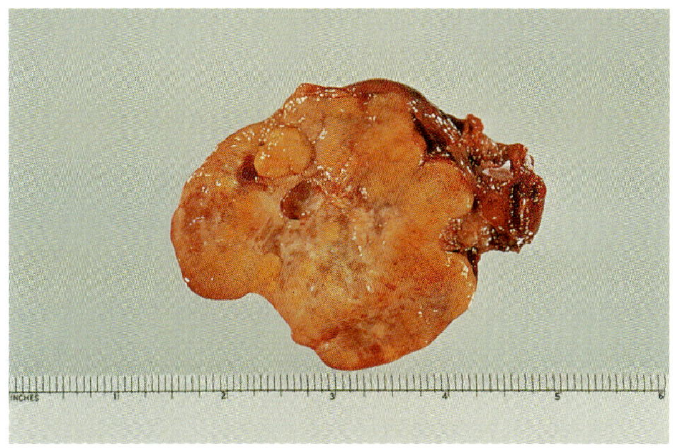

6.77 Thecoma of the ovary with solid yellow nodules.

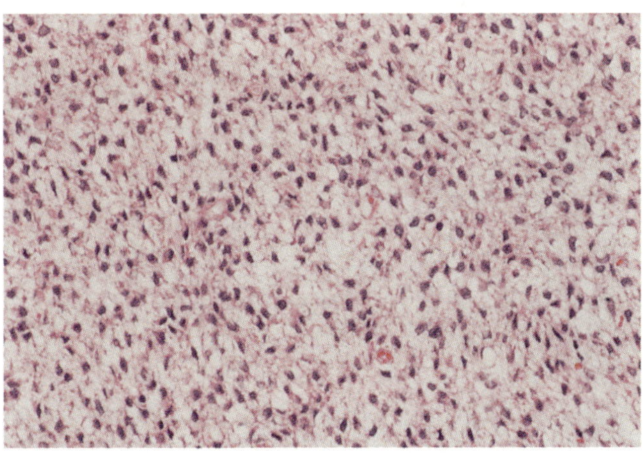

6.78 Thecoma of the ovary with vacuolated cells containing small round nuclei.

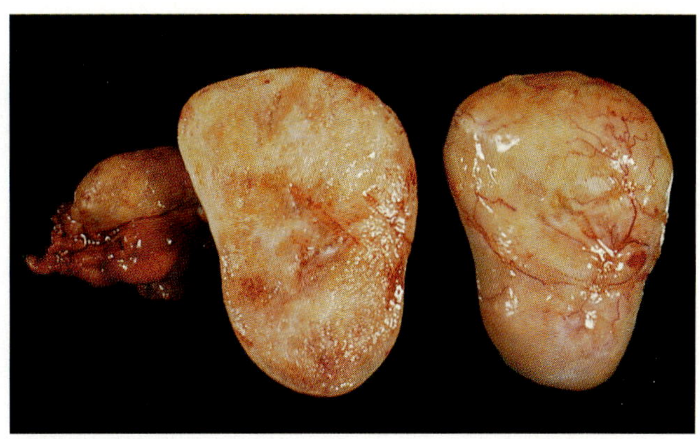

6.79 Fibrothecoma of the ovary with a lobulating, yellow-tan appearance.

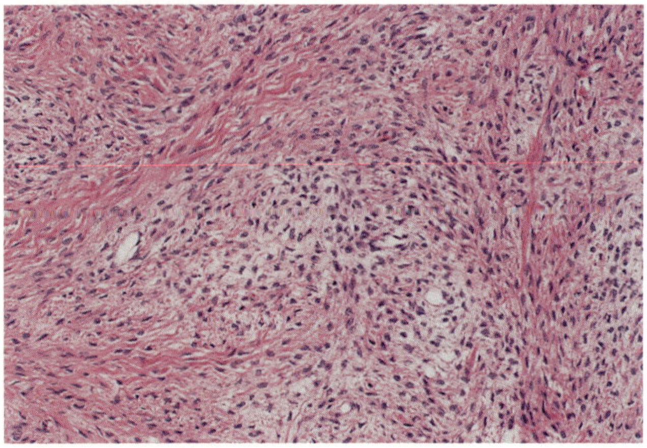

6.80 Fibrothecoma of the ovary with a mixed fibrous and vacuolated epithelial component.

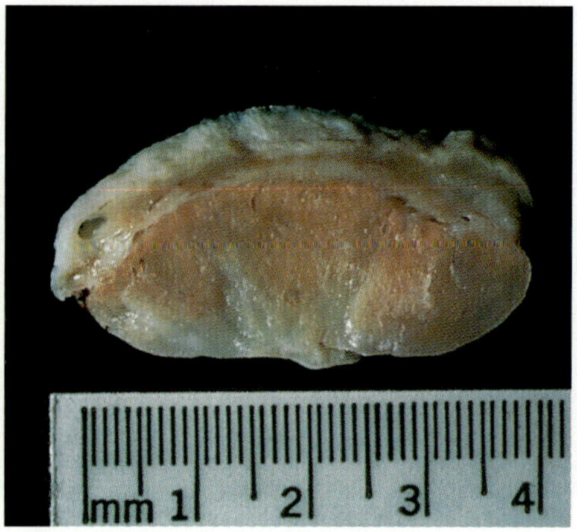

6.81 Sclerosing stromal tumor of the ovary composed of a well-circumscribed nodule containing fibrous septa.

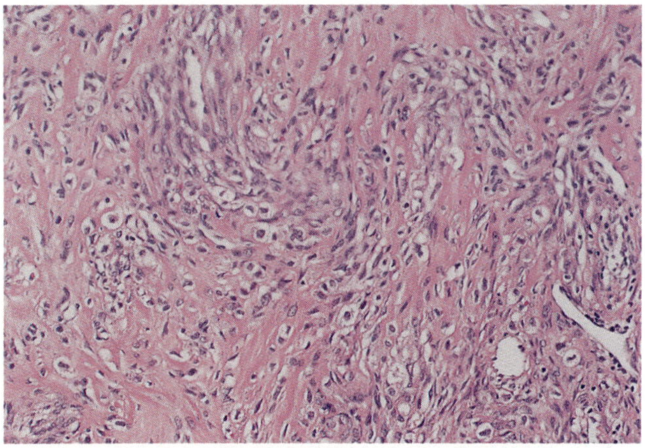

6.82 Sclerosing stroma tumor of the ovary with a mixture of spindle cells, which are focally vacuolated, and dense fibrous tissue.

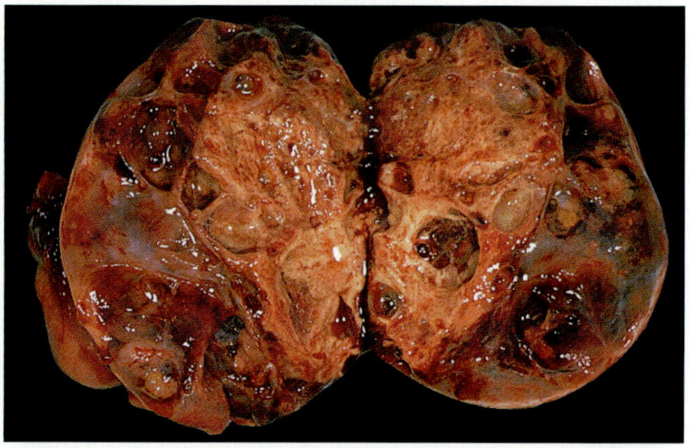

6.83 Sertoli-Leydig cell tumor of the ovary with solid and cystic areas containing focal hemorrhage.

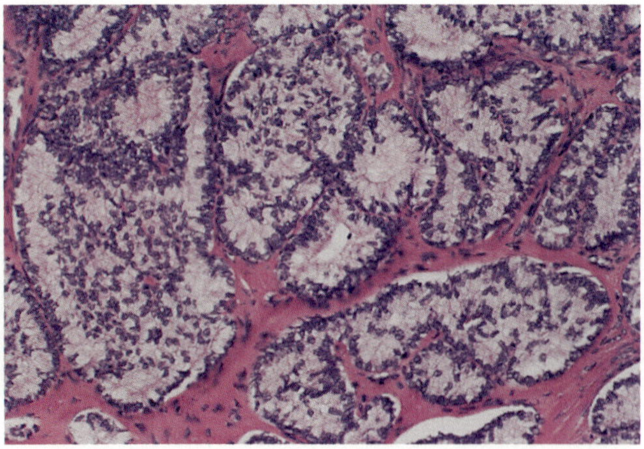

6.84 Sertoli cell tumor of the ovary consisting of well-differentiated Sertoli tubules.

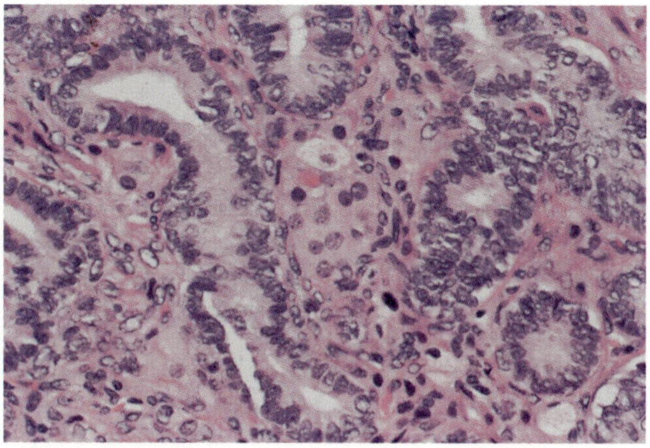

6.85 Well-differentiated Sertoli-Leydig cell tumor of the ovary containing Sertoli tubules admixed with Leydig cells.

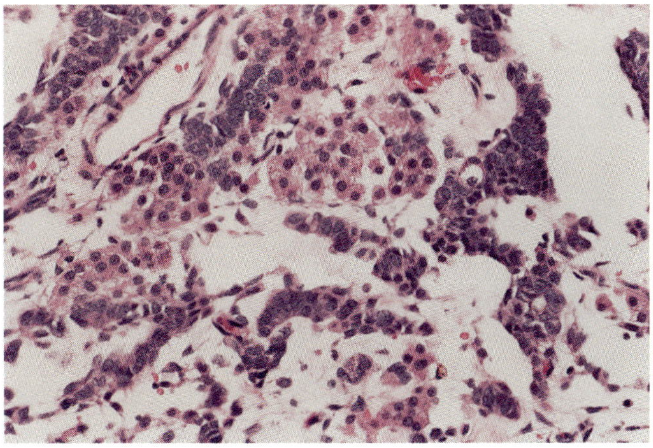

6.86 Sertoli-Leydig cell tumor of intermediate differentiation with trabeculated cords of Sertoli cells admixed with Leydig cells.

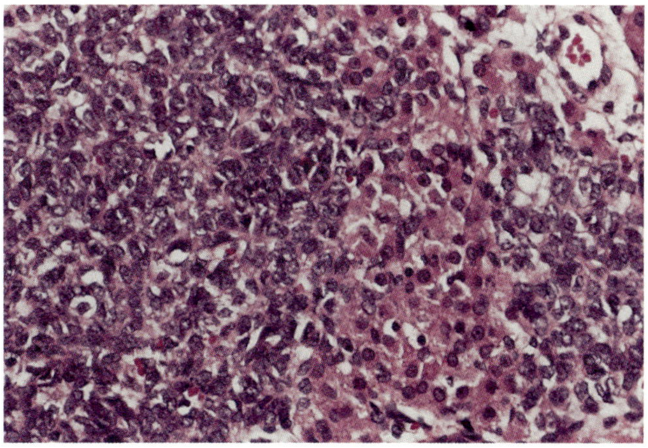

6.87 Sertoli-Leydig cell tumor, poorly differentiated, with a diffuse Sertoli cell pattern admixed with Leydig cells.

Intermediately and poorly differentiated Sertoli-Leydig cell tumors can have heterologous differentiation. This can be epithelial such as mucinous epithelium (Figures 6-88 and 6-89) or carcinoid tumor; or mesenchymal such as rhabdomyoblasts or cartilage.[73,74,117,118] There appears to be a better prognosis if the differentiation is epithelial.

Hilus cell tumors are similar to Leydig cell tumors and are identified by their anatomic location in the ovary (Figure 6-90).[97] They contain a uniform population of Leydig cells with crystals of Reinke (Figure 6-91). If Reinke crystals cannot be found, the tumor is placed in the more generic category of steroid (lipid) cell tumor (Figures 6-92 and 6-93).[34,35,103,130] Reinke crystals are reassuring signs of the benign nature of the tumor. In steroid cell tumors, the size of the tumor is prognostic. Tumors less than 8 cm in diameter have not been shown to behave in an aggressive fashion.

Gonadal stromal tumors may have minor components of another cell line (granulosa cell or Sertoli-Leydig). It is for this reason that the term gynandroblastoma (Figure 6-94) is reserved for tumors that have more than 10% differentiation of both the ovarian and testicular cell types.[12,120] Sex cord tumor with annular tubules is a special category of tumor with a distinctive cell pattern (Figure 6-95).[1,126] The precise cell lineage in this tumor has not yet been described. There is an association of these tumors with patients who have Peutz-Jeghers syndrome. These tumors contain complex tubules with prominent hyaline bodies (Figure 6-96).

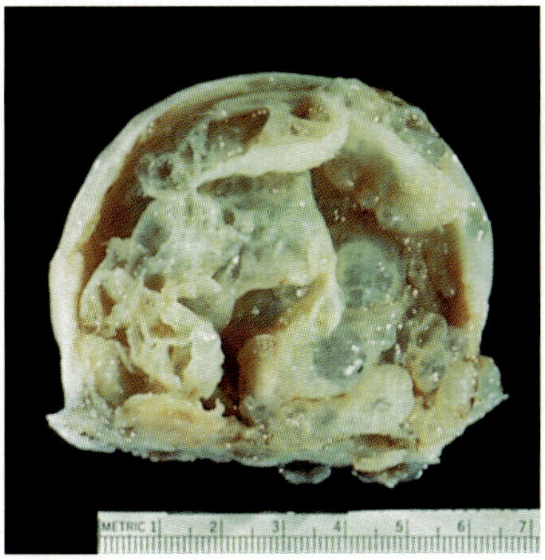

6.88 Sertoli-Leydig cell tumor of the ovary with heterologous differentiation containing multiloculated mucinous areas.

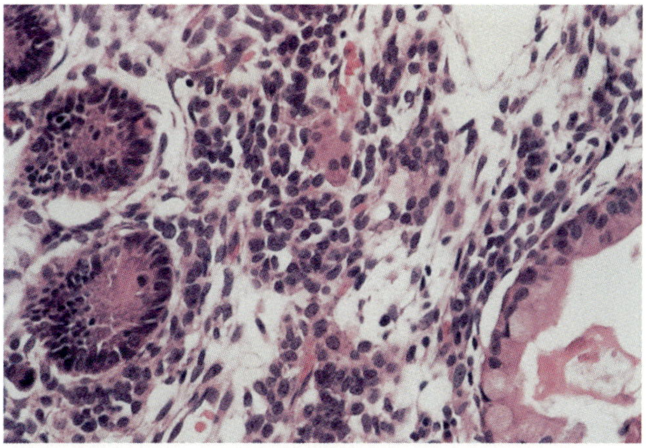

6.89 Sertoli-Leydig cell tumor with heterologous differentiation containing mucinous epithelium.

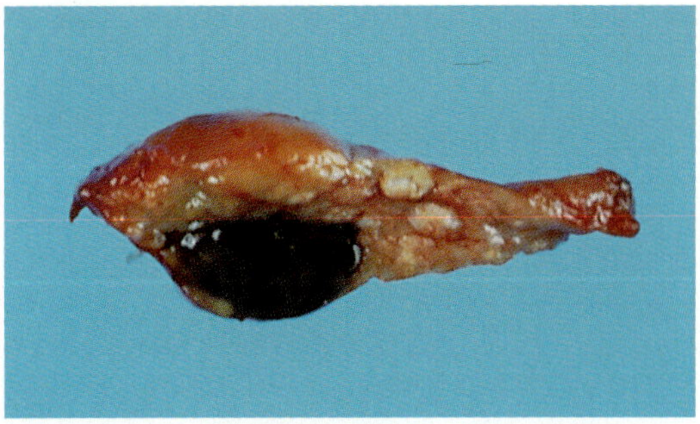

6.90 Leydig cell tumor in the hilum of the ovary (hilus cell tumor).

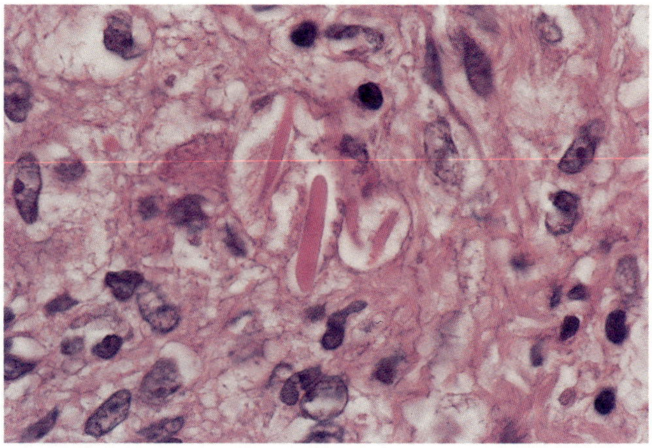

6.91 Leydig cell tumor of the ovary containing numerous crystals of Reinke.

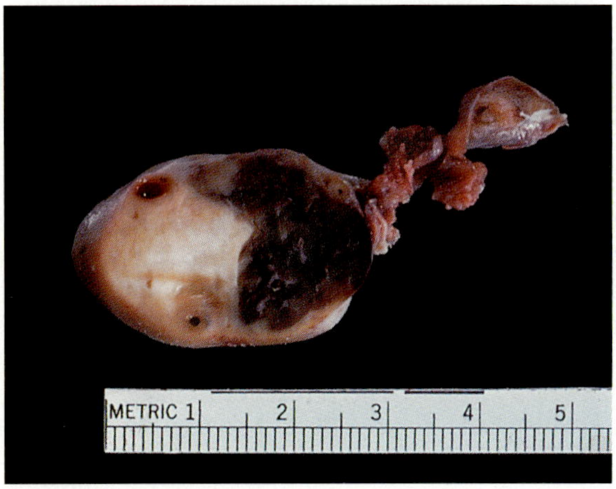

6.92 Steroid cell tumor of the ovary.

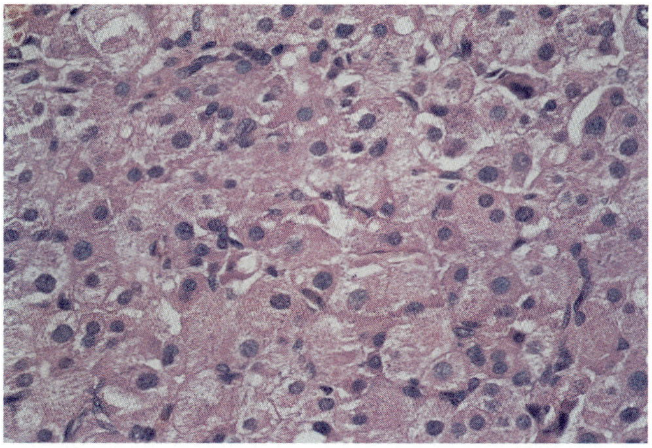

6.93 Steroid cell tumor of the ovary composed of steroid cells without Reinke crystals.

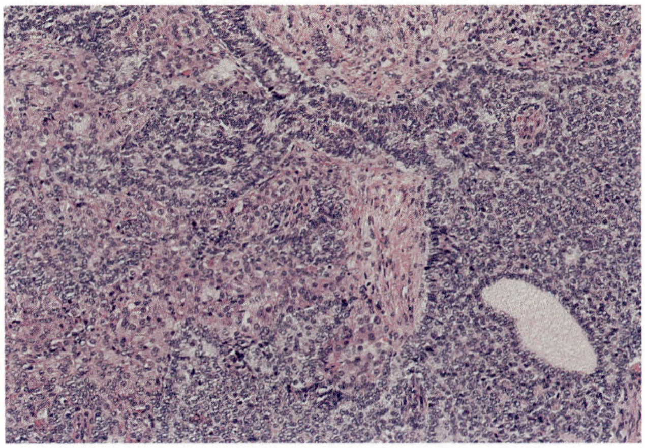

6.94 Gynandroblastoma of the ovary containing a mixture of Sertoli-Leydig cells and a granulosa cell differentiation.

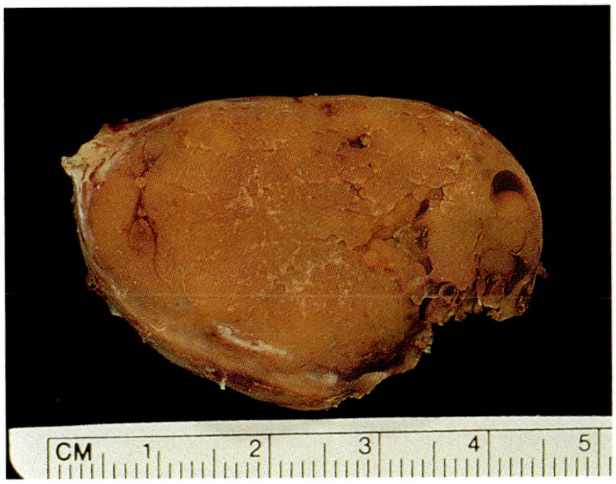

6.95 Sex cord tumor with annular tubules.

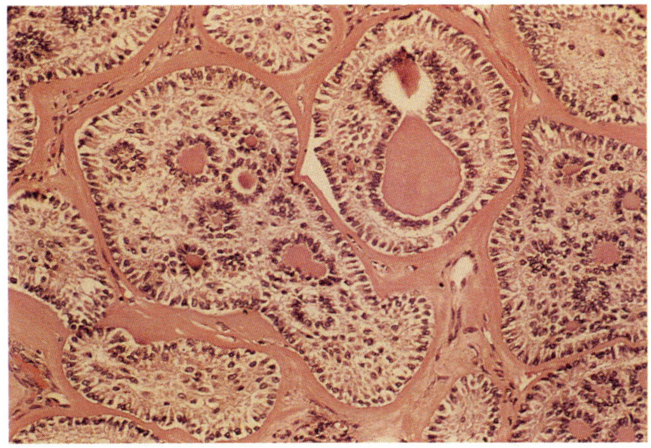

6.96 Sex cord tumor with annular tubules demonstrating a characteristic complex tubular pattern with a central eosinophilic material.

TUMORS OF GERM CELL ORIGIN

Dysgerminoma is a tumor of uniform germ cell proliferation that is probably the most undifferentiated of all the germ cell tumors.[11,30,38] Grossly, the tumor is solid with a smooth surface (Figure 6-97). It is characterized by a uniform population of primitive germ cells with prominent nucleoli and a clearing of the nuclear chromatin. There is also a characteristic fibrosis and lymphocytic infiltrate accompanying the tumor (Figure 6-98), with occasional granulomas (Figure 6-99). Benign syncytiotrophoblastic differentiation can occur, which may produce low levels of human chorionic gonadotropin (hCG) (Figure 6-100).[129]

The yolk sac or endodermal sinus tumor was originally designated as a mesonephroma by Schiller due to the presence of glomeruloid structures. Teilum subsequently recognized these structures to be similar in their appearance to the so-called endodermal sinuses in the rodent placenta. The yolk sac tumor is now considered a germ cell tumor that recapitulates the embryonic development of the yolk sac.[44,45,61] The human yolk sac is in direct continuity with the primitive gut, which has been referred to as the secondary yolk sac vesicle. Yolk sac differentiation may be of a parietal or visceral type, with most tumors exhibiting both patterns. Parietal yolk sac differentiation is characterized by an extracellular accumulation of basement membrane–like material which is alpha-fetoprotein (AFP) negative and is composed of laminin and Type IV collagen. This material is similar to that seen in the basement membrane of the parietal yolk sac cells in the rat (Reichert membrane). Visceral yolk sac differentiation is associated with the production of AFP and hyaline droplets. Enteric and hepatic differentiation in some yolk sac tumors indicates both embryonal and extraembryonal differentiation. These findings are consistent with the development of the hepatobiliary anlage from the primitive gut.

Yolk sac tumors are rare but are the second most common malignant germ cell tumor in the ovary. They occur most commonly in children and adolescents and are rare in individuals over the age of 40. Patients usually present with a recent onset of abdominal pain and swelling. Grossly the tumors are large, averaging around 15 cm. The external surface is predominantly smooth with frequent rupture. The tumor is soft and friable with areas of hemorrhage and necrosis (Figure 6-101). Cystic areas can be present, sometimes giving a honeycomb appearance to the cut surface. The tumors are usually unilateral, with bilateral involvement as a secondary process.

A variety of histologic patterns have been observed.[109] The most common type has been referred to as the reticular or microcystic pattern. It is characterized by a loose meshwork of spaces and channels lined with mitotically active cells producing hyaline droplets containing AFP (Figure 6-102). Schiller-Duval bodies (Figure 6-103), which are histologically similar to the endodermal sinuses in the rodent placenta, have been described in over half of yolk sac tumors. Parietal yolk sac differentiation is present in over 90% of tumors and is characterized by extracellular accumulation of basement membrane–like substance. This is usually a focal finding within areas demonstrating a reticular or solid pattern.

Visceral yolk sac differentiation may present in several ways.[106] A polyvesicular vitelline pattern is characterized by a dense spindle cell stroma containing cysts resembling the histologic appearance of the normal human yolk sac.[62] Foci of enteric differentiation present as well-defined glands lined by bland pseudostratified columnar cells.[18,19] A hepatoid pattern of yolk sac tumor resembles hepatocellular carcinoma (Figures 6-104 and 6-105).[39,56,68] An endometrioid variant resembles well-differentiated endometrial carcinoma (Figure 6-106).[17]

Embryonal carcinoma is extraordinarily rare, which distinguishes it from its testicular counterpart.[43] Embryonal carcinoma of the ovary can produce both AFP and hCG. The few tumors that have been reported are of a highly aggressive nature. The gross appearance is of hemorrhage and necrosis with a solid pattern. The tumor is primitive and undifferentiated (Figure 6-107). Polyembryoma is an extraordinarily rare tumor that is combined with numerous embryoid bodies of various stages of development. Choriocarcinoma of the ovary is a primary germ cell tumor, which distinguishes it from its gestational counterpart.[2,27,40] Choriocarcinoma of the ovary usually occurs in association with other germ cell tumors in a mixed pattern.[46] It is characterized by an admixture of both syncytial and cytotrophoblastic cells (Figure 6-108) and significant hemorrhage. Choriocarcinomas produce high levels of hCG.

Teratomas of the ovary are subdivided into immature, mature, and monodermal variants. Immature teratomas of the ovary are all considered to be of varying degrees of malignancy.[28,59,64] Grossly, they usually have a solid or solid and cystic appearance (Figure 6-109). Histologically, they are characterized by immature fetal tissue. The grading depends on the amount of immature fetal tissue present.[65] The most significant component of the immature fetal tissue is that of the immature neural-epidermal component (Figure 6-110). Glial implants can occur on the peritoneum, which can be of mature glial tissue (see Chapter 5, Figure 5-66). These glial implants may have been derived from an immature teratoma and then differentiated after the implantation.[60,77] The size of the tumor, the clinical stage and grade, and the grade of its metastasis are of value in determining the prognosis.

Grading of Ovarian Teratomas

Gynecologic Oncology Group

Grade 0 All tissues are mature and mitotic activity is rare or absent. Well-studied grade 0 primary teratomas are regarded as benign.

Grade 1 These are neoplasms with some immaturity but with neuroepithelium absent or limited to a rare low magnification (×40) field within the tumor, and not more than one such focus in any slide.

Grade 2 Immaturity and neuroepithelium are present to a greater degree than in Grade 1. Neuroepithelium is common but does not exceed three low-power microscopic fields in any one slide.

Grade 3 Immaturity and neuroepithelium are prominent, the latter occupying four or more low-magnification microscopic fields within individual sections.

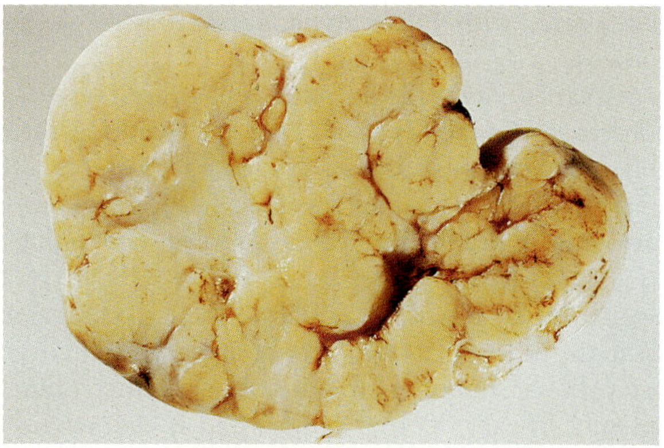

6.97 Dysgerminoma of the ovary with tan lobules separated by dense fibrous bands. (Courtesy Dr. Scot Milvanen, MD, Columbia Medical Center of Plano.)

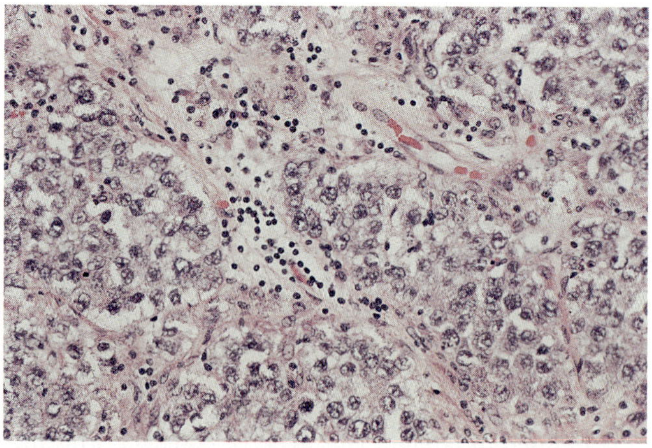

6.98 Dysgerminoma of the ovary demonstrating undifferentiated germ cells with scattered lymphocytes and fibrous septa.

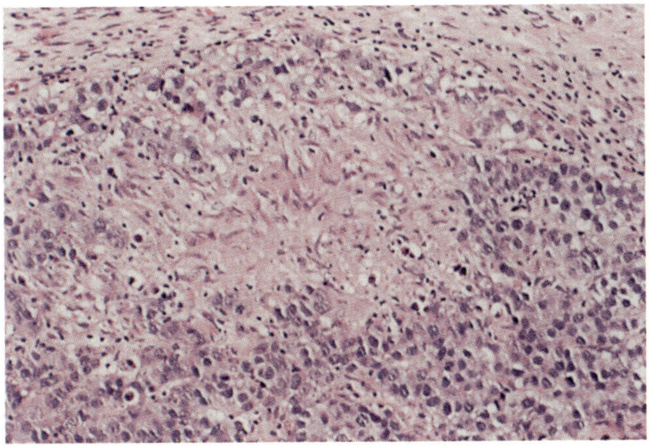

6.99 Dysgerminoma of the ovary with granuloma formation.

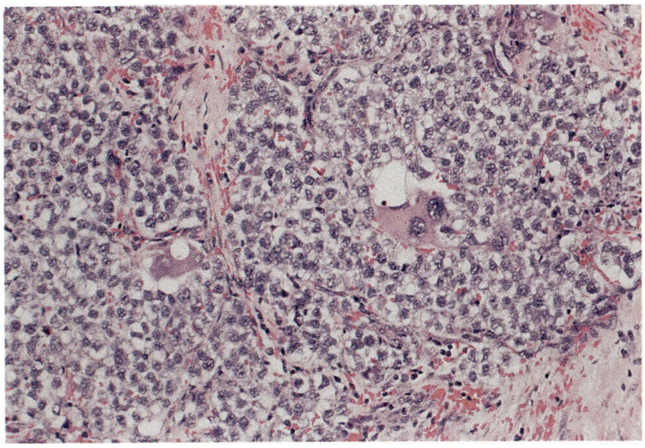

6.100 Dysgerminoma of the ovary with syncytiotrophoblastic giant cells.

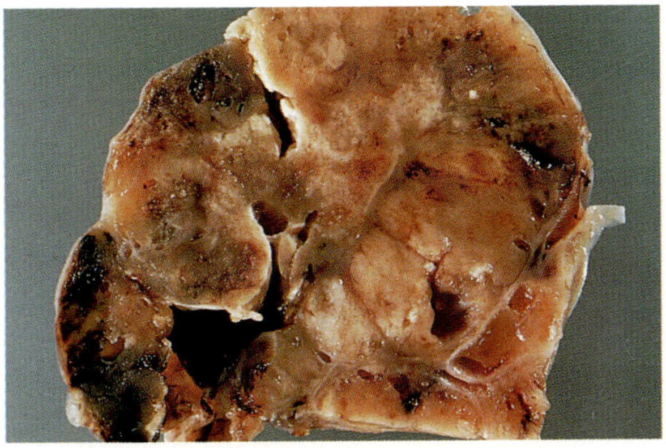

6.101 Yolk sac tumor of the ovary.

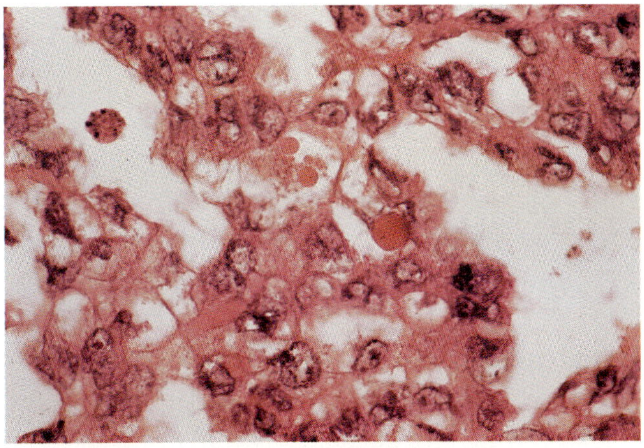

6.102 Yolk sac tumor of the ovary with endodermal sinus differentiation containing numerous hyaline droplets that contain alpha-fetoprotein.

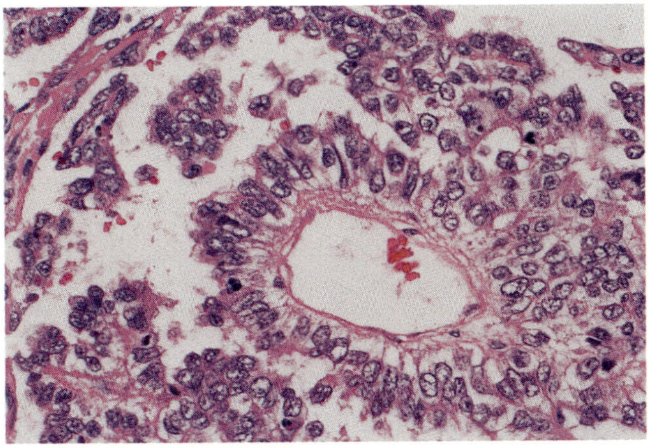

6.103 Yolk sac tumor of the ovary with endodermal sinus differentiation containing a Schiller-Duval body.

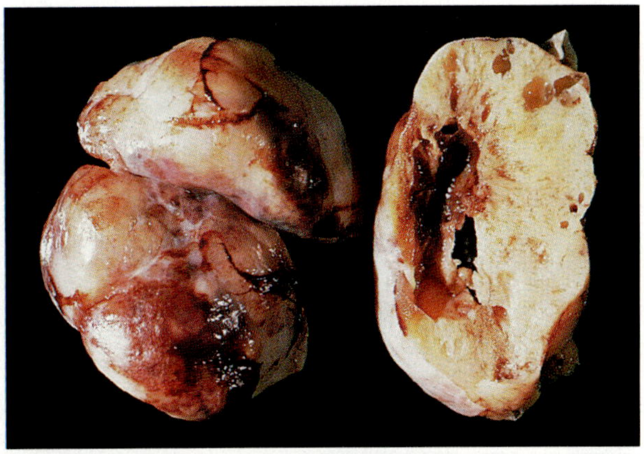

6.104 Yolk sac tumor of the ovary with hepatoid and glandular differentiation.

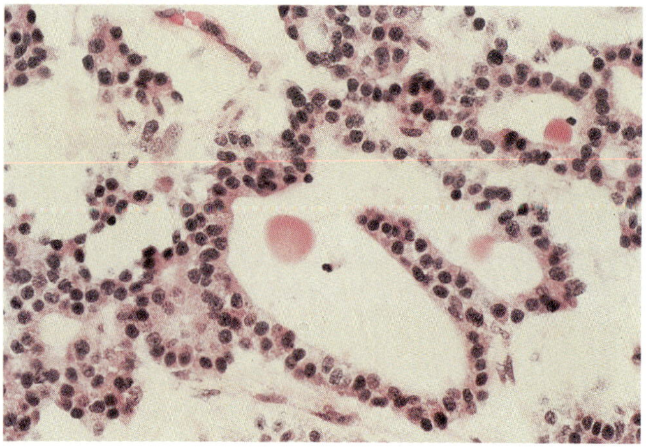

6.105 Yolk sac tumor of the ovary with glandular differentiation and scattered hyaline droplets.

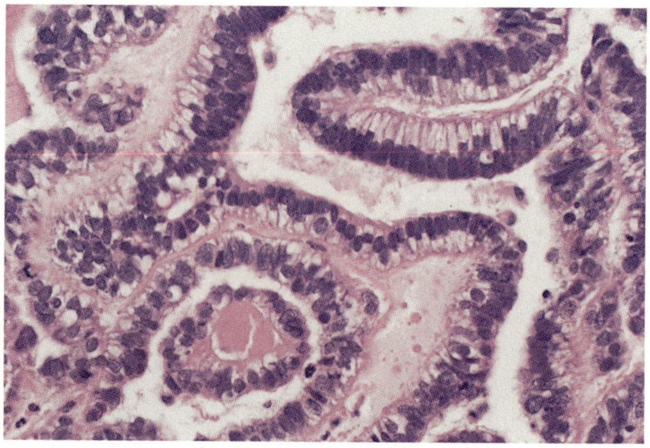

6.106 Yolk sac tumor of the ovary showing an endometrioid variant with areas of vacuolated epithelium similar to secretory endometrium.

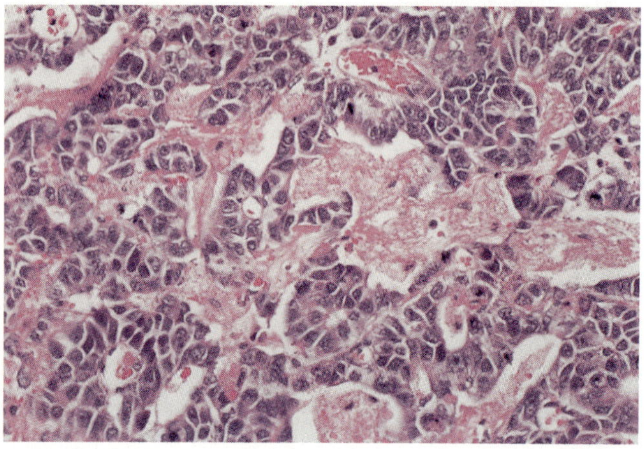

6.107 Embryonal carcinoma of the ovary with a primitive undifferentiated pattern of malignant cells.

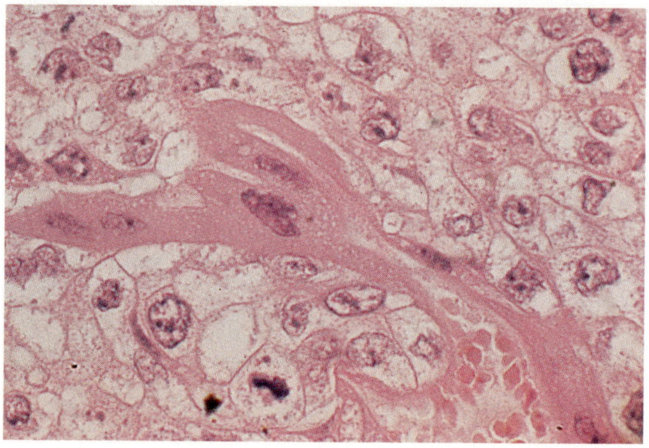

6.108 Choriocarcinoma of the ovary containing a mixture of syncytial and cytotrophoblastic cells.

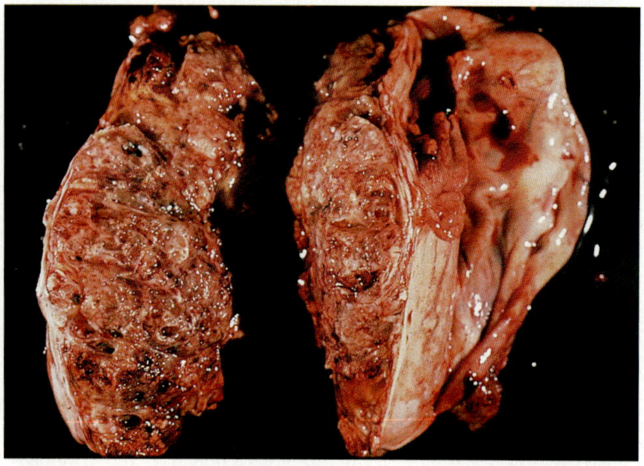

6.109 Immature teratoma of the ovary with a solid, partially microcystic pattern.

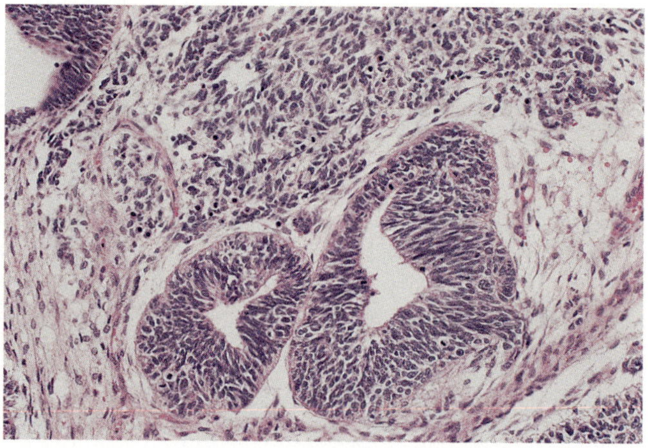

6.110 Immature teratoma of the ovary with primitive neural epithelium.

Mature teratomas of the ovary can be solid but are usually cystic (dermoid cysts). The gross appearance may show abundant hair and keratinous debris (Figure 6-111). Bone and well-formed teeth can also be identified in the central area known as the Rokitansky protuberance. It is in this solid area that generous samples should be taken to look for immature components and any malignant transformation that may occur. A variety of cell types from all three germ cell layers are present in dermoid cysts, with a predominance of squamous epithelium and related skin adnexal structures (Figure 6-112). Malignant transformation can occur in any of the components of the mature teratoma. The most common malignant transformation is that of squamous cell carcinoma (Figure 6-113).[104] Malignant melanomas and sarcomas have also been described as arising in mature teratomas. The mature teratoma (dermoid cyst) is the most common germ cell tumor; like most germ cell tumors, it occurs in women under the age of 30.

Monodermal differentiation in teratomas can occur as a single component or in combination with a mature teratoma. The most common monodermal differentiation is thyroid tissue. The term struma ovarii is used when thyroid tissue is seen grossly (Figure 6-114) or is a predominant component histologically (Figure 6-115).[67,100] Carcinoid tumors are the second most common monodermal differentiation (Figure 6-116). The insular pattern (Figure 6-117) resembles midgut carcinoids, is usually present in pure form, and is associated with carcinoid syndrome in about 30% of patients.[76] The trabecular pattern (Figure 6-118) resembles foregut and hindgut carcinoids, is usually mixed with other teratomatous components, and is not associated with carcinoid syndrome.[78] Struma carcinoid tumors (Figure 6-119) contain both thyroid and carcinoid components.[51] Epidermoid cysts, which are lined with squamous epithelium without other teratomatous components (Figures 6-120 and 6-121), may also be monodermal teratomas.[25,116]

Combined germ cell and sex cord–stromal tumors can occur; the most common type is the gonadoblastoma. This is a mixed tumor that contains cells resembling those of dysgerminoma and immature granulosa or Sertoli cells (Figure 6-122). This tumor often has marked calcification. Most of these tumors occur in patients with abnormal gonads, such as in gonadal dysgenesis. Gonadoblastoma can occur in combination with a more malignant type of germ cell tumor.

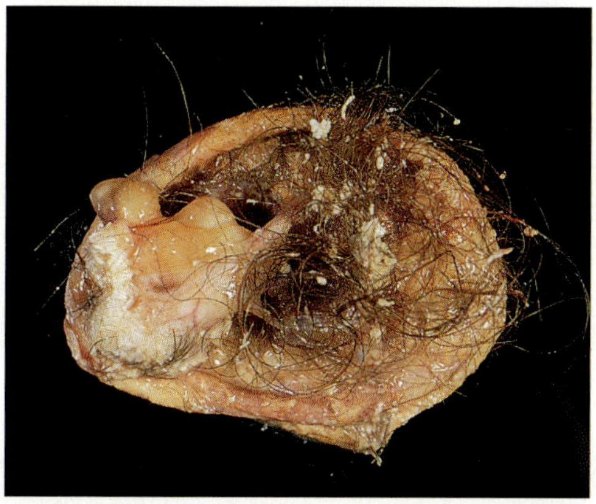

6.111 Mature cystic teratoma (dermoid cyst) filled with hair and keratinous debris with one solid nodular area (Rokitansky protuberance).

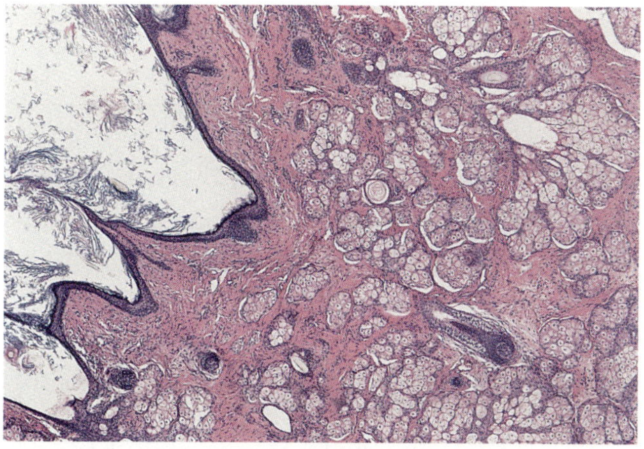

6.112 Mature cystic teratoma of the ovary with keratinizing squamous epithelium and numerous sebaceous glands.

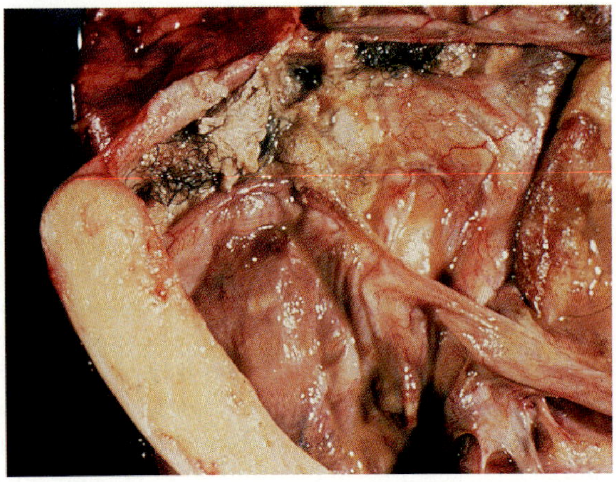

6.113 Mature cystic teratoma of the ovary with squamous carcinoma arising in the cyst wall.

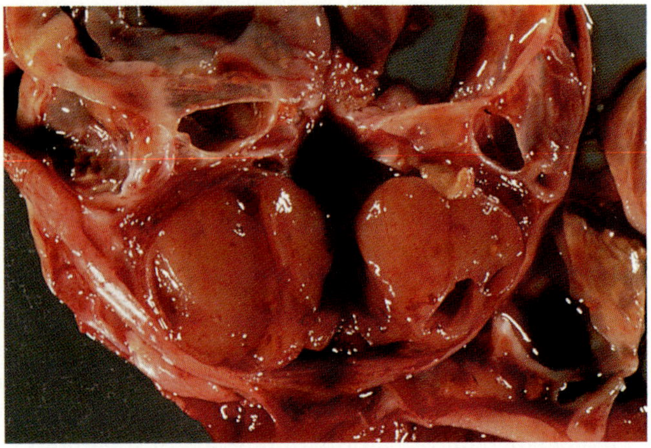

6.114 Struma ovarii characterized by tan nodular areas in a cystic teratoma.

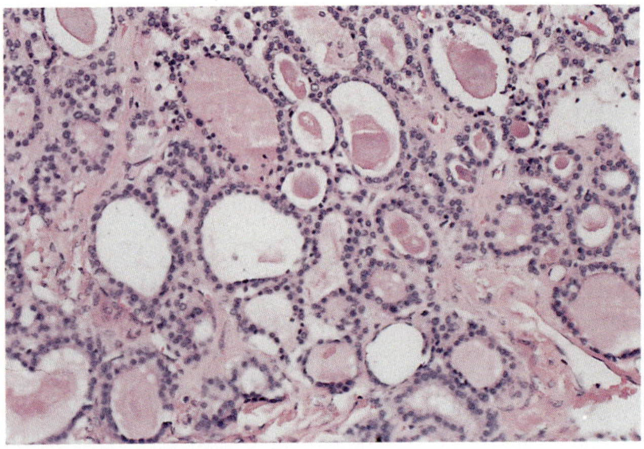

6.115 Struma ovarii with mature thyroid follicles.

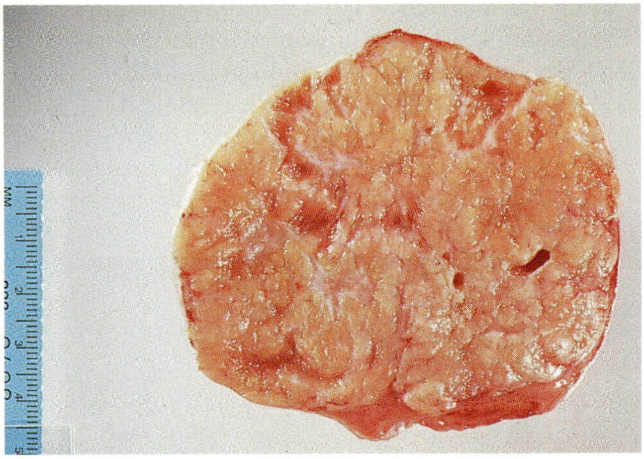

6.116 Carcinoid tumor of the ovary having a solid, yellow-tan, lobulated appearance. (Courtesy Dr. Scot Milvanen, MD, Columbia Medical Center of Plano.)

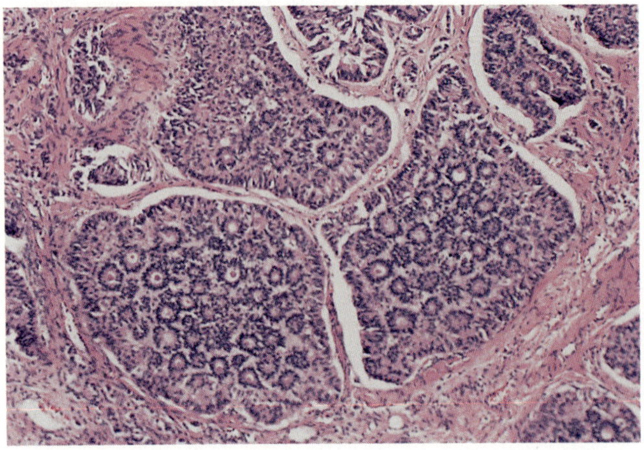

6.117 Carcinoid tumor of the ovary with an insular pattern.

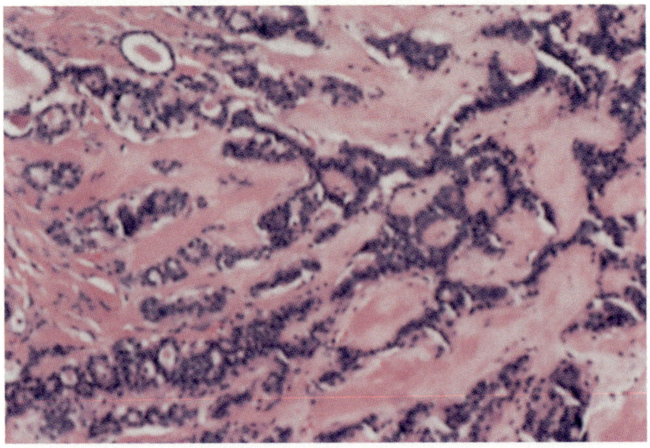

6.118 Carcinoid tumor of the ovary with a trabecular pattern.

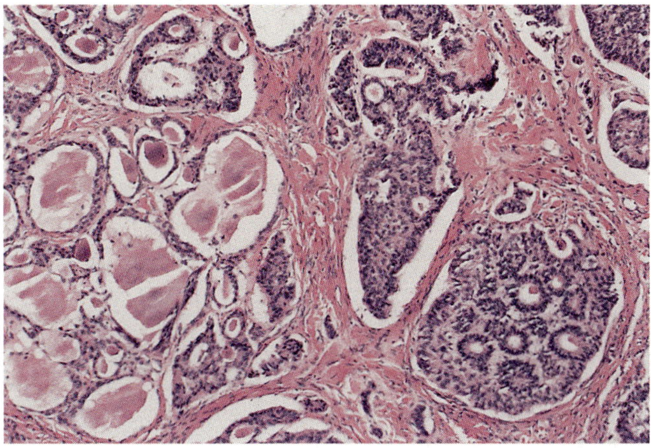

6.119 Strumal carcinoid with mixtures of thyroid follicles and carcinoid tumor.

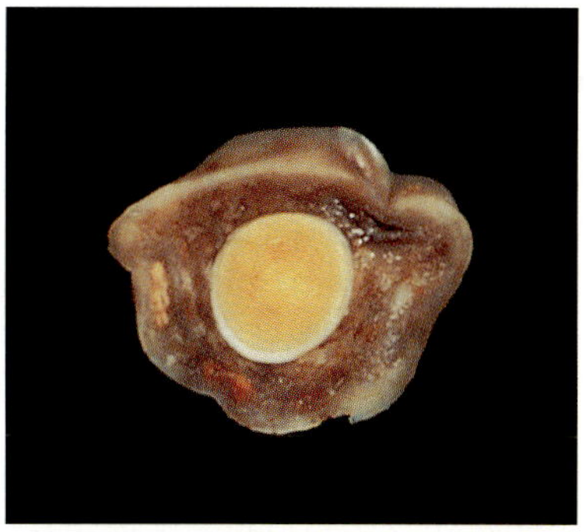

6.120 Epidermoid cyst of the ovary.

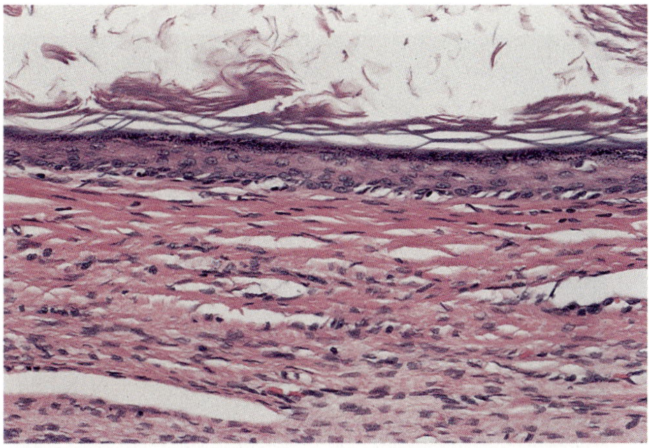

6.121 Epidermoid cyst of the ovary lined with keratinizing squamous epithelium and no other teratomatous component.

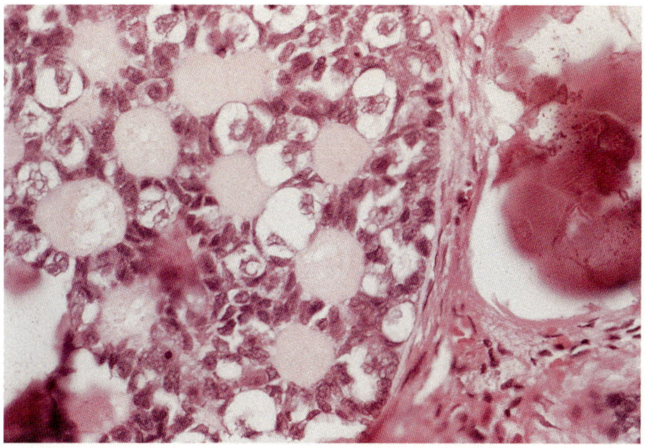

6.122 Gonadoblastoma of the ovary containing a mixture of hyalinized Call-Exner-like bodies and primitive germ cells with calcification.

MISCELLANEOUS TUMORS OF THE OVARY

Cysts of rete ovarii are usually seen in postmenopausal women.[89] They are unilocular and filled with clear fluid. They are lined with bland columnar epithelium and contain nests of hilus cells in the surrounding stroma (Figure 6-123). Lymphoma of the ovary is rare and is usually the result of metastatic disease (Figures 6-124 and 6-125).[55] Small cell carcinoma of the ovary associated with hypercalcemia (Figure 6-126) is a very aggressive tumor that presents in young women.[21,23,115] It contains undifferentiated cells that may form follicle-like structures (Figure 6-127) that may be confused with other tumors such as juvenile granulosa cell tumor.[121]

Metastatic carcinoma to the ovary can take several patterns.[107] The classic Krukenberg tumor is a metastatic carcinoma of the stomach that is usually bilateral (Figure 6-128).[36,108] Signet ring adenocarcinoma cells infiltrate a fibrous stroma (Figure 6-129). The signet ring cells are mucin positive (Figure 6-130) and the stroma may have luteinization. Patterns similar to that of the Krukenberg tumor can also be seen in metastasis from other parts of the gastrointestinal tract, especially the colon. Occasionally, metastatic breast carcinoma to the ovary can take the same pattern as a Krukenberg tumor. Breast carcinoma metastatic to the ovary usually presents as smaller, firm, white nodules consisting of glandular elements similar to a breast primary tumor. Metastatic carcinoma from the colon may be difficult to distinguish from primary mucinous adenocarcinoma of the ovary (Figure 6-131).[48] There is usually a distinctive pattern of "dirty" necrosis and segmental destruction of the glandular epithelium (Figure 6-132).

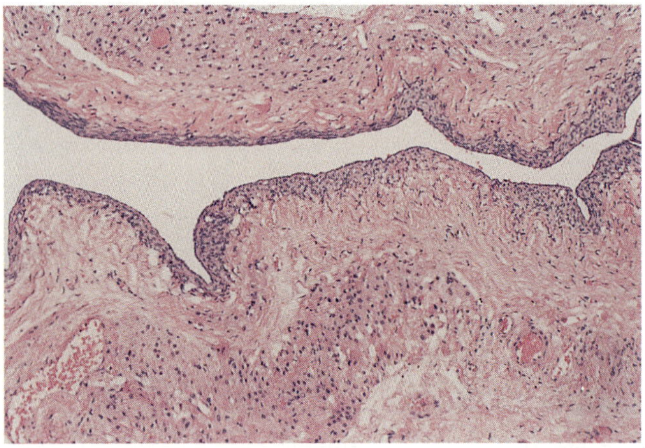

6.123 Rete ovarii cyst lined with flattened epithelium and containing clusters of hilus cells in the stroma.

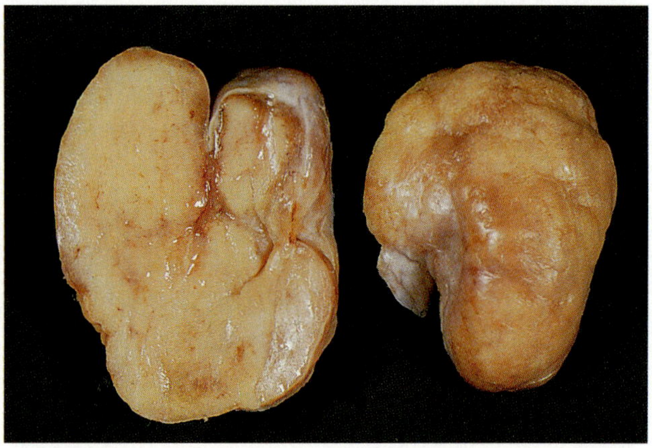

6.124 Lymphoma of the ovary.

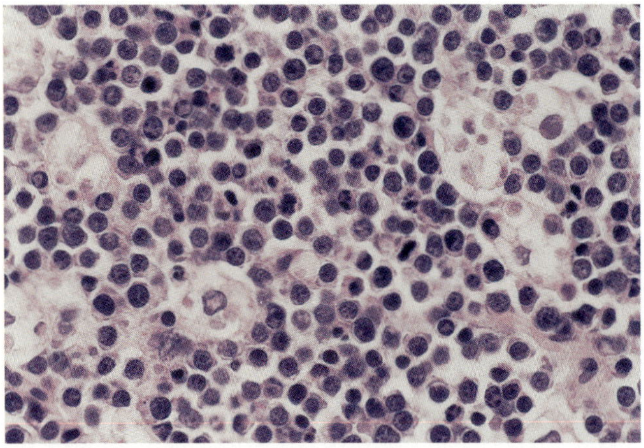

6.125 Burkitt lymphoma of the ovary showing the characteristic "starry sky" pattern.

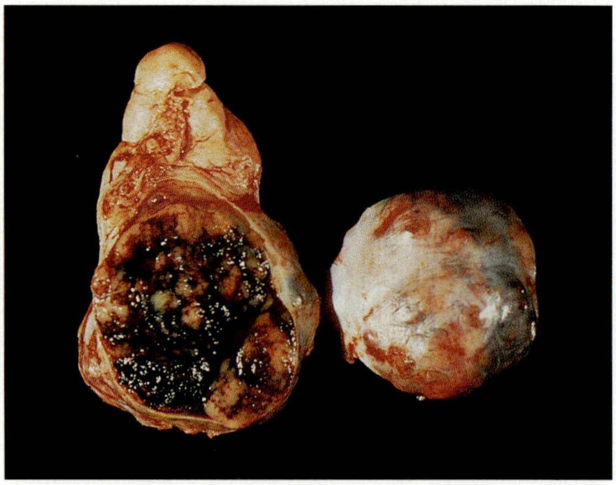

6.126 Small cell carcinoma of the ovary, hypercalcemic type.

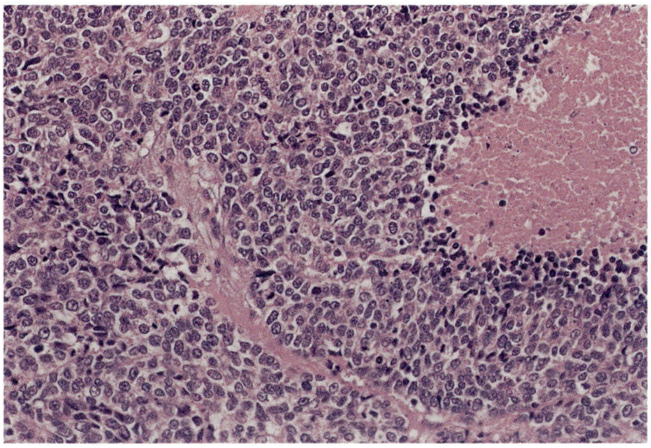

6.127 Small cell carcinoma of the ovary containing neoplastic undifferentiated cells with scant cytoplasm and scattered follicle-like structures.

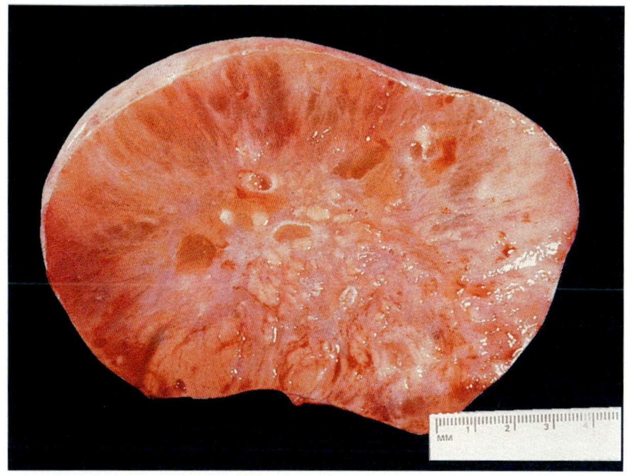

6.128 Krukenberg tumor of the ovary showing a smooth external surface and a solid, partially microcystic tumor with fibrous septa.

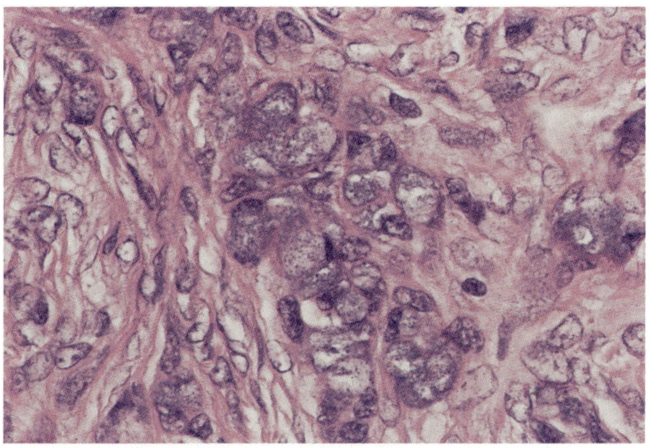

6.129 Krukenberg tumor of the ovary containing signet ring cells embedded in a densely fibrotic stroma.

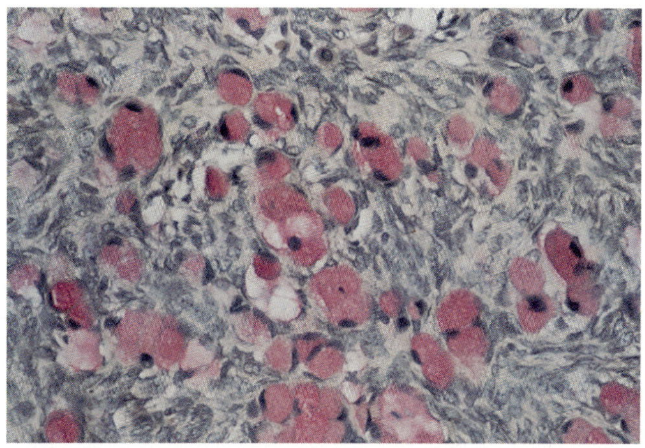

6.130 Krukenberg tumor of the ovary showing mucin-positive signet ring cells embedded in a densely cellular stroma.

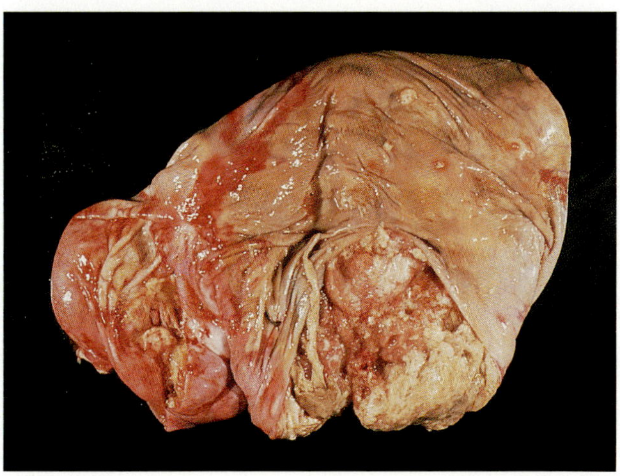

6.131 Adenocarcinoma of the colon metastatic to the ovary.

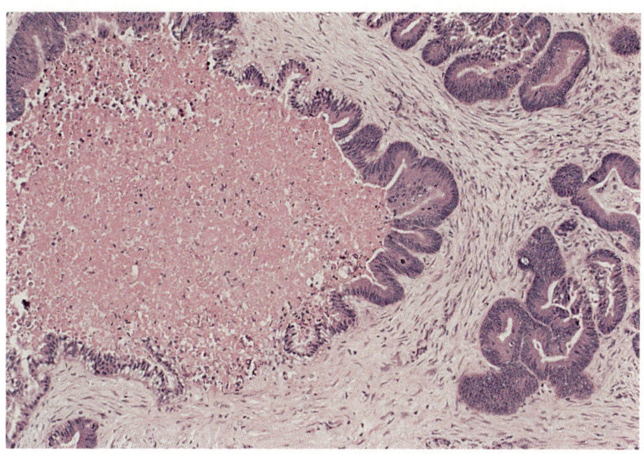

6.132 Metastatic adenocarcinoma from the colon showing areas of necrosis and segmental destruction of the glandular epithelium.

Histologic Classification of Ovarian Tumors

(Modified WHO and ISGYP Classification)

I. Surface epithelial-stromal tumors

- A. Serous tumors
  - 1. Benign
    - a. Cystadenoma and papillary cystadenoma
    - b. Surface papilloma
    - c. Adenofibroma and cystadenofibroma
  - 2. Of borderline malignancy (of low malignant potential)
    - a. Cystadenoma and papillary cystic tumor
    - b. Surface papillary tumor
    - c. Adenofibroma and cystadenofibroma
  - 3. Malignant
    - a. Adenocarcinoma, papillary adenocarcinoma, papillary cystadenocarcinoma
    - b. Surface papillary adenocarcinoma
    - c. Adenocarcinofibroma and cystadenocarcinofibroma (malignant adenofibroma and cystadenofibroma)
- B. Mucinous tumors, endocervical-like and intestinal-type
  - 1. Benign
    - a. Cystadenoma
    - b. Adenofibroma and cystadenofibroma
  - 2. Of borderline malignancy (of low malignant potential)
    - a. Cystic tumor
    - b. Adenofibroma and cystadenofibroma
  - 3. Malignant
    - a. Adenocarcinoma and cystadenocarcinoma
    - b. Adenocarcinofibroma and cystadenocarcinofibroma (malignant adenofibroma and cystadenofibroma)
- C. Endometrioid tumors
  - 1. Benign
    - a. Cystadenoma
    - b. Cystadenoma with squamous differentiation
    - c. Adenofibroma and cystadenofibroma
    - d. Adenofibroma and cystadenofibroma with squamous differentiation
  - 2. Of borderline malignancy (of low malignant potential)
    - a. Cystic tumor
    - b. Cystic tumor with squamous differentiation
    - c. Adenofibroma and cystadenofibroma
    - d. Adenofibroma and cystadenofibroma with squamous differentiation
  - 3. Malignant
    - a. Adenocarcinoma and cystadenocarcinoma
    - b. Adenocarcinoma and cystadenocarcinoma with squamous differentiation
    - c. Adenocarcinofibroma and cystadenocarcinofibroma (malignant adenofibroma and cystadenofibroma)
    - d. Adenocarcinofibroma and cystadenocarcinofibroma with squamous differentiation (malignant adenofibroma and cystadenofibroma with squamous differentiation)
  - 4. Epithelial-stromal and stromal
    - a. Adenosarcoma, homologous and heterologous
    - b. Mesodermal (müllerian) mixed tumor (carcinosarcoma), homologous and heterologous
    - c. Stromal sarcoma
- D. Clear cell tumors
  - 1. Benign
    - a. Cystadenoma
    - b. Adenofibroma and cystadenofibroma
  - 2. Of borderline malignancy (of low malignant potential)
    - a. Cystic tumor
    - b. Adenofibroma and cystadenofibroma
  - 3. Malignant
    - a. Adenocarcinoma and cystadenocarcinoma
    - b. Adenocarcinofibroma and cystadenocarcinofibroma (malignant adenofibroma and cystadenofibroma)
- E. Transitional cell tumors
  - 1. Brenner tumor
  - 2. Brenner tumor of borderline malignancy (proliferating)
  - 3. Malignant Brenner tumor
  - 4. Transitional cell carcinoma (non-Brenner type)
- F. Squamous cell tumors
- G. Mixed epithelial tumors (specify types)
  - 1. Benign
  - 2. Of borderline malignancy (of low malignant potential)
  - 3. Malignant
- H. Undifferentiated carcinoma

II. Sex cord–stromal tumors

- A. Granulosa cell tumor
  - 1. Adult type
  - 2. Juvenile type
- B. Tumors in the thecoma-fibroma group
  - 1. Thecoma
    - a. typical
    - b. luteinized
  - 2. Fibroma
  - 3. Cellular fibroma
  - 4. Fibrosarcoma
  - 5. Stromal tumor with minor sex cord elements
  - 6. Sclerosing stromal tumor
  - 7. Unclassified (fibrothecoma)
  - 8. Others
- C. Sertoli-Leydig cell tumors; androblastomas
  - 1. Well-differentiated
    - a. Sertoli cell tumor (tubular androblastoma)
    - b. Sertoli-Leydig cell tumor
    - c. Leydig cell tumor (hilus cell tumor)
  - 2. Intermediate differentiation
    - a. Variant—with heterologous elements (specify type)

Histologic Classification of Ovarian Tumors

(Modified WHO and ISGYP Classification)

3. Poorly differentiated (sarcomatoid)
    a. Variant—with heterologous elements (specify type)
4. Retiform
    a. Variant—with heterologous elements (specify type)

D. Sex cord tumor with annular tubules
E. Gynandroblastoma
F. Unclassified
G. Steroid (lipid) cell tumors
   1. Stromal luteoma
   2. Unclassified (not otherwise specified)

III. Germ cell tumors

A. Dysgerminoma
   1. Variant—with syncytiotrophoblast cells
B. Yolk sac tumor
   1. Endodermal sinus tumor
   2. Polyvesicular vitelline tumor variant
   3. Hepatoid variant
   4. Glandular variant
   5. Endometrioid variant
C. Embryonal carcinoma
D. Polyembryoma
E. Choriocarcinoma
F. Teratomas
   1. Immature
   2. Mature
      a. Solid
      b. Cystic (dermoid cyst)
      c. With secondary tumor (specify type)
      d. Fetiform (homunculus)
   3. Monodermal
      a. Struma ovarii
         (1) Variant—with secondary tumor (specify type)
      b. Carcinoid
         (1) Insular
         (2) Trabecular
      c. Strumal carcinoid
      d. Mucinous carcinoid
      e. Neuroectodermal tumors (specify type)
      f. Sebaceous tumors
      g. Others
G. Mixed forms (specify type)

IV. Gonadoblastoma

A. Variant—with dysgerminoma or other germ cell tumor

V. Germ cell and sex cord–stromal tumors

A. Variant—with dysgerminoma or other germ cell tumor

VI. Tumors of rete ovarii

A. Adenoma and cystadenoma
B. Carcinoma

VII. Mesothelial tumors

A. Adenomatoid tumor
B. Mesothelioma

VIII. Tumors of uncertain origin

A. Small cell carcinoma
   1. Hypercalcemic type
   2. Pulmonary type
B. Tumor of probable wolffian origin
C. Hepatoid carcinoma
D. Oncocytoma
E. Myxoma

IX. Gestational trophoblastic diseases
X. Soft tissue tumors not specific to the ovary
XI. Malignant lymphomas
XII. Unclassified tumors
XIII. Secondary (metastatic) tumors
XIV. Tumor-like lesions

A. Solitary follicle cyst
B. Multiple follicle cysts (polycystic ovarian disease, sclerocystic ovaries)
C. Large solitary luteinized follicle cyst of pregnancy and puerperium
D. Hyperreactio luteinalis (multiple luteinized follicle cysts)
   1. Variant—with corpora lutea
E. Corpus luteum cyst
F. Pregnancy luteoma
G. Ectopic pregnancy
H. Stromal hyperplasia
I. Stromal hyperthecosis
J. Massive edema
K. Fibromatosis
L. Endometriosis
M. Cyst, unclassified (simple cyst)
N. Inflammatory lesions
   1. Xanthogranuloma
   2. Malakoplakia
   3. Others

TNM Staging Classification for Ovarian Tumors

International Union Against Cancer (UICC)

Primary Tumor (T)—see corresponding FIGO stages

T1ai, 1aii, 1bi, 1bii, 1c
T2a, 2b, 2c
T3

Nodal Involvement (N)

NX	Minimum requirements to assess the regional nodes cannot be met
N0	No involvement of regional nodes
N1	Evidence of regional node involvement

Distant Metastasis (M)

MX	Minimum requirements to assess distant metastasis cannot be met
M0	No (known) distant metastasis
M1	Distant metastasis present—specify site

Residual Tumor (R)—postsurgical treatment

R0	No residual tumor
R1	Microscopic residual tumor
R2	Macroscopic residual tumor—specify site

FIGO Staging Classification for Ovarian Tumors

Stage I Growth limited to the ovaries

- Stage IA Growth limited to one ovary; no ascites. No tumor on the external surface; capsule intact.
- Stage IB Growth limited to both ovaries; no ascites. No tumor on the external surfaces; capsule intact.
- Stage IC* Tumor either Stage Ia or Stage Ib but with tumor on the surface of one or both ovaries; or with capsule ruptured; or with ascites present containing malignant cells or with positive peritoneal washings

Stage II Growth involving one or both ovaries with pelvic extension

- Stage IIA Extension and/or metastases to the uterus and/or tubes
- Stage IIB Extension to other pelvic tissues
- Stage IIC* Tumor either Stage IIa or Stage IIb but with tumor on the surface of one or both ovaries; or with capsule(s) ruptured; or with ascites present containing malignant cells or with positive peritoneal washings

Stage III Tumor involving one or both ovaries with peritoneal implants outside the pelvis and/or positive retroperitoneal or inguinal nodes. Superficial liver metastasis equals Stage III. Tumor is limited to the true pelvis but with histologically verified malignant extension to small bowel or omentum

- Stage IIIA Tumor grossly limited to the pelvis with negative nodes but with histologically confirmed microscopic seeding of abdominal peritoneal surfaces.
- Stage IIIB Tumor of one or both ovaries with histologically confirmed implants of abdominal peritoneal surfaces, none exceeding 2 cm in diameter. Nodes negative.
- Stage IIIC Abdominal implants >2 cm in diameter and/or positive retroperitoneal or inguinal nodes.

Stage IV Growth involving one or both ovaries with distant metastases. If pleural effusion is present, there must be positive cytologic test results to allot a case to Stage IV. Parenchymal liver metastasis equals Stage IV.

These categories are based on findings at clinical examination and/or surgical exploration. The histologic characteristics are to be considered in the staging, as are results of cytologic testing as far as effusions are concerned. It is desirable that a biopsy be performed on suspicious areas outside the pelvis.

**To evaluate the impact on prognosis of the different criteria for allotting cases to Stage IC or Stage IIC, it would be of value to know whether rupture of the capsule was (1) spontaneous or (2) caused by the surgeon, and if the source of malignant cells detected was (1) peritoneal washings or (2) ascites.*

Stage Grouping of Ovarian Carcinoma

The International Federation of Gynecology and Obstetrics (FIGO)
International Union Against Cancer (UICC)
American Joint Committee on Cancer (AJCC)

STAGE	TNM		
Stage IA1	T1ai	N0	M0
Stage IA2	T1aii	N0	M0
Stage IB1	T1bi	N0	M0
Stage IB2	T1bii	N0	M0
Stage IC	T1c	N0	M0
Stage IIA	T2a	N0	M0
Stage IIB	T2b	N0	M0
Stage IIC	T2c	N0	M0
Stage III	T3	N0	M0
	T1	N1	M0
	T2	N1	M0
	T3	N1	M0
Stage IV	Any T	Any N	M1

BIBLIOGRAPHY

General Reading

1a. Clement PB: Histology of the ovary, *Am J Surg Pathol* 11:277-303, 1987.

2a. Kurman RJ, editor: *Blaustein's pathology of the female genital tract,* ed 4, New York, 1994, Springer-Verlag.

3a. Scully RE: *Tumors of the ovary and maldeveloped gonads. Atlas of tumor pathology,* 2nd series, fascicle 16, Washington, DC, 1979, Armed Forces Institute of Pathology.

4a. Serov SF, Scully RE: *Histological typing of ovarian tumours (International Histological Classification of Tumours No. 9),* Geneva, 1973, World Health Organization.

5a. Young RH, Clement PB, Scully RE: *The ovary*. In Sternberg SS, editor: *Diagnostic surgical pathology,* ed 2, New York, 1994, Raven Press.

References

1. Ahn GH, Chi JG, Lee SK: Ovarian sex cord tumor with annular tubules, *Cancer* 57:1066-1073, 1986.
2. Axe SR, Klein VR, Woodruff JD: Choriocarcinoma of the ovary, *Obstet Gynecol* 66:111-114, 1985.
3. Baergen RN, Rutgers JL: Mural nodules in common epithelial tumors of the ovary, *Int J Gynecol Pathol* 13:62-72, 1994.
4. Bell DA: Mucinous adenofibromas of the ovary, *Am J Surg Pathol* 15:227-232, 1991.
5. Bell DA, Scully RE: Atypical and borderline endometrioid adenofibromas of the ovary. A report of 27 cases, *Am J Surg Pathol* 9:205-214, 1985.
6. Bell DA, Scully RE: Benign and borderline clear cell adenofibromas of the ovary, *Cancer* 56:2922-2931, 1985.
7. Bell DA, Scully RE: Ovarian serous borderline tumors with stromal microinvasion: a report of 21 cases, *Hum Pathol* 21:397-403, 1990.
8. Bell DA, Scully RE: Early de novo ovarian carcinoma, *Cancer* 73:1859-1864, 1994.
9. Bell DA, Weinstock MA, Scully RE: Peritoneal implants of ovarian serous borderline tumors, *Cancer* 62:2212-2222, 1988.
10. Boucher D, Tetu B: Morphologic prognostic factors of malignant mixed müllerian tumors of the ovary: a clinicopathologic study, *Int J Gynecol Pathol* 13:22-28, 1994.
11. Burkons DM, Hart WR: Ovarian germinomas (dysgerminomas), *Obstet Gynecol* 51:221-224, 1978.
12. Chalvardjian A, Derzko C: Gynandroblastoma, *Cancer* 50:710-721, 1982.
13. Chalvardjian A, Scully RE: Sclerosing stromal tumors of the ovary, *Cancer* 31:664-670, 1973.
14. Clement PB: Tumor-like lesions of the ovary associated with pregnancy, *Int J Gynecol Pathol* 12:108-115, 1993.
15. Clement PB, Scully RE: Large solitary luteinized follicle cyst of pregnancy and puerperium, *Am J Surg Pathol* 4:431-438, 1980.

16. Clement PB, Young RH, Hanna W, Scully RE: Sclerosing peritonitis associated with luteinized thecomas of the ovary, Am J Surg Pathol 18:1-13, 1994.
17. Clement PB, Young RH, Scully RE: Endometrioid-like variant of ovarian yolk sac tumor. A clinicopathological analysis of eight cases, *Am J Surg Pathol* 11:767-778, 1987.
18. Cohen MB, Friend DS, Molnar JJ: Gonadal endodermal sinus (yolk sac) tumor with pure intestinal differentiation: a new histologic type, *Pathol Res Pract* 182:609-616, 1987.
19. Cohen MB, Mulchahey KM, Molnar JJ: Ovarian endodermal sinus tumor with intestinal differentiation, *Cancer* 57:1580-1583, 1986.
20. Czernobilsky B: Endometrioid neoplasia of the ovary: a reappraisal, *Int J Gynecol Pathol* 1:203-210, 1982.
21. Dickersin GR, Kline IW, Scully RE: Small cell carcinoma of the ovary with hypercalcemia: a report of eleven cases, *Cancer* 49:188-197, 1982.
22. Dictor M: Malignant mixed mesodermal tumor of the ovary: a report of 22 cases, *Obstet Gynecol* 65:720-724, 1985.
23. Eichhorn JH, Young RH, Scully RE: Primary ovarian small cell carcinoma of pulmonary type, *Am J Surg Pathol* 16:926-938, 1992.
24. Evans AR, Gaffey TA, Malkasian GD, Annegers JF: Clinicopathologic review of 118 granulosa and 82 theca call tumors, *Obstet Gynecol* 55:231-238, 1980.
25. Fan LD, Zang HY, Zhang XS: Ovarian epidermoid cyst: report of eight cases, *Int J Gynecol Pathol* 15:69-71, 1996.
26. Garcia-Bunuel R, Berek JS, Woodruff JD: Luteomas of pregnancy, *Obstet Gynecol* 45:407-417, 1975.
27. Gerbie MV, Brewer JI, Tamimi H: Primary choriocarcinoma of the ovary, *Obstet Gynecol* 46:720-723, 1975.
28. Gershenson DM, Del Junco G, Silva EG, Copeland LJ, Wharton JT, Rutledge FN: Immature teratoma of the ovary, *Obstet Gynecol* 68:624-629, 1986.
29. Gershenson DM, Silva EG: Serous ovarian tumors of low malignant potential with peritoneal implants, *Cancer* 65:578-585, 1990.
30. Gordon A, Lipton D, Woodruff JD: Dysgerminoma: a review of 158 cases from the Emil Novak Ovarian Tumor Registry, *Obstet Gynecol* 58:497-504, 1981.
31. Hanselaar AGJM, Vooijs GP, Mayall B, Ras-Zeijlmans GJM, Chadha-Ajwani S: Epithelial markers to detect occult microinvasion in serous ovarian tumors, *Int J Gynecol Pathol* 12:20-27, 1993.
32. Hart WR: Ovarian epithelial tumors of borderline malignancy (carcinomas of low malignant potential), *Hum Pathol* 8:541-549, 1977.
33. Hart WR, Norris HJ: Borderline and malignant mucinous tumors of the ovary, *Cancer* 31:1031-1045, 1973.
34. Hayes MC, Scully RE: Ovarian steroid cell tumors (not otherwise specified), *Am J Surg Pathol* 11:835-845, 1987.
35. Hayes MC, Scully RE: Stroma luteoma of the ovary: a clinicopathological analysis of 25 cases, *Int J Gynecol Pathol* 6:313-321, 1987.
36. Holtz F, Hart WR: Krukenberg tumors of the ovary. A clinicopathologic analysis of 27 cases, *Cancer* 50:2438-2447, 1982.
37. Hughesdon PE: Benign endometrioid tumours of the ovary and the müllerian concept of ovarian epithelial tumours, *Histopathology* 8:977-990, 1984.
38. Hughesdon PE, Bennett MH: The oocytic origin of dysgerminoma, *Int J Gynecol Pathol* 5:52-62, 1986.
39. Ishikura H, Scully RE: Hepatoid carcinoma of the ovary, *Cancer* 60:2775-2784, 1987.
40. Jacobs AJ, Newland JR, Green RK: Pure choriocarcinoma of the ovary, *Obstet Gynecol Surv* 37:603-609, 1982.
41. Kao GF, Norris HJ: Unusual cystadenofibromas. Endometrioid, mucinous and clear cell types, *Obstet Gynecol* 54:729-736, 1979.
42. Kurman RJ, Craig JM: Endometrioid and clear cell carcinoma of the ovary, *Cancer* 29:1653-1664, 1972.
43. Kurman RJ, Norris HJ: Embryonal carcinoma of the ovary: a clinico-pathological entity distinct from endodermal sinus tumor resembling embryonal carcinoma of the adult testis, *Cancer* 38:2420-2433, 1976.
44. Kurman RJ, Norris HJ: Endodermal sinus tumor of the ovary. A clinical and pathologic analysis of 71 cases, *Cancer* 38:2404-2419, 1976.
45. Kurman RJ, Norris HJ: Malignant germ cell tumors of the ovary, *Hum Pathol* 8:551-564, 1977.
46. Kurman RJ, Norris HJ: Malignant mixed germ cell tumors of the ovary: a clinical and pathologic analysis of 30 cases, *Obstet Gynecol* 48:579-589, 1976.
47. Kurman RJ, Trimble CL: The behavior of serous tumors of low malignant potential: are they ever malignant?, *Int J Gynecol Pathol* 12:120-127, 1993.
48. Lash RH, Hart WR: Intestinal adenocarcinomas metastatic to the ovaries, *Am J Surg Pathol* 11:114-121, 1987.

49. Lawrence WD: The borderland between benign and malignant surface epithelial ovarian tumors, *Cancer* 76:2138-2142, 1995.
50. Lee W, Voet RL, Poliak J: Combined intrauterine and ovarian pregnancy. A case report, *J Reprod Med* 30:563-566, 1985.
51. Matias-Guiu X, Forteza J, Prat J: Mixed strumal and mucinous carcinoid tumor of the ovary, *Int J Gynecol Pathol* 14:179-183, 1995.
52. Michael H, Roth LM: Invasive and noninvasive implants in ovarian serous tumors of low malignant potential, *Cancer* 57:1240-1247, 1986.
53. Miles PA, Norris HJ: Proliferative and malignant Brenner tumors of the ovary, *Cancer* 30:174-186, 1972.
54. Montag AG, Jenison EL, Griffiths CT, Welch WR, Lavin PT, Knapp RC: Ovarian clear cell carcinoma, *Int J Gynecol Pathol* 8:85-96, 1989.
55. Monterroso V, Jaffe ES, Merino MJ, Medeiros LJ: Malignant lymphomas involving the ovary, *Am J Surg Pathol* 17:154-170, 1993.
56. Nakashima N, Fukatsu T, Nagasaka T, Sobue M, Takeuchi J: The frequency and histology of hepatic tissue in germ cell tumors, *Am J Surg Pathol* 11:682-692, 1987.
57. Nichols GE, Mills SE, Ulbright TM, Czernobilsky B, Roth LM: Spindle cell mural nodules in cystic ovarian mucinous tumors, *Am J Surg Pathol* 15:1055-1062, 1991.
58. Nictolis M, Montironi R, Tommasoni S, Valli M, Pisani E, Fabris G, Prat J: Benign, borderline and well-differentiated malignant intestinal mucinous tumors of the ovary: a clinicopathologic, histochemical, immunohistochemical and nuclear quantitative study of 57 cases, *Int J Gynecol Pathol* 13:10-21, 1994.
59. Nielsen SNJ, Gaffey TA, Malkasian GD Jr: Immature ovarian teratoma: a review of 14 cases, *Mayo Clin Proc* 61:110-115, 1986.
60. Nielsen SNJ, Scheithauer BW, Gaffey TA: Gliomatosis peritonei, *Cancer* 56:2499-2503, 1985.
61. Nogales FF: Embryologic clues to human yolk sac tumors: a review, *Int J Gynecol Pathol* 12:101-107, 1993.
62. Nogales FF, Matilla A, Nogales-Ortiz F, Galera-Davidson HL: Yolk sac tumors with pure and mixed polyvesicular vitelline patterns, *Hum Pathol* 9:553-566, 1978.
63. Norris HJ: Proliferative endometrioid tumors and endometrioid tumors of low malignant potential of the ovary, *Int J Gynecol Pathol* 12:134-140, 1993.
64. Norris HJ, Zirkin HJ, Benson WL: Immature (malignant) teratoma of the ovary. A clinical and pathologic study of 58 cases, *Cancer* 37:2359-2372, 1976.
65. O'Connor DM, Norris HJ: The influence of grade on the outcome of stage I ovarian immature (malignant) teratomas and the reproducibility of grading, *Int J Gynecol Pathol* 13:283-289, 1994.
66. Pace EH, Voet RL, Melancon JT: Xanthogranulomatous oophoritis: an inflammatory pseudotumor of the ovary, *Int J Gynecol Pathol* 3:398-402, 1984.
67. Pardo-Mindan JF, Vazquez JJ: Malignant struma ovarii, *Cancer* 51:337-343, 1983.
68. Prat J, Bhan AK, Dickersin RG, Robboy SJ, Scully RE: Hepatoid yolk sac tumor of the ovary (endodermal sinus tumor with hepatoid differentiation). A light microscopic, ultrastructural and immunohistochemical study of seven cases, *Cancer* 50:2355-2368, 1982.
69. Prat J, Scully RE: Ovarian mucinous tumors with sarcoma-like mural nodules, *Cancer* 44:1332-1344, 1979.
70. Prat J, Scully RE: Sarcomas in ovarian mucinous tumors. A report of two cases, *Cancer* 44:1327-1331, 1979.
71. Prat J, Scully RE: Cellular fibromas and fibrosarcomas of the ovary: a comparative clinicopathologic analysis of seventeen cases, *Cancer* 47:2663-2670, 1981.
72. Prat J, Scully RE: Cellular fibromas and fibrosarcomas of the ovary, *Cancer* 47:2663-2670, 1981.
73. Prat J, Young RH, Scully RE: Ovarian Sertoli-Leydig cell tumors with heterologous elements, *Cancer* 50:2465-2475, 1982.
74. Prat J, Young RH, Scully RE: Ovarian Sertoli-Leydig cell tumors with heterologous elements. II. Cartilage and skeletal muscle: a clinicopathologic analysis of twelve cases, *Cancer* 50:2465-2475, 1982.
75. Prayson RA, Hart WR: Primary smooth-muscle tumors of the ovary, *Arch Pathol Lab Med* 116:1068-1071, 1992.
76. Robboy SJ, Norris HJ, Scully RE: Insular carcinoid primary in the ovary, *Cancer* 36:404-418, 1975.
77. Robboy SJ, Scully RE: Ovarian teratoma with glial implants on the peritoneum. An analysis of 12 cases, *Hum Pathol* 1:643-653, 1970.
78. Robboy SJ, Scully RE, Norris HJ: Primary trabecular carcinoid of the ovary, *Obstet Gynecol* 49:202-207, 1977.

79. Roth LM, Anderson MC, Govan ADT, Langley FA, Gowing NFC, Woodcock AS: Sertoli-Leydig cell tumors: a clinicopathologic study of 34 cases, *Cancer* 48:187-191, 1981.
80. Roth LM, Czernobilsky B. Ovarian Brenner tumors. II. Malignant, *Cancer* 56:592-601, 1985.
81. Roth LM, Dallenbach-Hellweg G, Czernobilsky B: Ovarian Brenner tumors. I. Metaplastic, proliferating, and of low malignant potential, *Cancer* 56:582-591, 1985.
82. Roth LM, Gersell DJ, Ulbright TM: Ovarian Brenner tumors and transitional cell carcinoma: recent developments, *Int J Gynecol Pathol* 12:128-133, 1993.
83. Roth LM, Langley FA, Fox H, Wheeler JE, Czernobilsky B: Ovarian clear cell adenofibromatous tumors, *Cancer* 53:1156-1163, 1984.
84. Roth LM, Sternberg WH: Proliferating Brenner tumors, *Cancer* 27:687-693, 1971.
85. Roth LM, Sternberg WH: Ovarian stromal tumors containing Leydig cells. II. Pure Leydig cell tumor, non-hilar type, *Cancer* 32:952-960, 1973.
86. Rutgers JL, Bell DA: Immunohistochemical characterization of ovarian borderline tumors of intestinal and müllerian types, *Mod Pathol* 5:367-371, 1992.
87. Rutgers JL, Baergen RN: Mucin histochemistry of ovarian borderline tumors of mucinous and mixed-epithelial types, *Mod Pathol* 7:825-828, 1994.
88. Rutgers JL, Scully RE: Functioning ovarian tumors with peripheral steroid cell proliferation: a report of twenty-four cases, *Int J Gynecol Pathol* 5:319-337, 1986.
89. Rutgers JL, Scully RE: Cysts (cystadenomas) and tumors of the rete ovarii, *Int J Gynecol Pathol* 7:330-342, 1988.
90. Rutgers JL, Scully RE: Ovarian mixed-epithelial papillary cystadenomas of borderline malignancy of müllerian type, *Cancer* 61:546-554, 1988.
91. Rutgers JL, Scully RE: Ovarian müllerian mucinous papillary cystadenomas of borderline malignancy, *Cancer* 61:340-348, 1988.
92. Savargaonkar PR, Wells S, Graham I, Buckley CH: Ovarian hemangiomas and stroma luteinization, *Histopathology* 25:185-188, 1994.
93. Segal GH, Hart WR: Ovarian serous tumors of low malignant potential (serous borderline tumors), *Am J Surg Pathol* 16:577-583, 1992.
94. Seldenrijk CA, Willig AP, Baak JPA, Kuhnel R, Rao BR, Burger CW, vander Harten JJ, Dijkhuizen Meijer JLM: Malignant Brenner tumor. A histologic, morphometrical, immunohistochemical, and ultrastructural study, *Cancer* 58:754-760, 1986.
95. Siriaunkgul S, Robbins KM, McGowan L, Silverberg SG: Ovarian mucinous tumors of low malignant potential: a clinicopathologic study of 54 tumors of intestinal and müllerian types, *Int J Gynecol Pathol* 14:198-208, 1995.
96. Snyder RR, Norris HJ, Tavassoli F: Endometrioid proliferative and low malignant potential tumors of the ovary, *Am J Surg Pathol* 12:661-671, 1988.
97. Sohval AR, Churg J, Cobin RH, Katz N, Gabrilove JL: Histopathology and ultrastructure of ovarian hilus cell tumor. Report of two cases, *Gynecol Oncol* 7:79-101, 1979.
98. Stenwig JT, Hazekamp JT, Beecham JB: Granulosa cell tumors of the ovary. A clinicopathological study of 118 cases with long-term follow-up, *Gynecol Oncol* 7:136-152, 1979.
99. Sternberg WH, Roth LM: Ovarian stromal tumors containing Leydig cells. I. Stromal-Leydig cell tumor and non-neoplastic transformation of ovarian stroma to Leydig cells, *Cancer* 32:940-951, 1973.
100. Szyfelbein WM, Young RH, Scully RE: Struma ovarii simulating ovarian tumors of other types, *Am J Surg Pathol* 19:21-29, 1995.
101. Tavassoli FA: Serous tumor of low malignant potential with early stromal invasion (serous LMP with microinvasion), *Mod Pathol* 1:407-414, 1988.
102. Tavassoli FA, Norris HJ: Sertoli tumors of the ovary. A clinicopathologic study of 28 cases with ultrastructural observations, *Cancer* 46:2281-2297, 1980.
103. Taylor HB, Norris HJ: Lipid cell tumors of the ovary, *Cancer* 20:1953-1962, 1967.
104. Tetu B, Silva EG, Gershenson DM: Squamous cell carcinoma of the ovary, *Arch Pathol Lab Med* 111:864-866, 1987.
105. Tornos C, Silva EG, Ordonez NG, Gershenson DM, Young RH, Scully RE: Endometrioid carcinoma of the ovary with a prominent spindle-cell component, a source of diagnostic confusion, *Am J Surg Pathol* 19:1343-1353, 1995.
106. Ulbright TM, Roth LM, Brodhecker CA: Yolk sac differentiation in germ cell tumors. A morphologic study of fifty cases with emphasis on hepatic, enteric, and parietal yolk sac features, *Am J Surg Pathol* 10:151-164, 1986.
107. Ulbright TM, Roth LM, Stehman FB: Secondary ovarian neoplasia. A clinicopathological study of 35 cases, *Cancer* 53:1164-1174, 1984.

108. Wong PC, Ferenczy A, Fan LD, McCaughey E: Krukenberg tumors of the ovary. Ultrastructural, histochemical, and immunohistochemical studies of 15 cases, *Cancer* 57:751-760, 1986.
109. Young RH: New and unusual aspects of ovarian germ cell tumors, *Am J Surg Pathol* 17:1210-1224, 1993.
110. Young RH: Sertoli-Leydig cell tumors of the ovary: review with emphasis on historical aspects and unusual variants, *Int J Gynecol Pathol* 12:141-147, 1993.
111. Young RH, Dickersin GR, Scully RE: Juvenile granulosa cell tumor of the ovary, *Am J Surg Pathol* 8:575-596, 1984.
112. Young RH, Dickersin GR, Scully RE: Juvenile granulosa cell tumor of the ovary. A clinicopathological analysis of 125 cases, *Am J Surg Pathol* 8:576-596, 1984.
113. Young RH, Dudley AG, Scully RE: Granulosa cell, Sertoli-Leydig cell, and unclassified sex cord-stromal tumors associated with pregnancy: a clinicopathological analysis of thirty-six cases, *Gynecol Oncol* 18:181-205, 1984.
114. Young RH, Oliva E, Scully RE: Luteinized adult granulosa cell tumors of the ovary: a report of four cases, *Int J Gynecol Pathol* 13:302-310, 1994.
115. Young RH, Oliva E, Scully RE: Small cell carcinoma of the ovary, hypercalcemic type, *Am J Surg Pathol* 18:1102-1116, 1994.
116. Young RH, Prat J, Scully RE: Epidermoid cyst of the ovary, *Am J Clin Pathol* 73:272-276, 1980.
117. Young RH, Prat J, Scully RE: Ovarian Sertoli-Leydig cell tumors with heterologous elements. I. Gastrointestinal epithelium and carcinoid: a clinicopathologic analysis of thirty-six cases, *Cancer* 50:2448-2456, 1982.
118. Young RH, Prat J, Scully RE: Ovarian Sertoli-Leydig cell tumors with heterologous elements, *Cancer* 50:2248-2456, 1982.
119. Young RH, Scully RE: Ovarian Sertoli-Leydig cell tumors with a retiform pattern: a problem in histopathologic diagnosis, *Am J Surg Pathol* 7:755-771, 1983.
120. Young RH, Scully RE: Ovarian stromal tumors with minor sex cord elements: a report of seven cases, *Int J Gynecol Pathol* 2:227-234, 1983.
121. Young RH, Scully RE: Ovarian tumors of probable wolffian origin, *Am J Surg Pathol* 7:125-135, 1983.
122. Young RH, Scully RE: Fibromatosis and massive edema of the ovary, possibly related entities: a report of 14 cases of fibromatosis and 11 cases of massive edema, *Int J Gynecol Pathol* 3:153-178, 1984.
123. Young RH, Scully RE: Ovarian Sertoli cell tumors: a report of 10 cases, *Int J Gynecol Pathol* 2:349-363, 1984.
124. Young RH, Scully RE: Ovarian Sertoli-Leydig cell tumors. A clinicopathological analysis of 207 cases, *Am J Surg Pathol* 9:543-569, 1985.
125. Young RH, Scully RE: Ovarian Sertoli-Leydig cell tumors. A clinicopathological analysis of 207 cases. *Am J Surg Pathol* 9:543-569, 1985.
126. Young RH, Welch WR, Dickersin GR, Scully RE: Ovarian sex cord tumor with annular tubules. Review of 74 cases including 27 with Peutz-Jeghers syndrome and four with adenoma malignum of the cervix, *Cancer* 50:1384-1402, 1982.
127. Zaloudek C, Norris HJ: Granulosa tumors of the ovary in children. A clinical and pathologic study of 32 cases, *Am J Surg Pathol* 6:503-512, 1982.
128. Zaloudek C, Norris HJ: Sertoli-Leydig tumors of the ovary. A clinicopathologic study of 64 intermediate and poorly differentiated neoplasms, *Am J Surg Pathol* 8:405-418, 1984.
129. Zaloudek CJ, Tavassoli FA, Norris HJ: Dysgerminoma with syncytiotrophoblastic giant cells. A histologically and clinically distinctive subtype of dysgerminoma, *Am J Surg Pathol* 5:361-367, 1981.
130. Zhang J, Young RH, Arseneau J, Scully RE: Ovarian stromal tumors containing lutein or Leydig cells (luteinized thecomas and stromal Leydig cell tumors)—a clinicopathological analysis of fifty cases, *Int J Gynecol Pathol* 1:270-285, 1982.

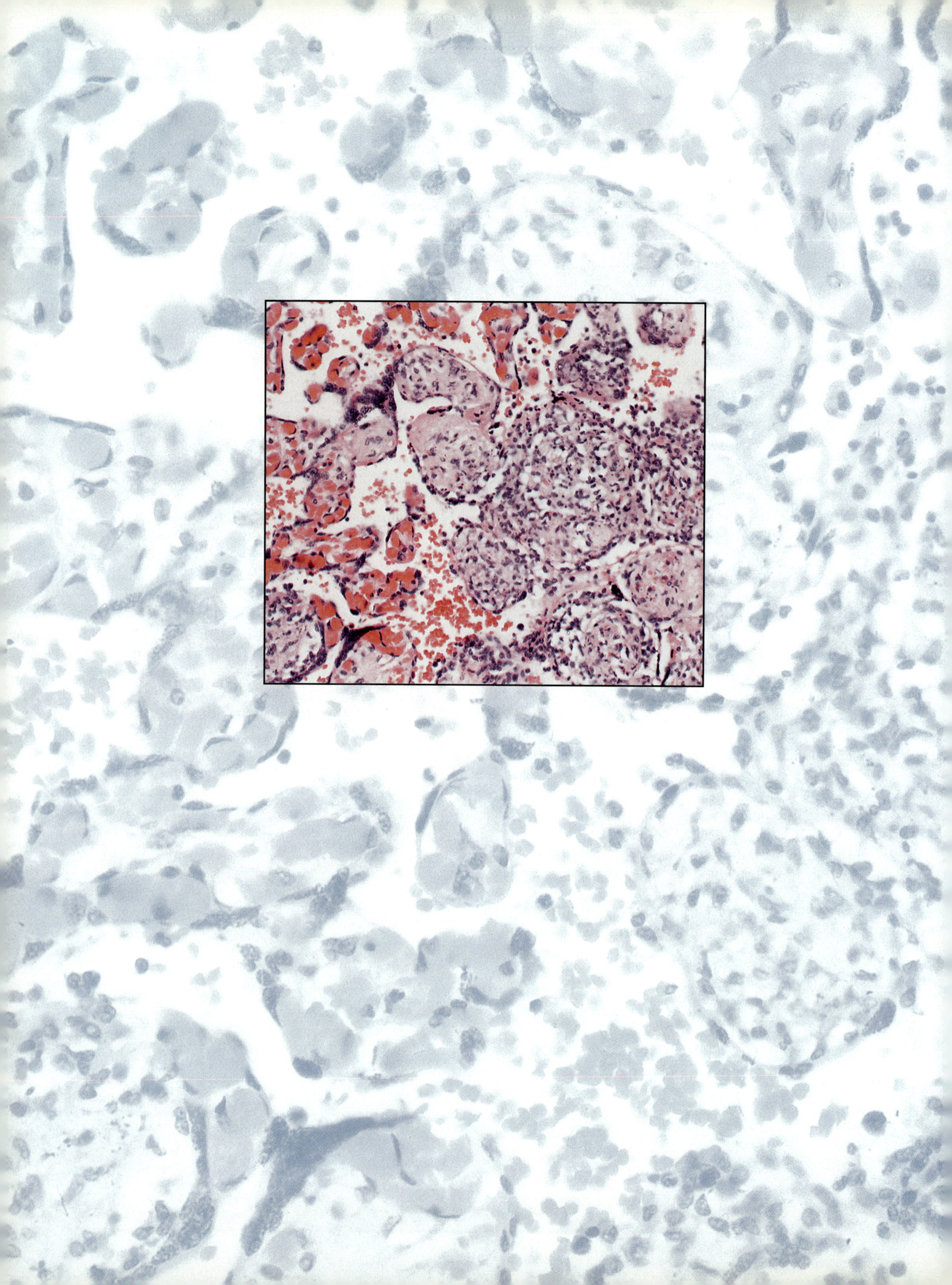

Chapter 7

Pathology of the Placenta and Trophoblastic Disease

PLACENTAL PATHOLOGY

Examination of the placenta has become more important because of current medicolegal issues.[24,60,64,73] Indications for placental examination (Table 7-1) and standard techniques have been the topic of numerous articles in recent years.[12-14,17,26,27,50] Many excellent reference tests are available for a more complete review of the subject.[1–10]

TABLE 7-1 Indications for Pathologic Examination of the Placenta[12]

MATERNAL CONDITIONS
Diabetes mellitus (or glucose intolerance)
Hypertension (chronic or pregnancy induced)
Prematurity (34 weeks' gestation or less)
Postmaturity (longer than 42 weeks)
History of reproductive failure
Oligohydramnios
Fever
Infection
Substance abuse
Repetitive bleeding
Abruptio placentae
FETAL AND NEONATAL CONDITIONS
Stillbirth or neonatal death
Multiple birth
Congenital abnormalities
Fetal growth retardation
Prematurity
Hydrops
Meconium
Admission to neonatal intensive care unit
Low Apgar score
Neurologic problems
Suspected infection
PLACENTAL CONDITIONS
Any gross abnormality of the placenta, its membranes, or the umbilical cord.
OTHER INDICATIONS
Any case in which there is reason to suspect abnormal pregnancy, abnormal delivery, an abnormal infant, or the potential for litigation

Umbilical Cord

The umbilical cord has two arteries and a vein. The cord usually twists to the left, but it is the absence of twists that may correlate with a poor outcome.[75] Embryonic remnants of the umbilical cord are frequently seen. Allantoic duct remnants are usually seen between the two umbilical arteries and consist of a cystic space lined by flattened epithelium. Omphalomesenteric (vitelline) duct remnants consist of tubular structures lined with a mucinous epithelium (Figure 7-1). These remnants may form cysts, but most cystic lesions of the cord are pseudocysts due to edema (Figure 7-2). A single umbilical artery (Figure 7-3) occurs in about 1% of deliveries and is associated with an increased incidence of fetal anomalies.[16,19,59,66] The umbilical cord usually inserts eccentrically into the placenta but may insert at the margin (battledore placenta) (Figure 7-4). A velamentous insertion occurs when the vessels separate prior to a marginal insertion (Figure 7-5). A furcate insertion occurs when the vessels separate prior to a normal insertion (Figure 7-6). True knots in the cord (Figure 7-7) must be distinguished from false knots, which are redundant folds (Figure 7-8). True knots and prolapse are more common with long umbilical cords (longer than 72 cm). Short umbilical cords (shorter than 32 cm) are associated with decreased fetal movement. Inflammation of the cord (funisitis) is usually associated with acute chorioamnionitis.[37] The inflammatory cells are of fetal origin and often aggregate in a targetoid pattern around the vessels (Figure 7-9). Necrotizing funisitis has been associated with, but is not diagnostic of, congenital syphilis.[25,35,43]

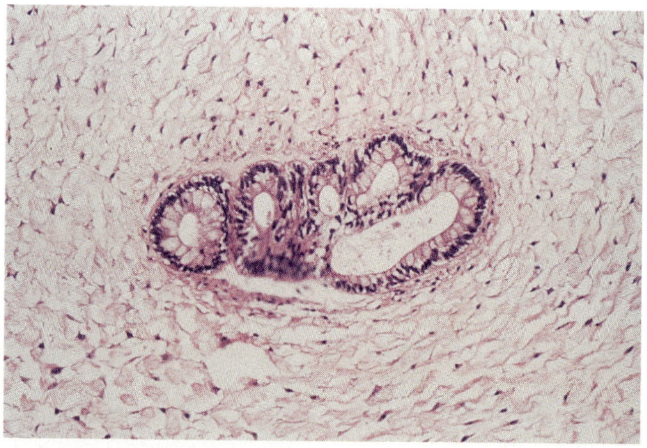

7.1 Omphalomesenteric vitelline duct remnant in the umbilical cord. The remnant is usually found between the two umbilical arteries and often has intestinal-type mucinous differentiation.

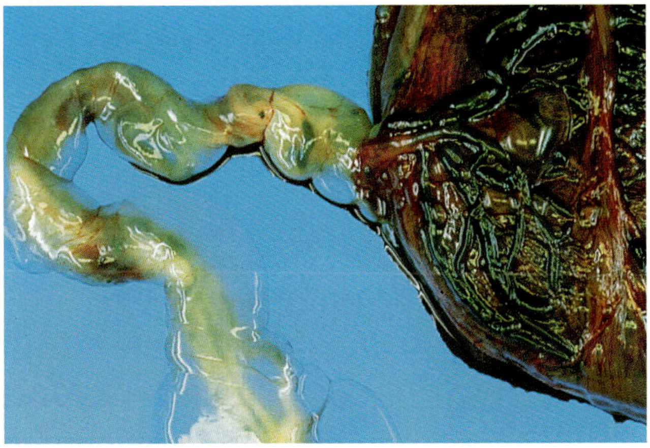

7.2 Umbilical cord edema forming a pseudocyst.

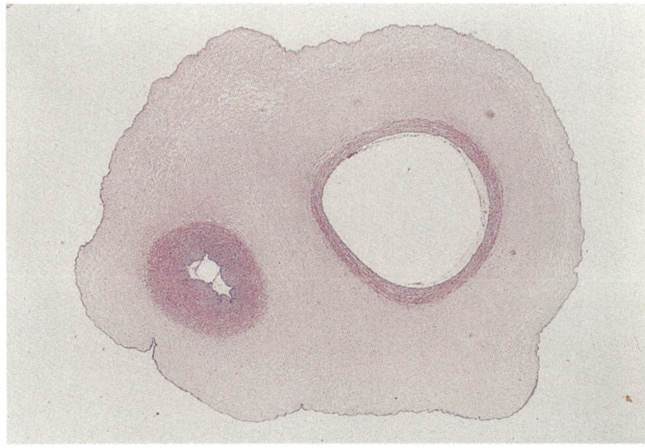

7.3 Umbilical cord with a single umbilical artery.

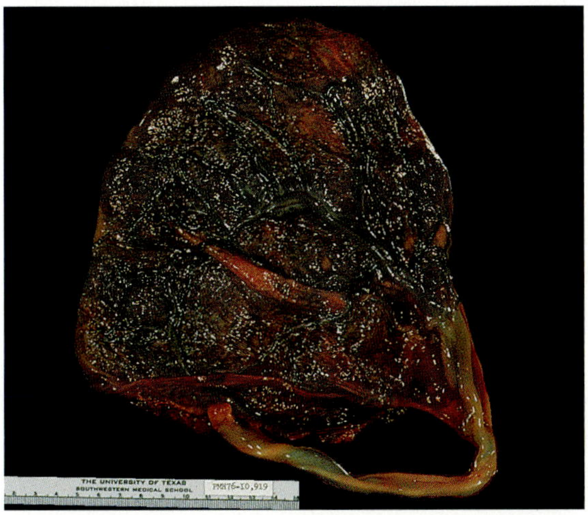

7.4 Marginal insertion of the umbilical cord (battledore placenta).

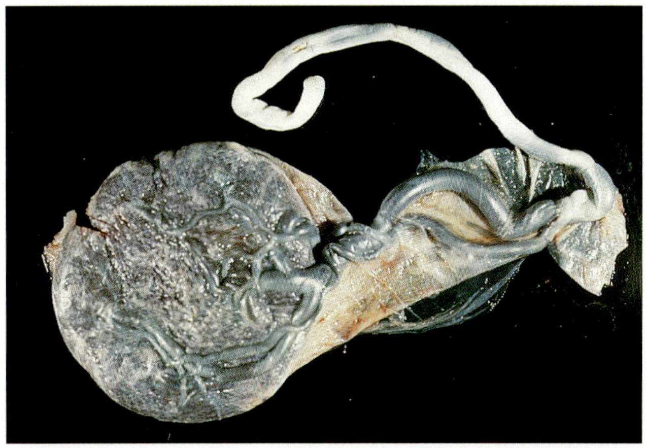

7.5 Velamentous insertion of the umbilical cord demonstrating separation of the vessels traversing the membranes before insertion into the placenta.

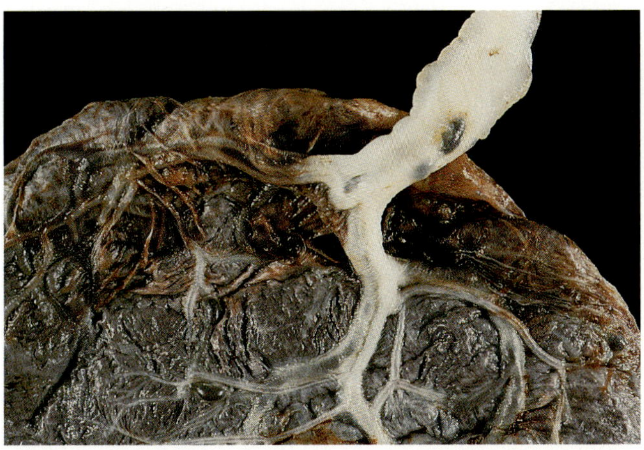

7.6 Furcate insertion of the umbilical cord. The vessels separate before insertion into the placenta.

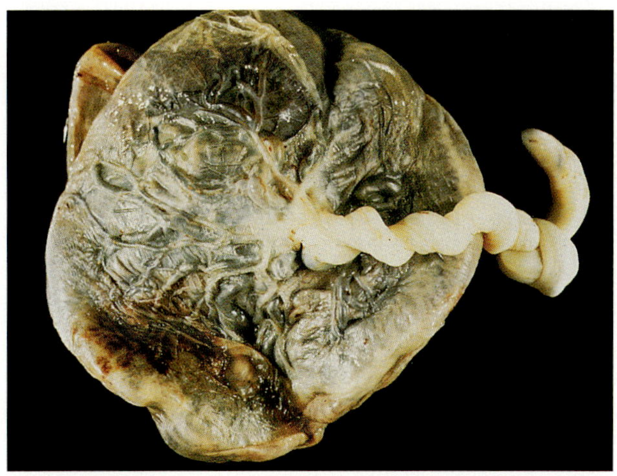

7.7 True knot of the umbilical cord.

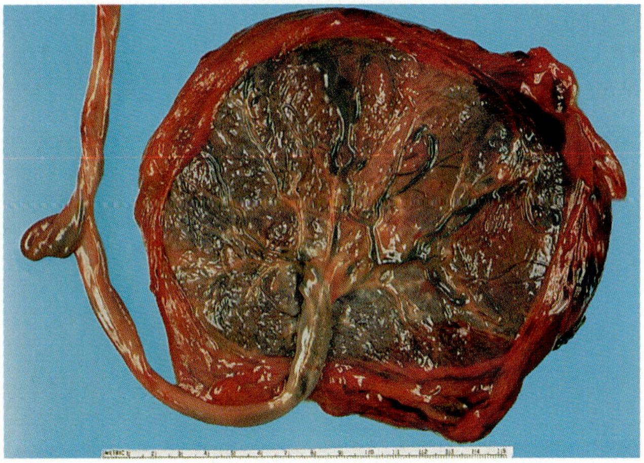

7.8 False knot of the umbilical cord.

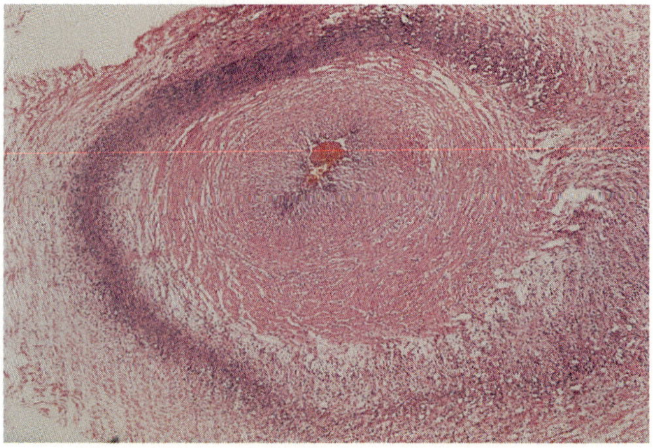

7.9 Acute funisitis of the umbilical cord. The fetal leukocytes form a dense, bandlike infiltrate surrounding the fetal vessels.

Placental Membranes

Placenta membranacea is a rare condition in which most of the fetal membranes are covered by placental tissue. A circummarginate placenta occurs when there is lateral extension of the villous tissue beyond the reflection of the chorion laeve. A circumvallate placenta is similar but contains a redundant membrane fold (Figure 7-10). Succenturiate, or accessory, lobes are single or multiple masses of placental tissue separated from the main body of the placenta and supported usually by a single artery and vein.

Acute chorioamnionitis is usually the result of ascending infection after rupture of the membranes.[70,72,86] Histologically, there is an acute inflammatory infiltrate in the chorion with extension to the amnion (Figure 7-11). In amnion nodosum, there are multiple, detachable nodules on the fetal surface of the placenta (Figure 7-12). The nodules are composed of fetal squamous cells embedded in the amnion (Figure 7-13). Amnion nodosum is associated with oligohydramnios. In contrast, squamous metaplasia of the amnion (Figure 7-14) is not detachable and has no clinical significance. The passage of fetal meconium into the amnionic fluid causes staining of the membranes (Figure 7-15). Histologically, meconium induces a reactive hyperplasia in the amnion and is deposited in macrophages (Figure 7-16). Since meconium passage may be associated with fetal distress,[21] there have been attempts to time the passage by examining the membranes.[62] Meconium-induced vasoconstriction may occur in postmature pregnancies with a poor outcome.[15] Amnionic bands are associated with early amnionic rupture. The bands may constrict the developing fetus, causing a variety of anomalies. Umbilical cord constriction may also occur (Figure 7-17).

Gross and microscopic examination of membranes in multiple gestations may be useful to determine the zygosity. A monochorionic, monoamniotic twin placenta has a single sac with no dividing membranes (Figure 7-18). There is an increased incidence of cord entanglement and fetal morbidity and mortality in this condition. Most twin pregnancies have two sacs with dividing membranes (Figure 7-19). Diamniotic, monochorionic twin placentas have two dividing membranes, each lined by cuboidal amnionic cells (Figure 7-20). Diamniotic, dichorionic placentas contain four dividing membranes that include both chorionic membranes fused between the two amnionic membranes (Figure 7-21). If one twin dies, the other may develop normally. The dead twin may be seen as a compressed, macerated fetus papyraceus (Figure 7-22).[18,30-32,46]

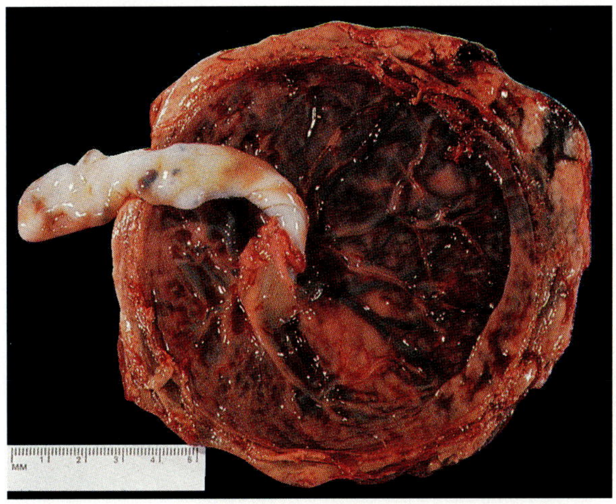

7.10 Circumvallate placenta demonstrating the membranes extending beyond the placental edge.

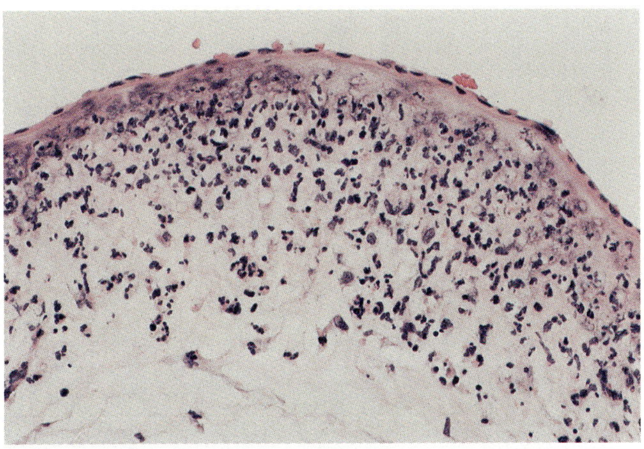

7.11 Acute chorioamnionitis with numerous neutrophils at the subamnionic region.

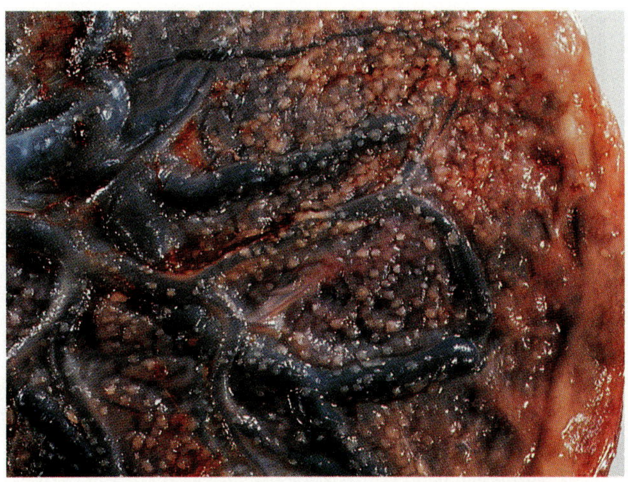

7.12 Amnion nodosum with numerous small tan nodules on the fetal surface of the placenta.

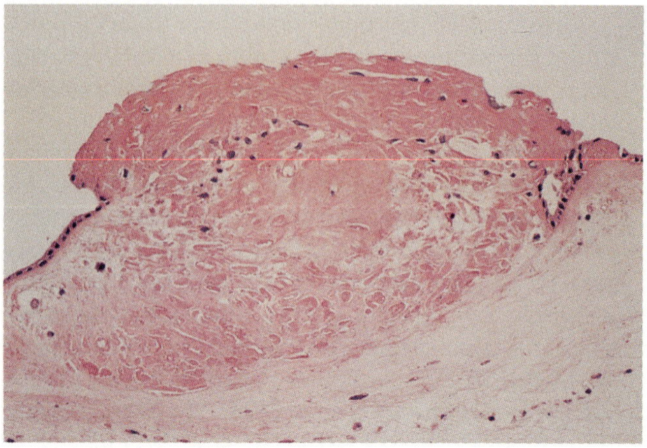

7.13 Amnion nodosum demonstrating fetal squames implanted on the amnion.

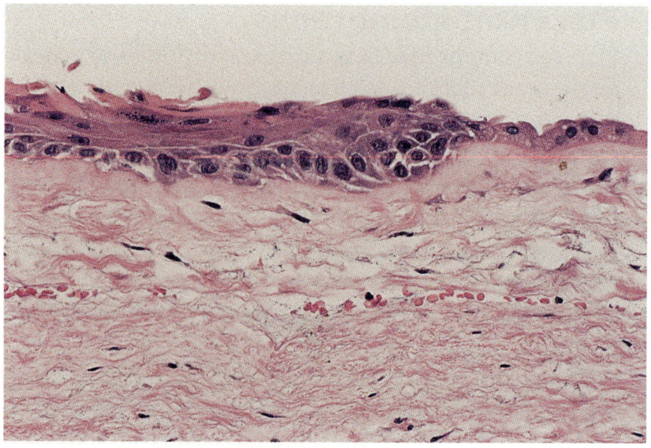

7.14 Squamous metaplasia of the amnion.

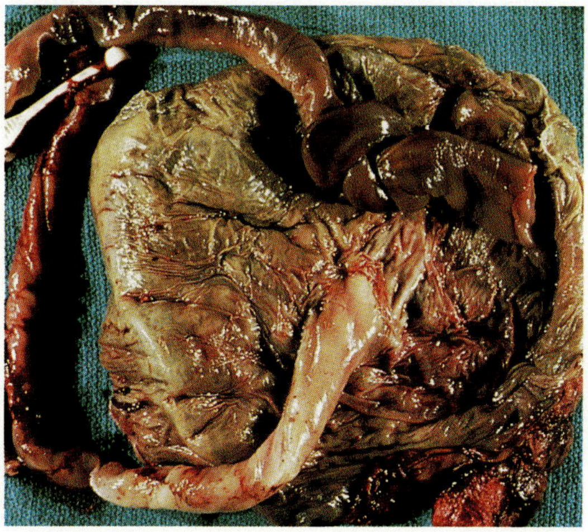

7.15 Meconium-stained placenta with true knot of the umbilical cord.

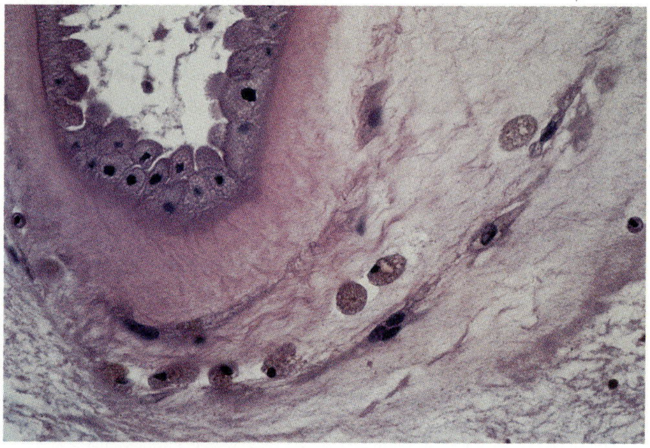

7.16 Meconium staining with reactive hyperplastic amnion and pigmented macrophages in the subamnionic tissue.

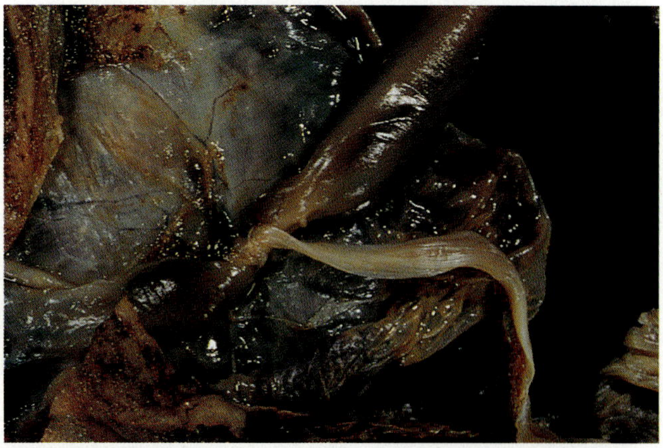

7.17 Amnionic band constricting the umbilical cord.

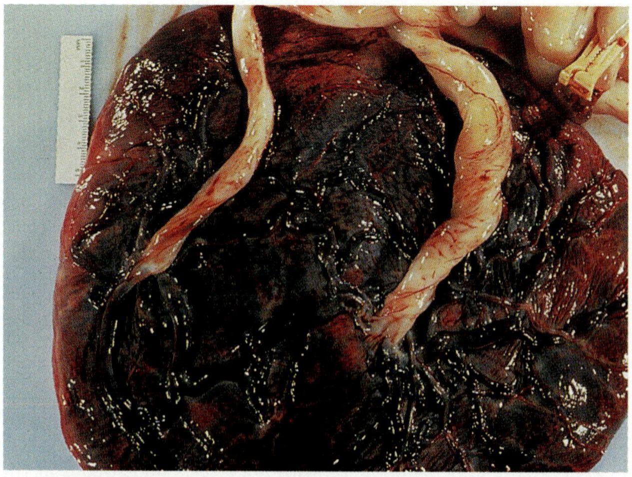

7.18 Monoamniotic, monochorionic twin placenta with no dividing membranes.

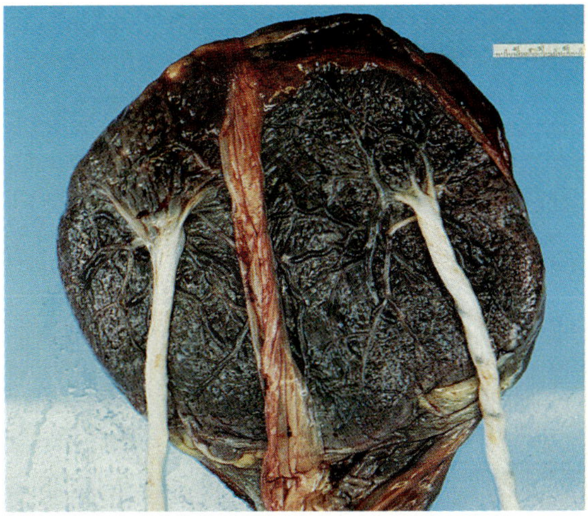

7.19 Diamniotic, monochorionic twin placenta with dividing membranes separating the gestational sacs.

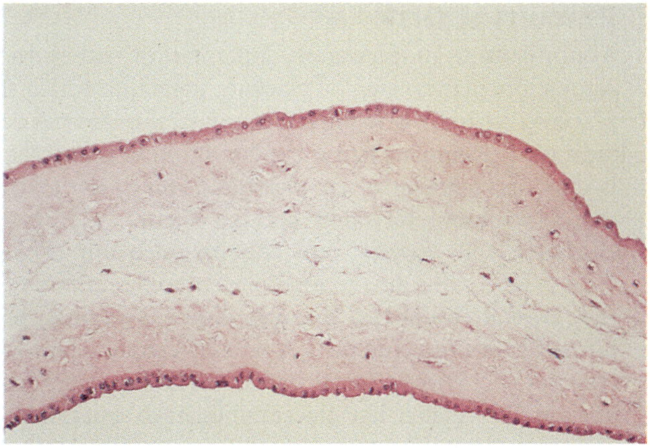

7.20 Dividing membranes of diamniotic, monochorionic placenta. The dividing membranes contain amnion on both sides with no central chorion.

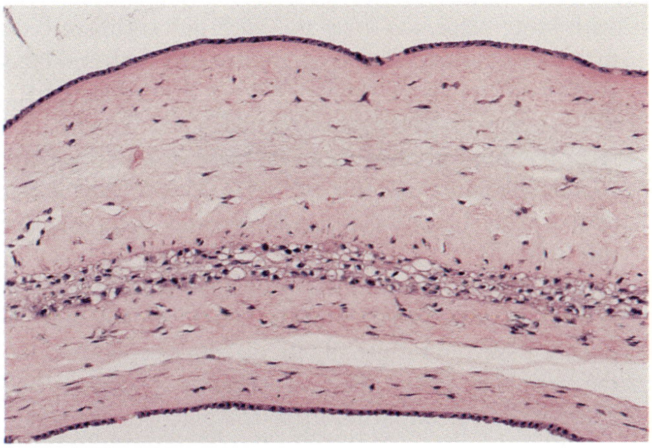

7.21 Dividing membranes of a diamniotic, dichorionic placenta. The dividing membranes contain amnion on both sides with a central fused chorion.

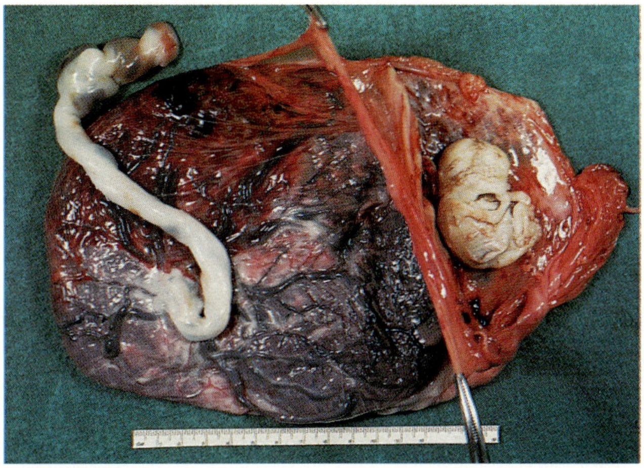

7.22 Diamniotic, dichorionic twin placenta. There is an early intrauterine fetal demise of one twin forming a fetus papyraceus.

Placental Disk

Abnormalities of placental implantation, other than ectopic pregnancy, include placenta previa, in which the placenta partially or completely covers the internal cervical os. Placenta accreta is the condition in which there is direct attachment of the chorionic villi to the uterine muscle without intervening decidua (Figure 7-23). If the chorionic villi extend into the myometrium (Figure 7-24), the condition is termed placenta increta,[45] and if they extend completely through the myometrium, it is termed placenta percreta.[22] A retroplacental hematoma (Figures 7-25 and 7-26) occurs in association with abruptio placentae. The placenta begins to separate prematurely from its uterine attachment, with resultant hemorrhage. The separation may be partial or focal, leaving a scalloped area of indentation in the maternal surface (Figure 7-27).

The placenta can be affected by infectious diseases due to a variety of organisms.[40,49,63] However, the placenta can react in only a limited fashion to a variety of stimuli. Nonspecific changes occur in the placenta as the result of many different infections. Many infections of the placenta contain a chronic villitis with lymphocytes, plasma cells, and histiocytes. In cytomegalovirus infection, characteristic intranuclear inclusions may be found. Syphilitic placentitis (Figures 7-28 and figure 7-29) demonstrates a proliferative endarteritis, and spirochetal organisms as well as granulomas may be found.[67,71,82] *Listeria monocytogenes* is characterized by an acute villitis with microabscesses (Figure 7-30).[81] Villous edema (Figure 7-31) is nonspecific and may be seen in a variety of disorders, including fetal cardiovascular anomalies and genetic abnormalities. Nonspecific chronic villitis composed of lymphocytes and histiocytes (Figure 7-32) is often referred to as villitis of unknown etiology (VUE). This may be related to an immune host-versus-graft reaction.[33,44,68]

Erythroblastosis fetalis results from the hemolysis of fetal red blood cells by maternal antibodies across the placenta. These placentas are markedly edematous and the fetal vessels usually contain nucleated fetal red blood cells (Figure 7-33). Laminated intervillous thrombi (Figure 7-34) are common and are thought to be the result of small fetal-to-maternal hemorrhages. Placental infarctions (Figure 7-35) are common findings and are not clinically significant if they occupy less than 5% of the placental parenchyma.[52,69] They are more frequent in pregnancy-induced hypertension (PIH). Decidual vasculopathy (Figure 7-36) and acute atherosis (Figure 7-37) may be found in the maternal vessels of these patients.[51] PIH is also associated with an appearance of premature aging of the placenta with increased syncytial knots (Figure 7-38). Maternal diabetes is associated with large placentas (over the 90th percentile) and dysmaturity characterized by a mixture of mature (Figure 7-39) and immature (Figure 7-40) villi. Chorangiosis is also seen with increased frequency in diabetes. This term has been applied to an increase in fetal capillaries within chorionic villi (Figure 7-41). This finding is associated with high-risk pregnancies and increased fetal morbidity.[11]

The most common tumor of the placenta is a chorioangioma. It consists of a proliferation of vascular and fibrous tissue and is usually localized to a solid nodule at the periphery of the placenta (Figures 7-42 and 7-43). Maternal metastatic tumors to the placenta are rare.[34]

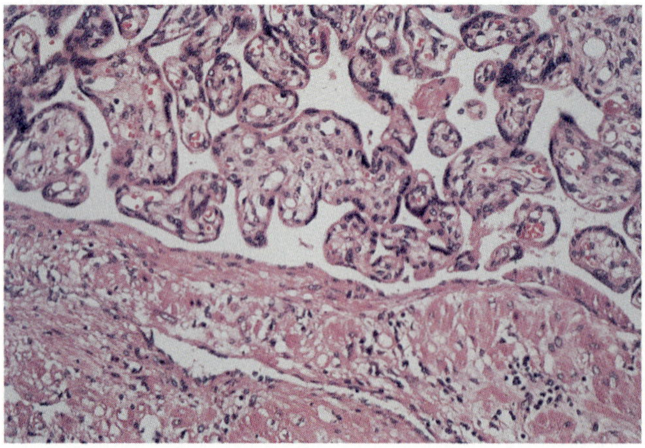

7.23 Placenta accreta demonstrating the implantation of chorionic villi directly into myometrial tissue.

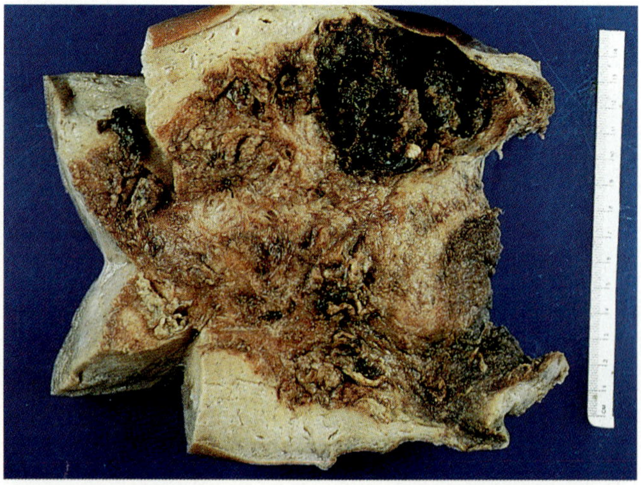

7.24 Placenta increta demonstrating the implantation site with retained placenta infiltrating the myometrium.

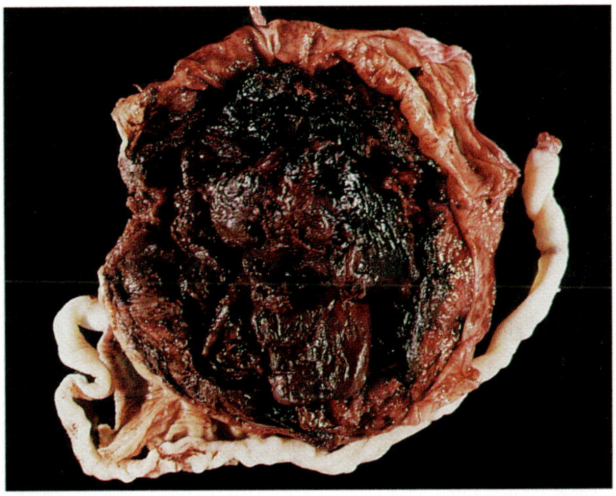

7.25 Retroplacental hematoma with adherent clot over 90% of the maternal surface.

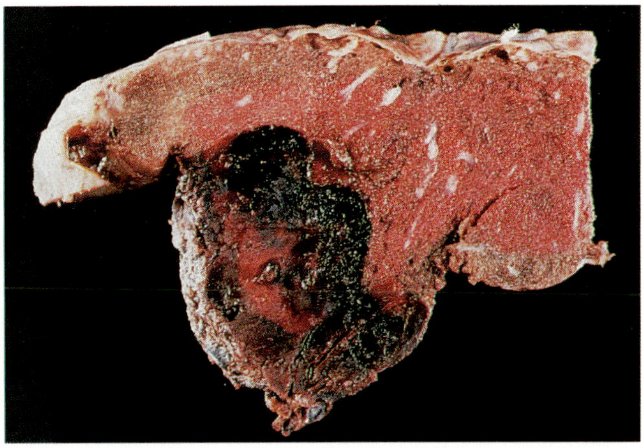

7.26 Cross-section of a retroplacental hematoma with organizing clot.

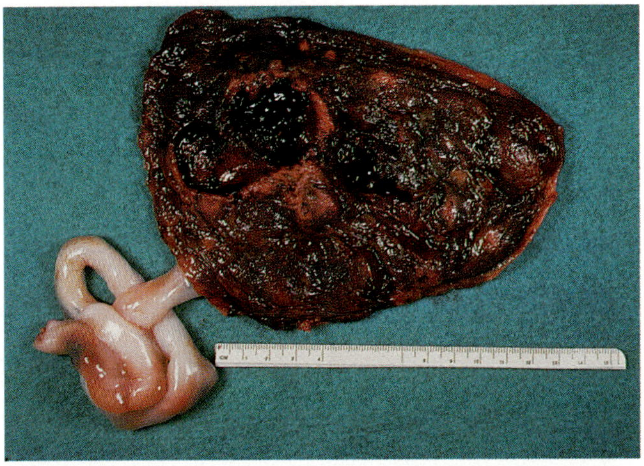

7.27 Retroplacental hematoma with an indented scalloped area of the maternal surface occupying approximately 20% of the placenta.

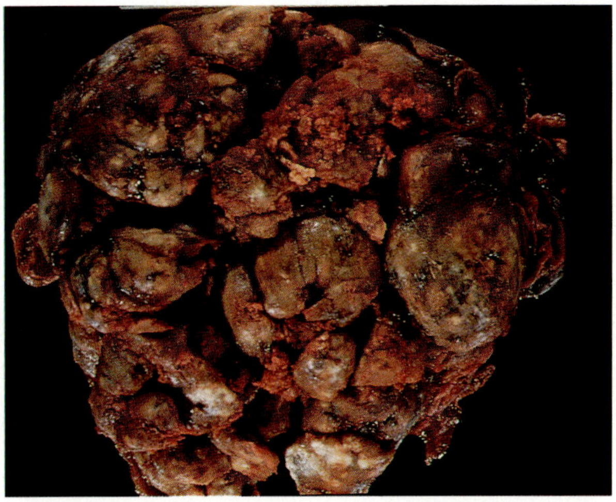

7.28 Syphilitic placenta demonstrating a large placenta with numerous tan-yellow necrotic foci.

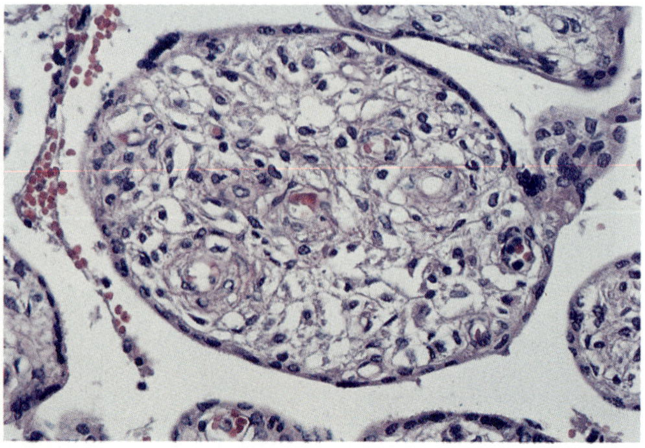

7.29 Chorionic villi from a term placenta in a patient with syphilis. There is an increase in the fibrous stroma of the villi and a proliferative thickening with subsequent narrowing of the fetal vessels.

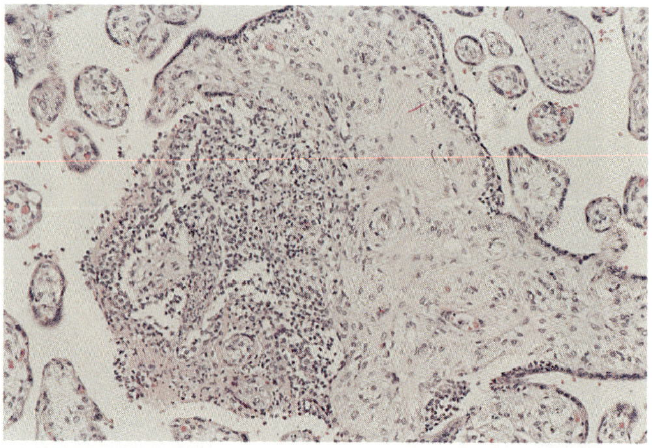

7.30 Acute villitis in a patient with *Listeria monocytogenes* forming microabscesses.

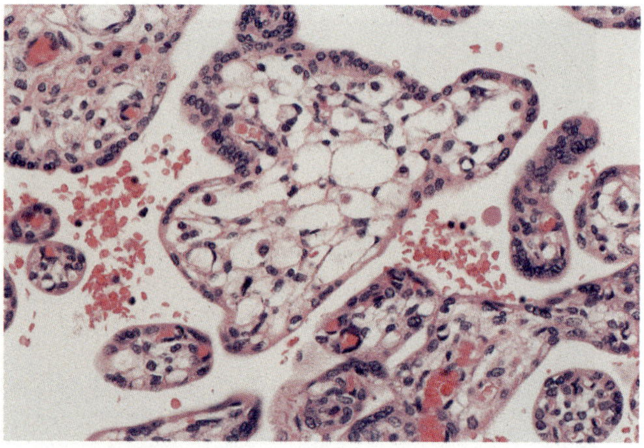

7.31 Villous edema in a 26-week placenta from a patient with acute chorioamnionitis.

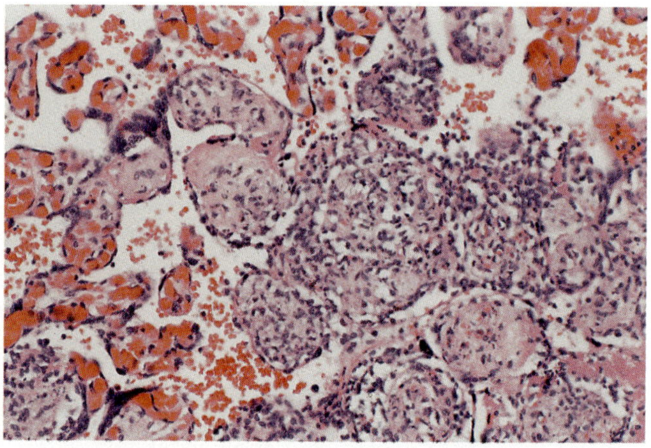

7.32 Villitis of uncertain etiology (VUE). The villi focally contain a proliferation of lymphocytes and histiocytes.

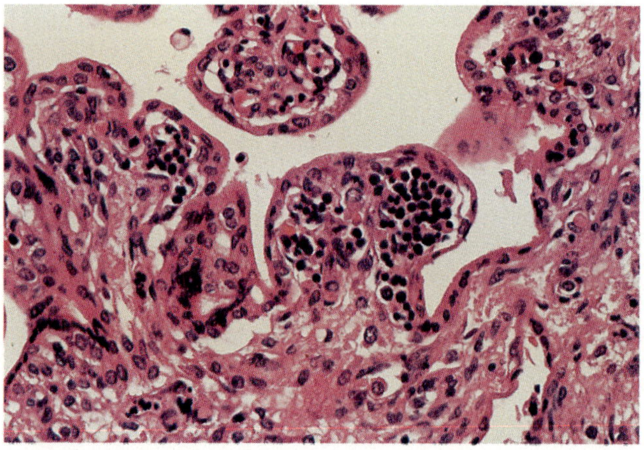

7.33 Numerous nucleated fetal red blood cells in a placenta in a patient with erythroblastosis.

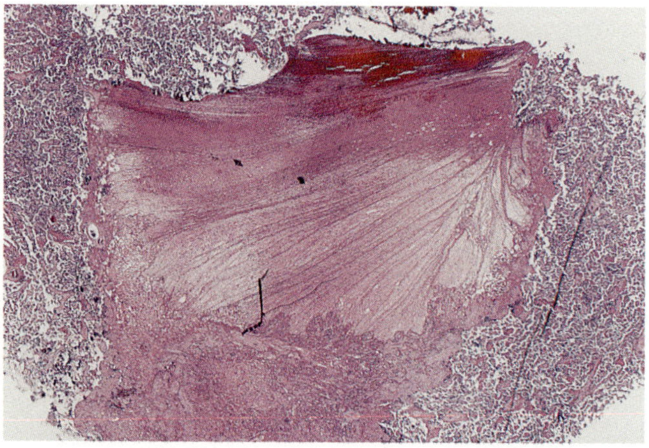

7.34 Intervillous thrombus with a laminated organizing clot.

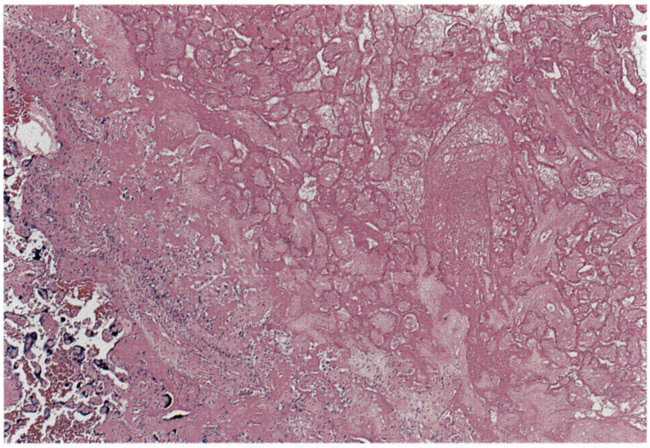

7.35 Placental infarction with ghost chorionic villi.

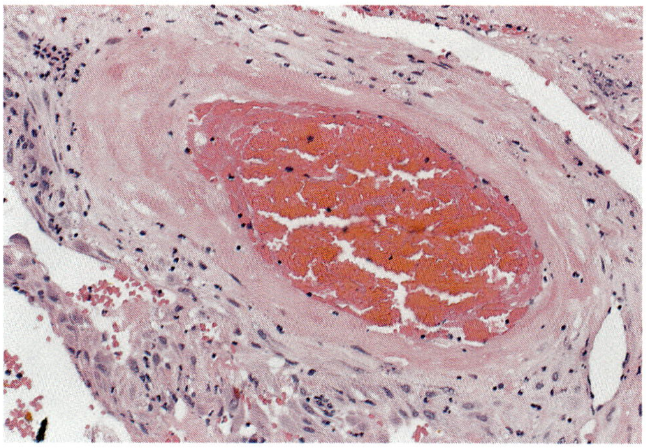

7.36 Decidual vasculopathy in a patient with severe pregnancy-induced hypertension. The maternal decidual vessels are thickened with fibrinoid necrosis.

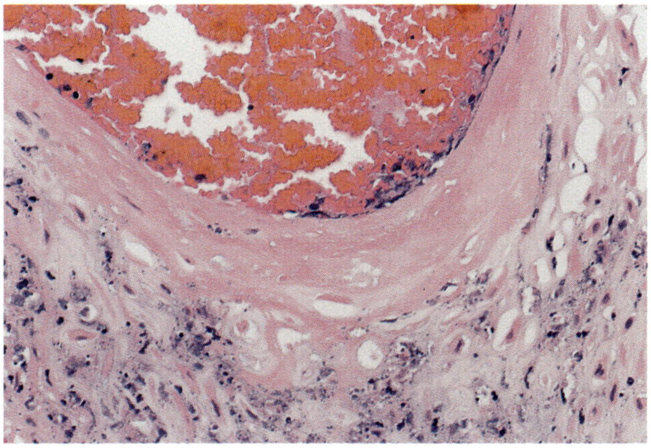

7.37 Focal acute atherosis with foamy histiocytes in the fibrinoid wall of the vessel.

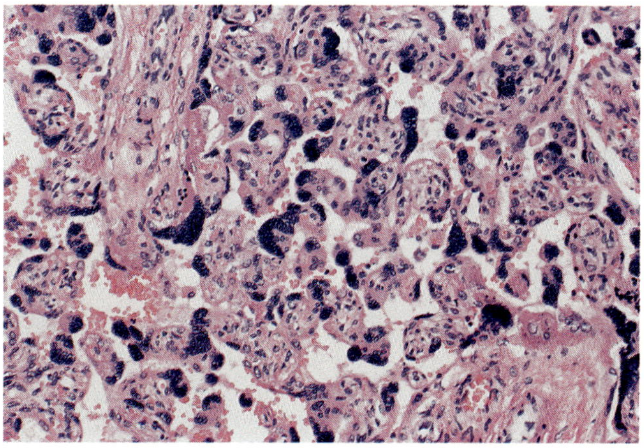

7.38 A 35-week placenta with accelerated maturation containing an increase in syncytial knots.

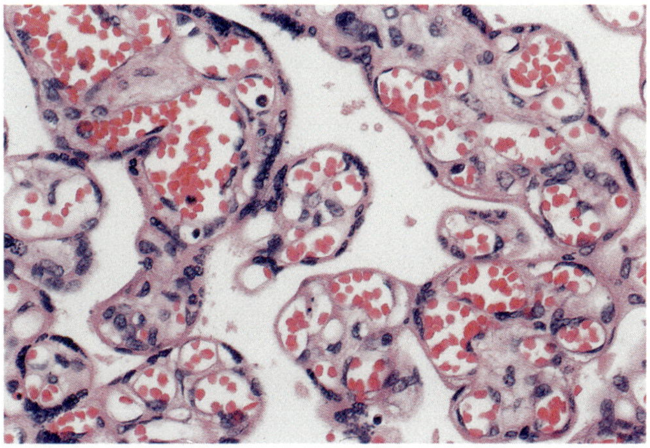

7.39 Third-trimester placenta at 40 weeks showing well-formed vascular syncytial membranes.

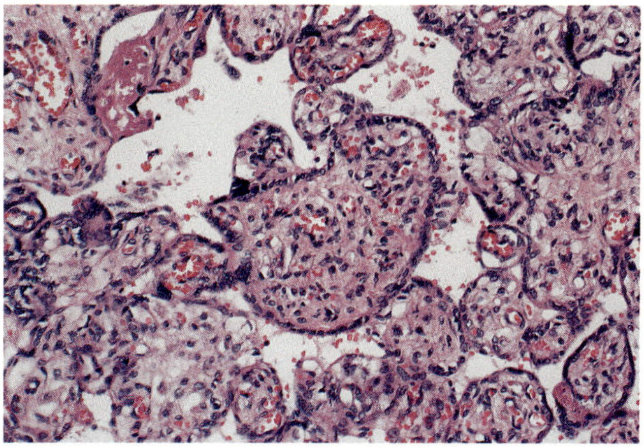

7.40 Dysmature placenta at 40 weeks containing an increase in the stromal tissue of the villi, small fetal vessels, and decreased vascular syncytial membranes.

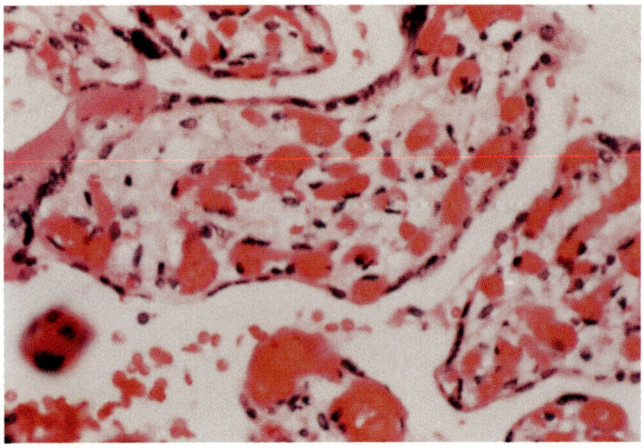

7.41 Chorioangiosis characterized by increased numbers of dilated fetal vessels.

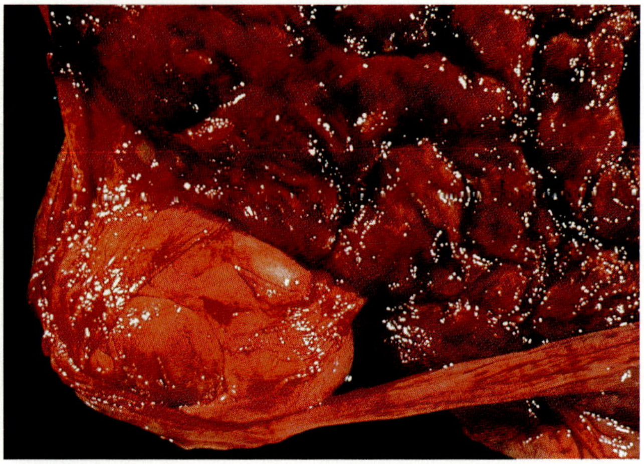

7.42 Chorioangioma presenting as a solid nodule at the edge of the placenta.

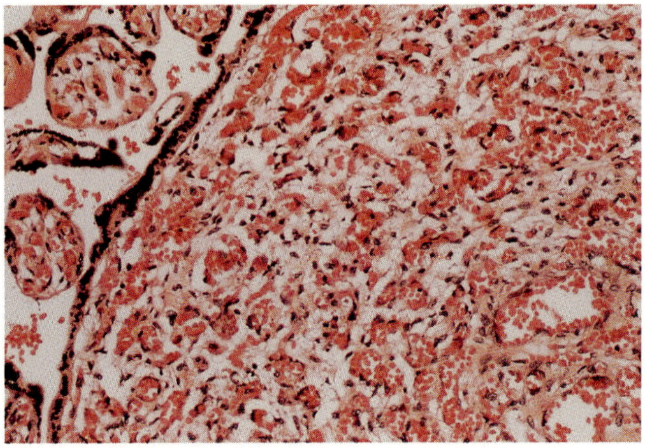

7.43 Chorioangioma containing numerous small vessels.

GESTATIONAL TROPHOBLASTIC DISEASE

Molar Trophoblastic Lesions

Features shared by complete and partial hydatidiform mole and the common abortus include: edematous enlargement of chorionic villi (hydropic change) and disappearance of villous vessels. A hydropic abortus usually does not manifest gross villous swelling. The embryo or fetus is absent in most cases. The important differences between complete and partial mole and the hydropic abortus reside in the trophoblast. Swollen villi of the common abortus are typically surrounded by attenuated trophoblast (Figure 7-44). When trophoblastic proliferation occurs under these circumstances, it is orderly, centrifugal, and polar. Trophoblastic atypia is not a feature of a hydropic abortus, and when present, it is strongly suggestive of trophoblastic neoplasia.[23]

Complete hydatidiform mole (complete mole) more accurately describes most lesions that have previously been termed hydatidiform mole. The complete mole is characterized by gross hydropic swelling of most of the chorionic villi (Figures 7-45 and 7-46) with loss of intravascular vascularity and absence of a fetus. Trophoblastic hyperplasia of varying degree involves most of the chorionic villi (Figures 7-47 and 7-48). The trophoblastic population is composed of all three types of trophoblastic cells (cytotrophoblasts, syncytiotrophoblasts, and intermediate trophoblasts) in varying proportions. Most complete moles develop from fertilization of an empty egg by a single spermatozoon (23,X) that duplicates to become 46,XX.[42,48,74] These are more aggressive than partial moles. Invasive hydatidiform mole (invasive mole) is characterized by hydropic chorionic villi within the myometrium (Figures 7-49 and 7-50) or its vascular spaces, or at distant sites, e.g., vagina or lung. Except under unusual circumstances when curettings contain myometrium with invasive molar villi, the diagnosis of an invasive mole can only be made on a hysterectomy specimen. Most invasive moles are complete moles.

Partial hydatidiform mole (partial mole) is an abnormal conceptus that is usually triploid.[41,57,65,76-80,83] A fetus is nearly always present but may require careful examination to detect, since early fetal demise may result in degeneration.[47] In contrast to complete mole, partial mole is characterized by two populations of chorionic villi, one of normal size and one showing hydropic swelling. Compared with complete mole, the hydropic swelling is more focal and much less pronounced. The chorionic villi of partial mole have a scalloped outline compared with the rounded, distended appearance of the villi in complete mole. The invagination that results forms trophoblastic inclusions (Figure 7-51). In addition, the villous stroma of partial mole frequently undergoes fibrosis in contrast to complete mole in which mesenchymal degeneration is accompanied by cistern formation. Another distinguishing feature of partial mole is the persistence of villous capillaries, frequently containing fetal nucleated red blood cells. The trophoblastic covering the villi is only focally and mildly hyperplastic. The cellular population is composed of cytotrophoblasts and syncytiotrophoblasts; intermediate trophoblasts are rarely encountered.

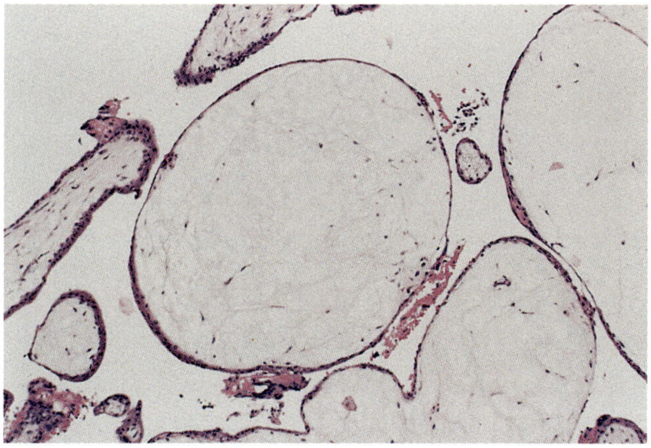

7.44 Hydropic degeneration in chorionic villi, which are evenly round with a thin rim of flattened trophoblastic tissue.

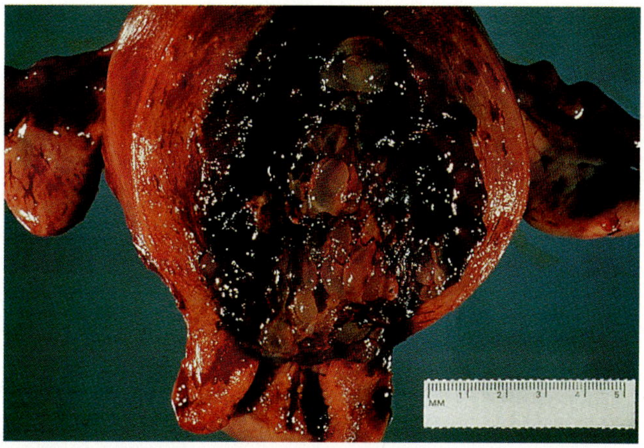

7.45 Gross view of a uterus containing a complete hydatidiform mole.

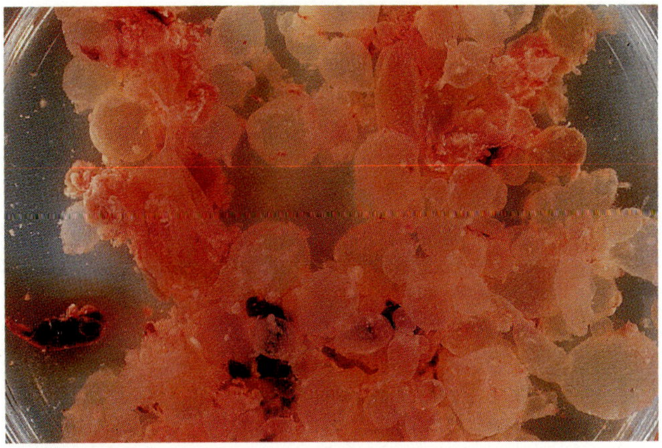

7.46 Complete hydatidiform mole demonstrating numerous enlarged villi.

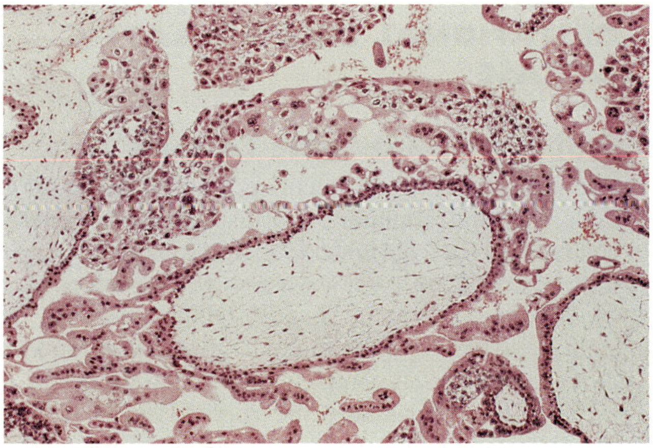

7.47 Complete hydatidiform mole with circumferential trophoblastic proliferation.

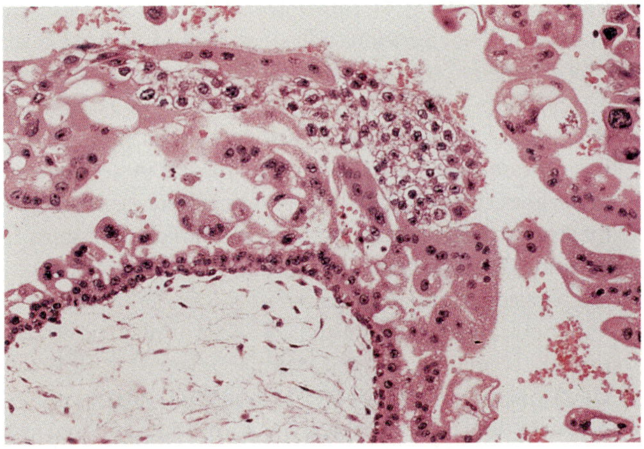

7.48 Complete hydatidiform mole demonstrating an admixture of syncytial and cytotrophoblastic proliferation.

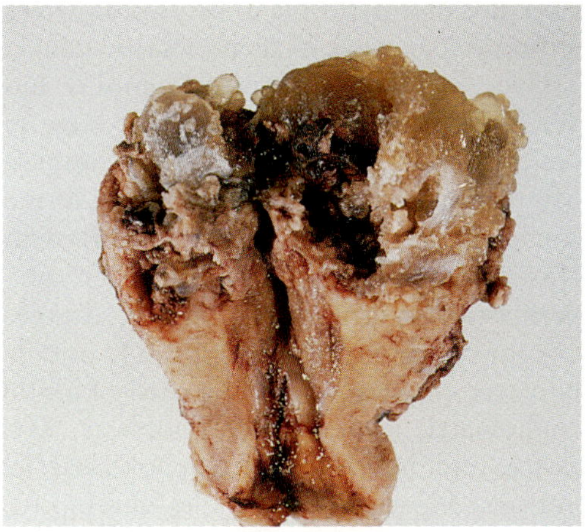

7.49 Invasive hydatidiform mole infiltrating the myometrium.

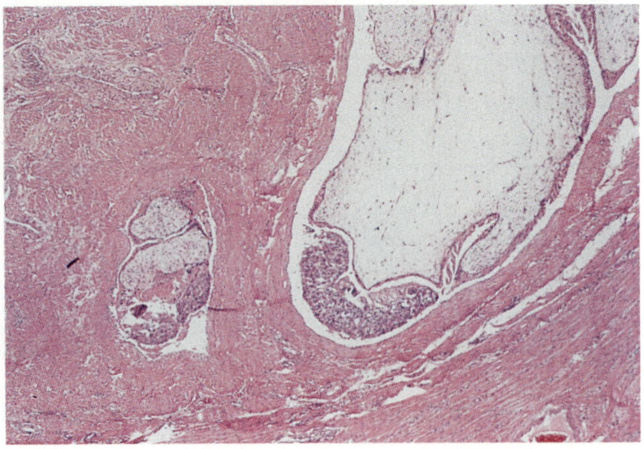

7.50 Invasive hydatidiform mole demonstrating abnormal villi infiltrating the myometrium.

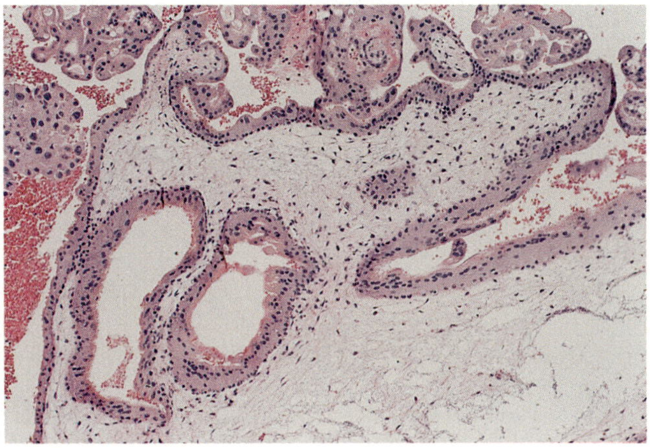

7.51 Partial hydatidiform mole with a scalloped outline, trophoblastic inclusions, and mild trophoblastic proliferation consisting predominantly of syncytial trophoblastic cells.

Nonmolar Trophoblastic Lesions

Gestational choriocarcinoma[20,58] is a malignant neoplasm derived from the trophoblastic epithelium that lacks chorionic villi (Figure 7-52). The tumor is characterized by masses and sheets of cells that invade surrounding tissue and permeate vascular spaces. Generally it grows in an expansile, centrifugal fashion, often accompanied by marked central hemorrhage and necrosis, with viable tumor limited to the interface with the myometrium. The tumor grows in a pattern that recapitulates the growth of the early previllous trophoblast, but it may display a wide variety of patterns. All types of trophoblastic cells are present in varying proportion.

The placental site trophoblastic tumor forms a variably cellular mass occupying the endometrium and myometrium (Figure 7-53). The predominant cellular population consists of intermediate trophoblasts (Figure 7-54), with cytotrophoblasts and syncytiotrophoblasts present to a lesser degree.[36,55,61,85] Most of the intermediate trophoblastic cells are mononucleate, but binucleate, trinucleate, and multinucleate cells are usually present.[53,54,56] As in the normal placental site, the cells at the periphery of the tumor typically infiltrate as single cells and small groups of cells between muscle fibers and bundles without producing extensive necrosis. This bland type of infiltration is also exemplified by the pattern of vascular invasion characterized by mononucleate intermediate trophoblastic cells migrating through and replacing the walls of arteries. Highly cellular areas of placental site trophoblastic tumor form solid masses that destroy the involved endometrium and myometrium.

In most cases the placental site trophoblastic tumor is benign, but occasionally it may behave in a highly malignant fashion.[28,29,38] The differential diagnosis is therefore extremely important, but, in certain instances, may prove to be very difficult because criteria to distinguish the placental site trophoblastic tumor from the placental site trophoblastic reaction are imprecise and poorly delineated. The distinction is particularly critical in dealing with curettings. If the process is focal, admixed with fragments of normal endometrium and myometrium, and if chorionic villi are present, it should be considered a placental site trophoblastic reaction. In contrast, a lesion with features of the placental site reaction that is composed of massive preponderance of trophoblasts with more than just occasional mitotic figures should be classified as a placental site trophoblastic tumor.

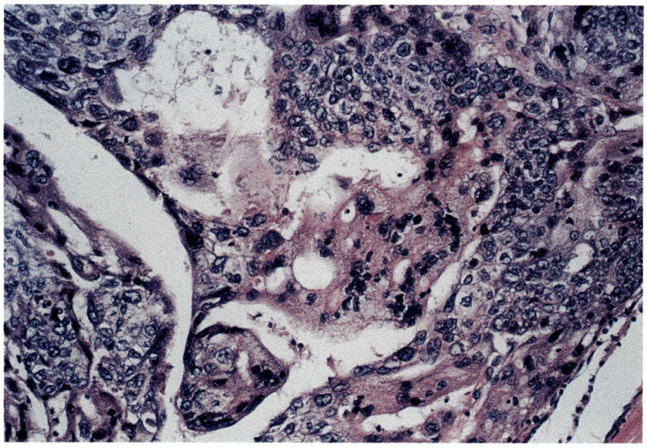

7.52 Choriocarcinoma containing a mixture of syncytial and cytotrophoblastic cells with no chorionic villi.

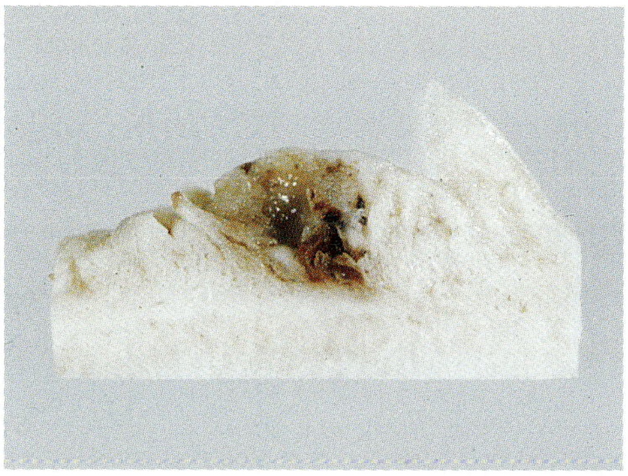

7.53 Gross view of a placental site trophoblastic tumor showing a gross nodule in the endometrium and myometrium.

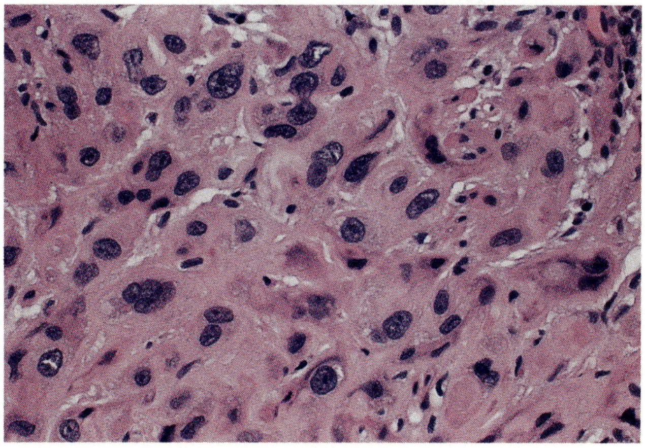

7.54 Placental site trophoblastic tumor with a solid confluent proliferation of intermediate trophoblastic cells showing scattered nuclear atypia.

Miscellaneous Trophoblastic Lesions

This term is used to describe those lesions previously diagnosed as trophoblastic neoplasms, that do not have the typical appearance of choriocarcinoma or placental site trophoblastic tumor. An exaggerated placental site reaction (Figure 7-55) and placental site nodule or plaques (Figure 7-56) are the lesions currently in this category.[39,84]

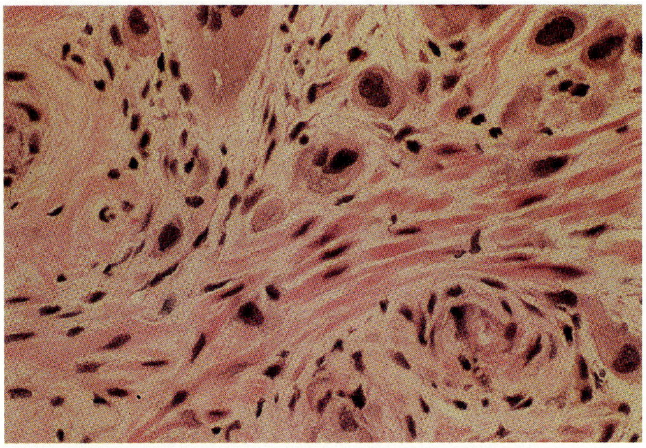

7.55 Exaggerated placental site reaction with scattered intermediate trophoblasts infiltrating myometrial fibers.

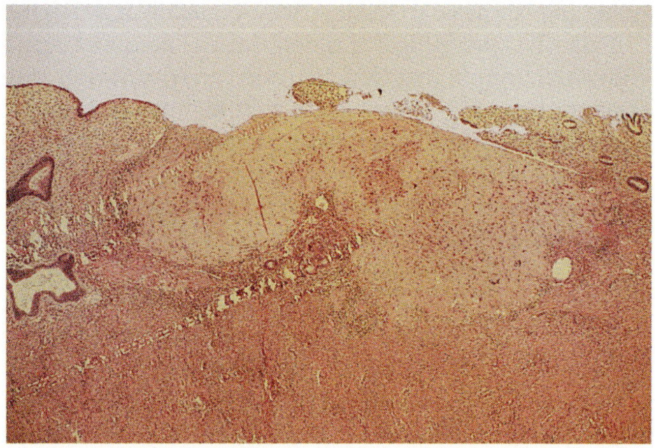

7.56 Placental site plaque forming a superficial plaquelike area from a previous implantation.

World Health Organization (WHO) Histologic Classification of Gestational Trophoblastic Disease[9]

(with associated SNOMED codes)

	SNOMED
I. Hydatidiform Mole	91000
A. Complete	91000
B. Partial	91030
II. Invasive Hydatidiform Mole (chorioadenoma destruens)	91001
III. Choriocarcinoma	91003
IV. Placental Site Trophoblastic Tumor	91041
V. Miscellaneous Trophoblastic Lesions	
A. Exaggerated placental site	79420
B. Placental site nodule or plaque	
VI. Unclassified Trophoblastic Lesions	

Clinical Staging for Gestational Trophoblastic Disease

The International Federation of Gynecology and Obstetrics (FIGO)

Stage I Disease confined to the uterus
- IA. Disease confined to the uterus with no risk factors
- IB. Disease confined to the uterus with one risk factor
- IC. Disease confined to the uterus with two risk factors

Stage II Gestational trophoblastic tumor (GTT) extends outside of the uterus but is limited to the genital structures (adnexa, vagina, broad ligament)
- IIA. GTT involving genital structures without risk factors
- IIB. GTT extends outside of the uterus but is limited to the genital structures with one risk factor
- IIC. GTT extends outside of the uterus but is limited to the genital structures with two risk factors

Stage III GTT extends to the lungs with or without known genital tract involvement
- IIIA. GTT extends to the lungs with or without genital tract involvement and with no risk factor
- IIIB. GTT extends to the lungs with or without genital tract involvement and with one risk factor
- IIIC. GTT extends to the lungs with or without genital tract involvement and with two risk factors

Stage IV All other metastatic sites
- IVA. All other metastatic sites without risk factors
- IVB. All other metastatic sites with one risk factor
- IVC. All other metastatic sites with two risk factors

Risk factors affecting staging include the following:
1. Human chorionic gonadotropin >100,000 mIU/ml
2. Duration of disease >6 months from termination of the antecedent pregnancy

The following factors should be considered and noted in reporting:
1. Prior chemotherapy for known GTT
2. Placental site tumors should be reported separately
3. Histologic verification of disease is not required

Notes to the Staging

The staging should be based on actual clinical examination, chest radiography, and other appropriate studies. It should be performed before any definitive therapy is begun. It is desirable that the evaluation be conducted by experienced physicians.

The clinical stage must under no circumstances be changed on the basis of subsequent findings. Those cases that do not fulfill the criteria for any given stage should be listed separately as "unstaged."

Physicians may dictate which findings should serve as a basis for clinical staging of gestational trophoblastic tumors. The Cancer Committee of FIGO considers it important that such examinations that can be carried out at any hospital by the physicians and surgeons be used exclusively. The following examinations fulfill this requirement: palpation, inspection, cystoscopy, intravenous pyelography, electroencephalography, x-ray examinations of the lungs, pelvic examinations, computed tomographic scan of the brain, liver function tests, liver scan, curettage. findings by examinations such as arteriography, laparoscopy, hysteroscopy, and hysterography are of value for planning of therapy but should have no influence on the staging. They are not carried out on a routine basis and the interpretation of the results is not uniform.

The clinical staging of gestational trophoblastic tumors should be based on the examination methods mentioned above. Hysterectomy and dilatation and curettage should also be regarded as a clinical examination.

BIBLIOGRAPHY

General Reading

1. Altshuler G: *The placenta.* In Steinberg SS, editor: *Diagnostic surgical pathology,* ed 2, New York, 1994, Raven Press.
2. Benirschke K, Kaufman P: *Pathology of the human placenta,* ed 3, New York, 1995, Springer-Verlag.
3. Joshi VV: *Handbook of placental pathology,* New York, 1994, Igaku-Shoin.
4. Kaplan CG: *Color atlas of gross placental pathology,* ed 2, New York, 1994, Springer-Verlag.
5. Kurman RJ, editor: *Blaustein's pathology of the female genital tract,* ed 4, New York, 1994, Springer-Verlag.
6. Mazur MT, Kurman RJ: *Gestational trophoblastic disease,* In Sternberg SS, editor: *Diagnostic surgical pathology,* ed 2, New York, 1994, Raven Press.
7. Naeye RL: *Disorders of the placenta, fetus, and neonate: Diagnosis and clinical significance,* St Louis, 1992, Mosby-Year Book.
8. Silverberg SG, Kurman RJ: *Tumors of the uterine corpus and gestational trophoblastic disease. Atlas of tumor pathology,* 3rd series, fascicle 3, Washington, DC, 1992, Armed Forces Institute of Pathology.
9. Scully RE, Bonfiglio TA, Kurman RJ, Silverberg SG, Wilkinson EJ: *World Health Organization. Histological classification of tumors of the female genital tract,* New York, 1994, Springer-Verlag.
10. Woodruff JD, Angtuaco TL, Parmley TH: *Atlas of gynecologic pathology,* ed 2, New York, 1993, Raven Press.

References

11. Altshuler G: Chorangiosis. An important placental sign of neonatal morbidity and mortality, *Arch Pathol Lab Med* 108:71-74, 1984.
12. Altshuler G. College of American Pathologists Conference XIX on the examination of the placenta: report of the working group on indications for placental examination, *Arch Pathol Lab Med* 115:701-703, 1991.
13. Altshuler G: Placenta within the medicolegal imperative, *Arch Pathol Lab Med* 115:688-695, 1991.
14. Altshuler G: A conceptual approach to placental pathology and pregnancy outcome, *Semin Diagn Pathol* 10:204-221, 1993.
15. Altshuler G, Hyde S: Meconium induced vasoconstriction: a potential cause of cerebral and other fetal hypoperfusion and of poor pregnancy outcome, *Child Neurol* 4:137-142, 1989.
16. Altshuler G, Tsang RC, Ermocilla R: Single umbilical artery. Correlation of clinical status and umbilical cord histology, *Am J Dis Child* 129:697-700, 1975.
17. Benirschke K: The placenta in the context of history and modern medical practice, *Arch Pathol Lab Med* 115:663-667, 1991.
18. Benirschke K: Intrauterine death of a twin: mechanisms, implications for surviving twin, and placental pathology, *Semin Diagn Pathol* 10:222-231, 1993.
19. Benirschke K: Obstetrically important lesions of the umbilical cord, *J Reprod Med* 39:262-272, 1994.
20. Berkowitz RS, Goldstein DP: Gestational trophoblastic disease, *Cancer* 76:2079-2085, 1995.
21. Berkus MD, Langer O, Samueloff A, Xenakis EM, Field NT, Ridgway LE: Meconium-stained amniotic fluid: increased risk for adverse neonatal outcome, *Obstet Gynecol* 84:115-120, 1994.
22. Breen JL, Neubecker R, Gregori CA, Franklin JE Jr: Placenta accreta, increta, and percreta. A survey of 40 cases, *Obstet Gynecol* 49:43-47, 1977.
23. Conran RM, Hitchcock CL, Popek EJ, Norris HJ, Griffin JL, Geissel A, McCarthy WF: Diagnostic considerations in molar gestations, *Hum Pathol* 24:41-48, 1993.
24. Cordry RD: Placental evidence in malpractice litigation: plaintiff's case, *Arch Pathol Lab Med* 115:682-684, 1991.
25. Craver RD, Baldwin VJ: Necrotizing funisitis, *Obstet Gynecol* 79:64-70, 1992.
26. Driscoll SG: Placental examination in a clinical setting, *Arch Pathol Lab Med* 115:668-671, 1991.
27. Driscoll SG, Langston C: College of American Pathologists Conference XIX on the examination of the placenta: report of the working group on methods for placental examination, *Arch Pathol Lab Med* 115:704-708, 1991.
28. Fukunaga M, Ushigome S: Malignant trophoblastic tumors: immunohistochemical and flow cytometric comparison of choriocarcinoma and placental site trophoblastic tumors, *Hum Pathol* 24:1098-1106, 1993.
29. Fukunaga M, Ushigome S: Metastasizing placental site trophoblastic tumor: an immunohistochemical and flow cytometric study of two cases, *Am J Surg Pathol* 17:1003-1010, 1993.
30. Genest DR: Estimating the time of death in stillborn fetuses: II. Histologic evaluation of the placenta; a study of 71 stillborns, *Obstet Gynecol* 80:585-592, 1992.

31. Genest DR, Williams MA, Greene MF: Estimating the time of death in stillborn fetuses: I. Histologic evaluation of fetal organs; an autopsy study of 150 stillborns, *Obstet Gynecol* 80:575-584, 1992.
32. Genest DR, Singer DB: Estimating the time of death in stillborn fetuses: III. External fetal examination; a study of 86 stillborns, *Obstet Gynecol* 80:593-600, 1992.
33. Gersell DJ: Chronic villitis, chronic chorioamnionitis, and maternal floor infarction, *Semin Diagn Pathol* 10:251-266, 1993.
34. Greenberg J, Collins JD, Voet RL, Jariwala L: Ewing's sarcoma metastatic to placenta, *Placenta* 3:191-196, 1982.
35. Heifetz SA, Bauman M: Necrotizing funisitis and herpes simplex infection of placental and decidual tissues: study of four cases, *Hum Pathol* 25:715-722, 1994.
36. Heintz APM, Schaberg A, Engelsman E, van Hall EV: Placental-site trophoblastic tumor: diagnosis, treatment, and biological behavior, *Int J Gynecol Pathol* 4:75-82, 1985.
37. Hood IC, Desa DJ, Whyte RK: The inflammatory response in candidal chorioamnionitis, *Hum Pathol* 14:984-990, 1983.
38. Hopkins M, Nunez C, Murphy JR, Wentz WB: Malignant placental site trophoblastic tumor, *Obstet Gynecol* 66:95S-100S, 1985.
39. Huettner PC, Gersell DJ: Placental site nodule: a clinicopathologic study of 38 cases, *Int J Gynecol Pathol* 13:191-198, 1994.
40. Hyde SR, Giacoia GP: Congenital herpes infection: placental and umbilical cord findings, *Obstet Gynecol* 81:852-855, 1993.
41. Jacobs PA, Szulman AE, Funkhouser J, Matsura JS, Wilson CC: Human triploidy: relationship between parental origin of the additional haploid complement and development of partial hydatidiform mole, *Ann Hum Genet* 46:223-231, 1982.
42. Jacobs PA, Wilson CM, Sprenkle JA, Rosenshein NB, Migeon BR: Mechanism of origin of complete hydatidiform moles, *Nature* 286:714-716, 1980.
43. Jacques SM, Qureshi F: Necrotizing funisitis: a study of 45 cases, *Hum Pathol* 23:1278-1283, 1992.
44. Jacques SM, Qureshi F: Chronic intervillositis of the placenta, *Arch Pathol Lab Med* 117:1032-1035, 1993.
45. Jacques SM, Qureshi F, Trent VS, Ramirez NC: Placenta accreta: mild cases diagnosed by placental examination, *Int J Gynecol Pathol* 15:28-33, 1996.
46. Jauniaux E, Elkazen N, Leroy F, Wilkin P, Rodesch F, Hustin J: Clinical and morphologic aspects of the vanishing twin phenomenon, *Obstet Gynecol* 72:577-581, 1988.
47. Jefers MD, O'Dwyer P, Curran B, Leader M, Gillan JE: Partial hydatidiform mole: a common but underdiagnosed condition, *Int J Gynecol Pathol* 12:315-323, 1993.
48. Kajii T, Ohama K: Androgenic origin of hydatidiform mole, *Nature* 268:633-634, 1978.
49. Kaplan C: The placenta and viral infections, *Semin Diagn Pathol* 10:232-250, 1993.
50. Kaplan C, Lowell DM, Salafia C: College of American Pathologists Conference XIX on the examination of the placenta: report of the working group on the definition of structural changes associated with abnormal function in the maternal/fetal/placental unit in the second and third trimesters, *Arch Pathol Lab Med* 115:709-716, 1991.
51. Khong TY: Acute atherosis in pregnancies complicated by hypertension, small-for-gestational-age infants, and diabetes mellitus, *Arch Pathol Lab Med* 115:722-725, 1991.
52. Kraus FT: Placental thrombi and related problems, *Semin Diagn Pathol* 10:275-283, 1993.
53. Kurman RJ: The morphology, biology and pathology of intermediate trophoblast: a look back to the present, *Hum Pathol* 22:847-855, 1991.
54. Kurman RJ, Main CS, Chen H: Intermediate trophoblast: a distinctive form of trophoblast with specific morphologic, biochemical, and functional features, *Placenta* 5:349-369, 1984.
55. Kurman RJ, Scully RE, Norris HJ: Trophoblastic pseudotumor of the uterus, *Cancer* 38:1214-1226, 1976.
56. Kurman RJ, Young RH, Norris HJ, Main CS, Lawrence WD, Scully RE: Immunocytochemical localization of placental lactogen and chorionic gonadotropin in the normal placenta and trophoblastic tumors, with emphasis on intermediate trophoblast and the placental site trophoblastic tumor, *Int J Gynecol Pathol* 3:101-121, 1984.
57. Lage JM, Popek EJ: The role of DNA flow cytometry in evaluation of partial and complete hydatidiform moles and hydropic abortions, *Semin Diagn Pathol* 10:267-274, 1993.
58. Lage JM, Roberts DJ: Choriocarcinoma in a term placenta: pathologic diagnosis of tumor in an asymptomatic patient with metastatic disease, *Int J Gynecol Pathol* 12:80-85, 1993.

59. Leung AK, Robson WL: Single umbilical artery. A report of 159 cases, *Am J Dis Child* 143:108-111, 1989.
60. Macpherson T: Fact and fancy: what can we really tell from the placenta?, *Arch Pathol Lab Med* 115:672-681, 1991.
61. Maymon R, Maymon B, Shulman A, Pomeranz M, Bahary C: Placental site trophoblastic tumors (trophoblastic pseudotumors): pathology and clinical importance, *Obstet Gynecol Surv* 45:654-655, 1990.
62. Miller PW, Coen RW, Benirschke K: Dating the time interval from meconium passage to birth, *Obstet Gynecol* 66:459-462, 1985.
63. Muhlemann K, Miller RK, Metlay L, Menegus MA: Cytomegalovirus infection of the human placenta: an immunocytochemical study, *Hum Pathol* 23:1234-1237, 1992.
64. Naeye R, Travers H: College of American Pathologists Conference XIX on the examination of the placenta: report of the working group on the role of the pathologist in malpractice litigation involving the placenta, *Arch Pathol Lab Med* 115:717-719, 1991.
65. Ohama K, Ueda K, Okamoto E, Takenaka M, Fujiwara A: Cytogenetic and clinicopathologic studies of partial moles, *Obstet Gynecol* 68:259-262, 1986.
66. Parilla VB, Tamura RK, MacGregor N, Beibel LK, Sabbagha RE: The clinical significance of a single umbilical artery as an isolated finding on prenatal ultrasound, *Obstet Gynecol* 85:570-572, 1995.
67. Qureshi F, Jacques SM, Reyes MP: Placental histopathology in syphilis, *Hum Pathol* 24:779-784, 1993.
68. Redline RW, Patterson P: Villitis of unknown etiology is associated with major infiltration of fetal tissue by maternal inflammatory cells, *Am J Pathol* 143:473-479, 1993.
69. Redline RW, Patterson P: Patterns of placental injury. Correlations with gestational age, placental weight, and clinical diagnoses, *Arch Pathol Lab Med* 118:698-701, 1994.
70. Russel P: Inflammatory lesions of the human placenta. I. Clinical significance of acute chorioamnionitis, *Am J Diagn Gynecol Obstet* 1:127-137, 1979.
71. Russel P, Altshuler G: Placental abnormalities of congenital syphilis, *Am J Dis Child* 128:160-163, 1974.
72. Salafia CM, Weigl C, Silberman L: The prevalence and distribution of acute placental inflammation in uncomplicated term pregnancies, *Obstet Gynecol* 73:383-389, 1989.
73. Schindler NR: Importance of the placenta and cord in the defense of neurologically impaired infant claims, *Arch Pathol Lab Med* 115:685-687, 1991.
74. Steller MA, Genest DR, Bernstein MR, Lage JM, Goldstein DP, Berkowitz RS: Natural history of twin pregnancy with complete hydatidiform mole and coexisting fetus, *Obstet Gynecol* 83:35-42, 1994.
75. Strong TH, Elliott JP, Radin TG: Non-coiled umbilical blood vessels: a new marker for the festus at risk, *Obstet Gynecol* 81:409-411, 1993.
76. Szulman AE: Examination of the early conceptus, *Arch Pathol Lab Med* 115:696-700, 1991.
77. Szulman AE, Phillipe E, Boue JG, Boue A: Human triploidy: association with partial hydatidiform moles and nonmolar conceptuses, *Hum Pathol* 12:1016-1021, 1981.
78. Szulman AE, Surti U: The syndromes of hydratidiform mole: I. Cytogenetic and morphologic correlations, *Am J Obstet Gynecol* 131:665-671, 1978.
79. Szulman AE, Surti U: The syndromes of hydatidiform mole: II. Morphologic evolution of the complete and partial mole, *Am J Obstet Gynecol* 132:20-27, 1978.
80. Szulman AE, Surti U: The syndromes of partial and complete molar gestation, *Clin Obstet Gynecol* 27:172-180, 1984.
81. Topalovski M, Yang SS, Boonpasat Y: Listeriosis of the placenta: clinicopathologic study of seven cases, *Am J Obstet Gynecol* 169:616-620, 1993.
82. Walter P, Blot P, Ivanoff B: The placental lesions in congenital syphilis. A study of six cases, *Virchows Arch (Pathol Anat)* 397:313-326, 1982.
83. Watson EJ, Hernandez E, Miyazawa K: Partial hydatidiform moles: a review, *Obstet Gynecol Surv* 42:540-544, 1987.
84. Young RH, Kurman RJ, Scully RE: Placental site nodules and plaques: a clinicopathologic analysis of 20 cases, *Am J Surg Pathol* 14:1001-1009, 1990.
85. Young RH, Scully RE: Placental-site trophoblastic tumor: current status, *Clin Obstet Gynecol* 27:248-258, 1984.
86. Zhang J, Kraus FT, Aquino TI: Chorioamnionitis: a comparative histologic, bacteriologic, and clinical study, *Int J Gynecol Pathol* 4:1-10, 1985.

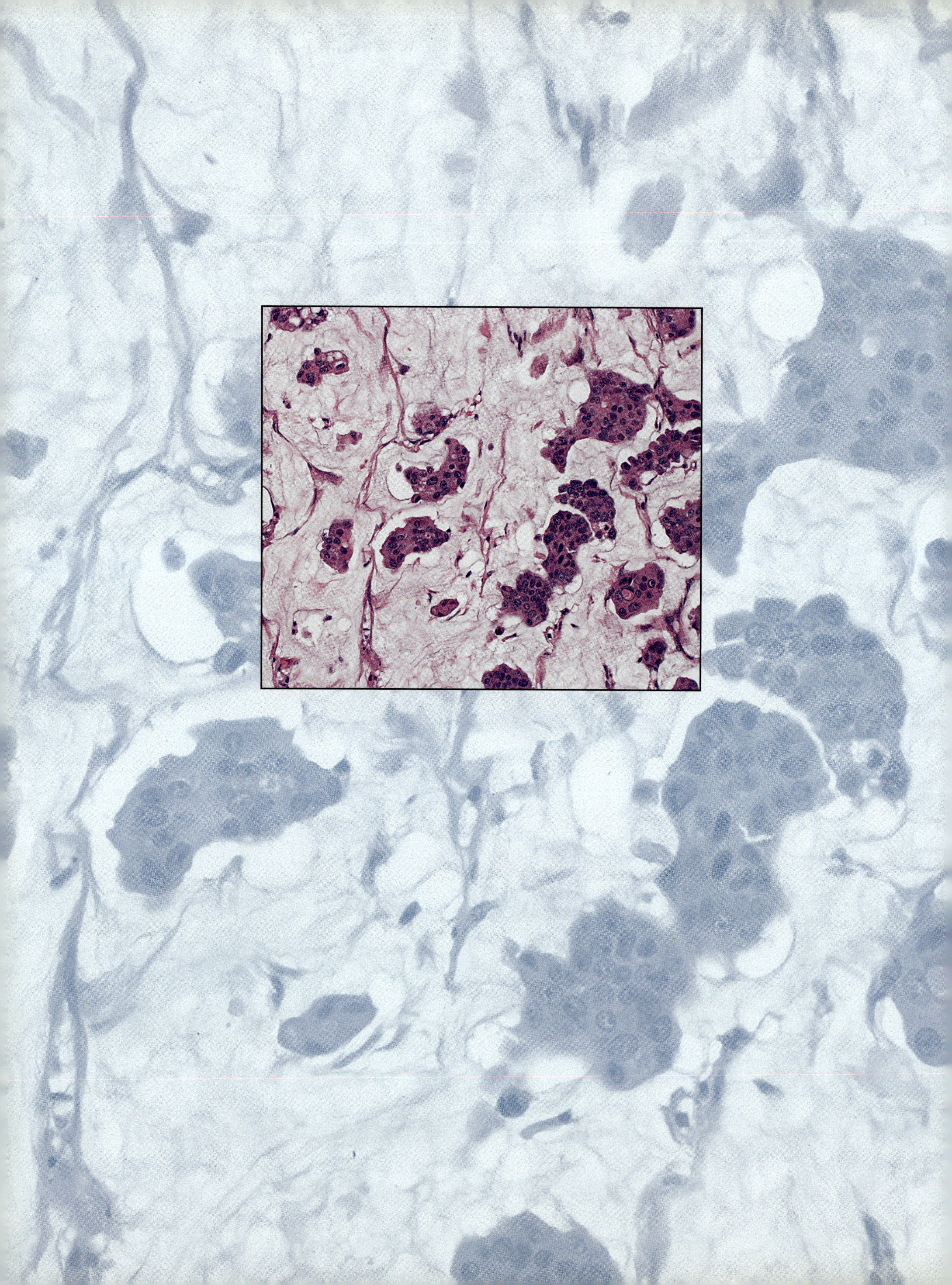

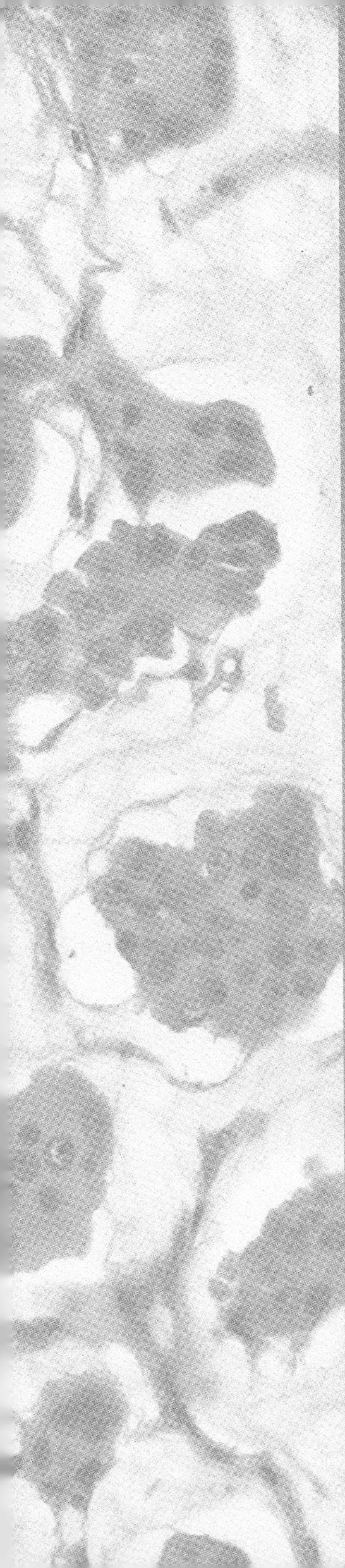

Chapter 8

Pathology of the Breast

Gynecologists are often the first physicians consulted when the patient has a problem in the breast, especially with their increasing role as primary care physicians. This role also places the gynecologist in a position of follow-up care for women who have had a diagnosis of breast cancer and a variety of premalignant breast lesions. A working knowledge of the terminology used to describe a variety of breast lesions and of the techniques available for diagnosis is essential for the practicing clinician responsible for women's healthcare. In addition, medicolegal issues, especially related to the failure to diagnose breast cancer, are a major concern in the delivery of women's healthcare.[25,48] A variety of references are available for a more in-depth study of breast pathology.[1-10]

REACTIVE AND INFLAMMATORY LESIONS

Acute mastitis may be seen in association with pregnancy and lactation and may proceed to the development of an abscess. A subareolar abscess may develop in women of all ages, unrelated to pregnancy. Granulomatous mastitis (Figure 8-1) is often idiopathic and usually presents as a palpable nodule in a patient without a history of specific infection, a foreign body, or evidence of sarcoidosis. Fat necrosis (Figure 8-2) is usually seen after trauma to the breast. Mammary duct ectasia is a specific lesion apart from fibrocystic changes. There is dilatation of the major ducts with an associated inflammatory reaction and varying degrees of fibrosis, producing a palpable mass (Figure 8-3). The lesion is usually in the subareolar area and occurs more often in patients over the age of 50.

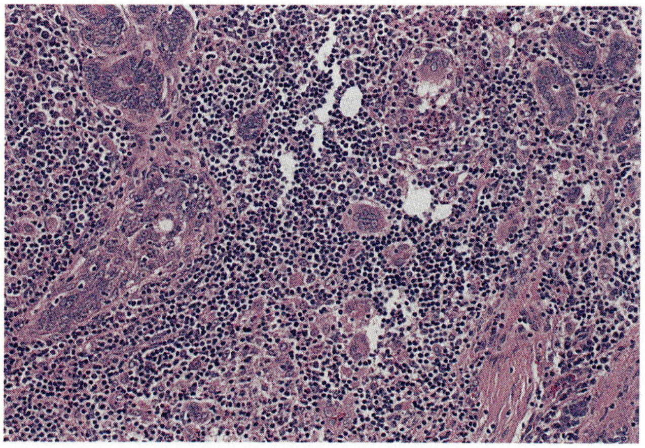

8.1 Granulomatous mastitis containing a lymphoplasmacytic infiltrate with multinucleated giant cells.

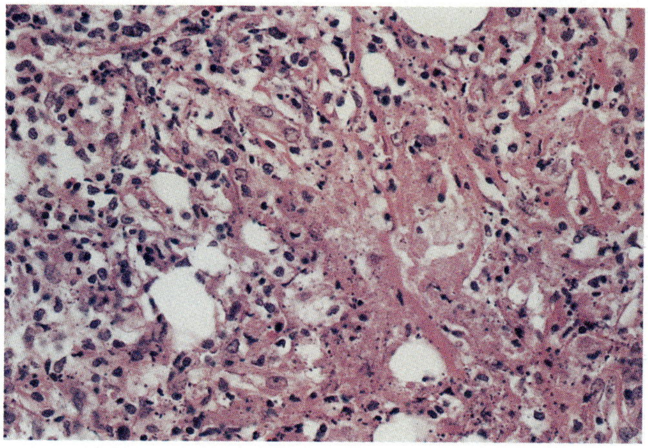

8.2 Fat necrosis with fibrosis, acute inflammation, and degenerating fat cells with vacuolation.

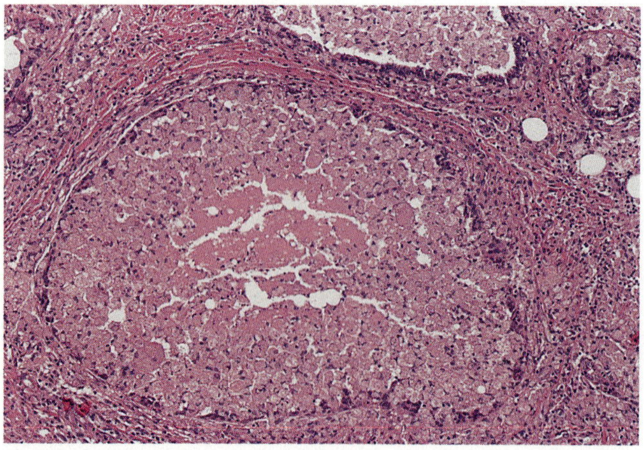

8.3 Mammary duct ectasia characterized by ductal dilatation filled with foamy histiocytes.

PROLIFERATIVE CHANGES

The term fibrocystic change encompasses a variety of changes in the breast. The Cancer Committee of the College of American Pathologists has subdivided various patterns of fibrocystic changes into major risk categories (Table 8-1).[27,28] Some modifications have been suggested, such as including sclerosing adenosis and fibroadenoma in the "slightly increased risk" category.[17,33] Macroscopic cysts (Figure 8-4) are often seen with surrounding fibrosis. Histologically, varying degrees of ductal dilatation and adenosis (Figure 8-5) and often apocrine metaplasia (Figure 8-6) are seen. Sclerosing adenosis is characterized by elongated glandular tubules compressed by the fibrous stroma (Figure 8-7). The glands retain the two cell layers, which should be useful in distinguishing this lesion from a tubular carcinoma. Varying degrees of hyperplasia are seen in fibrocystic changes. Mild hyperplasia exists when there are two to four cell layers of proliferation. Moderate and florid hyperplasia (Figure 8-8) has a more extensive epithelial proliferation that often includes solid nests protruding into the lumen. Atypical ductal hyperplasia has been poorly defined, and recent studies have attempted to more clearly define lesions that fall into this category. This category includes those lesions containing both architectural and cytologic features that are similar to, but fall short of, the diagnosis of a ductal carcinoma in situ (DCIS) (Figure 8-9).

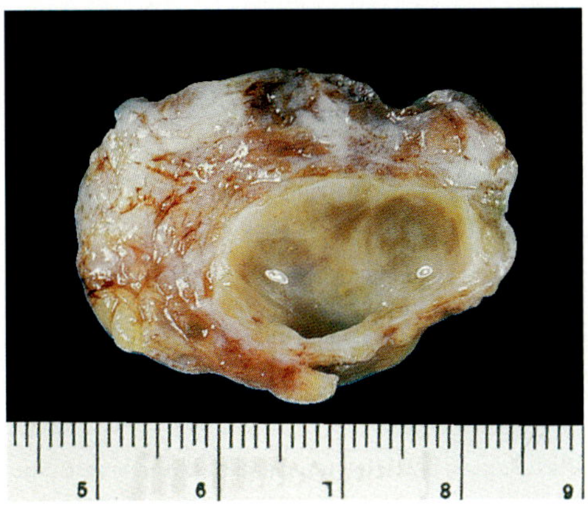

8.4 Fibrocystic changes of the breast with a macroscopic cyst.

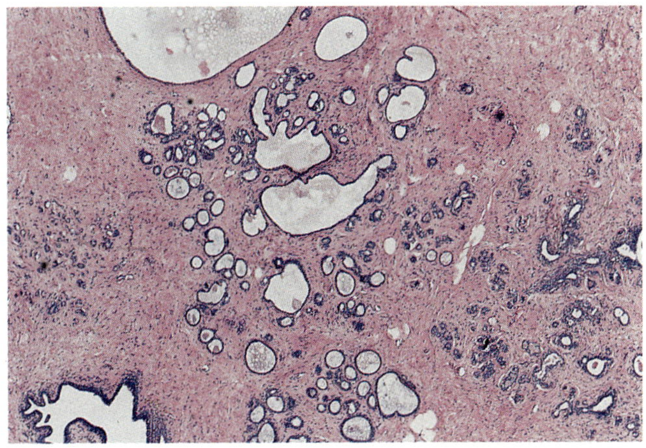

8.5 Fibrocystic changes of the breast containing ductal dilatation, fibrosis, and adenosis.

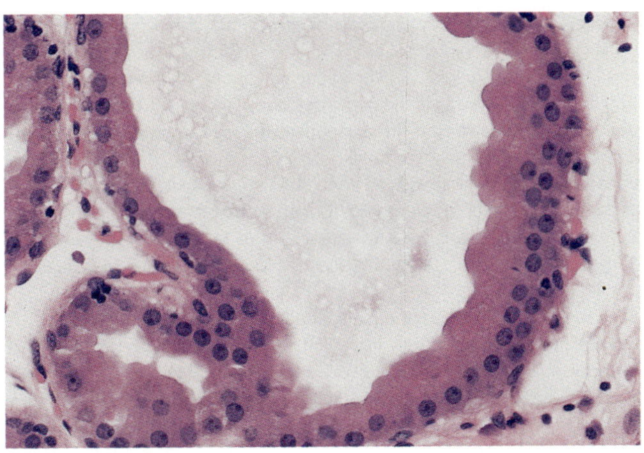

8.6 Fibrocystic changes with apocrine metaplasia.

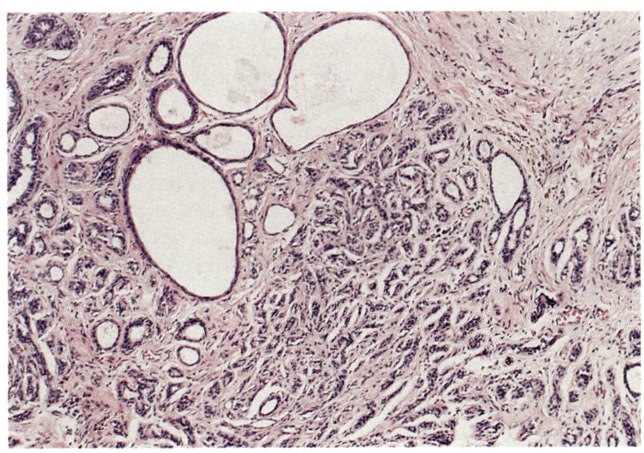

8.7 Sclerosing adenosis composed of tubules compressed by fibrous stroma.

TABLE 8-1 Relative Risk for Invasive Breast Carcinoma Based on Pathologic Examination of Benign Breast Tissue[27]

NO INCREASED RISK

Women with any lesion specified below in a biopsy specimen are at no greater risk for invasive breast carcinoma than comparable women who have had no breast biopsy:

- Adenosis, sclerosing,* or florid
- Apocrine metaplasia
- Cysts, macro- and/or micro-
- Duct ectasia
- Fibroadenoma*
- Fibrosis
- Hyperplasia, mild (more than two but not more than four epithelial cells in depth)
- Mastitis (inflammation)
- Periductal mastitis
- Squamous metaplasia

SLIGHTLY INCREASED RISK (1.5 - 2×)

Women with any lesion specified below in a biopsy specimen are at slightly increased risk for invasive breast carcinoma relative to comparable women who have had no breast biopsy:

- Hyperplasia, moderate or florid, solid or papillary
- Papilloma with fibrovascular core

MODERATELY INCREASED RISK (5×)

Women with any lesion specified below in a biopsy specimen are at moderately increased risk for invasive breast carcinoma relative to comparable women who have had no breast biopsy:

- Atypical hyperplasia (borderline lesion)
  - Ductal
  - Lobular

**Sclerosing adenosis and fibroadenoma have been shown by some authors to have a slightly increased risk.*[17,33]

From Hunter RVP, Consensus Meeting: Cancer Committee of the College of American Pathologists: Is "fibrocystic disease" of the breast precancerous? *Arch Pathol Lab Med* 110:171-173, 1986, American Medical Association, with permission.

Explanatory Notes and Supplements to the Consensus Statement

During the consensus development and by subsequent communication to the Chairman, it was recommended that the following explications be included with the consensus statement:

1. After a general discussion of epidemiologic risk factors for breast cancer, the participants agreed to limit the consensus statement to only those risk factors derived from the pathologic examination of benign breast tissue.
2. The indications for breast biopsy were not discussed. Nothing in this report suggests that a clinical diagnosis of "fibrocystic disease" must be followed by a biopsy to assess the risk for invasive carcinoma, in the absence of a usual indication for biopsy.
3. The use of the diagnostic term "fibrocystic *disease*" is discouraged; the terms "fibrocystic changes" or "fibrocystic condition" are preferred. However, when any of the above diagnostic terms is used, the component lesions should be specified so that the pathology consultation can be used, along with other relevant epidemiologic data, to estimate the relative risk for subsequent invasive cancer. The component lesions can be specified either in the body of the report or in the diagnosis.
4. Epithelial hyperplasias were discussed and assigned to risk categories. Ducts of ductules (lobules) with an epithelial lining no more than two cells deep are normal. *Mild hyperplasia* exists when the epithelium is greater than two but not more than four cells deep. *Moderate* and *florid hyperplasia* refers to more extensive degrees of epithelial proliferation. In the absence of atypical hyperplasia, mild hyperplasia is not associated with increased risk for invasive carcinoma. Moderate or florid hyperplasia without atypical hyperplasia is associated with a slightly increased risk (1.5 to 2 times) for invasive carcinoma.
5. *Atypical hyperplasia* (ductal or lobular) as used here refers to lesions that have some features of carcinoma in situ but not enough to make an unequivocal diagnosis of carcinoma in situ–the so-called borderline lesion. While there is a moderately increased risk for invasive cancer for women with atypical hyperplasia (approximately 5 times the risk of control populations in various studies), the relative risk of lesser degrees of atypia (mild, moderate) has not yet been established. Carcinoma in situ was considered during the discussion only to establish the end point for atypical hyperplasia. Of course, women with carcinoma in situ (ductal or lobular) in a breast biopsy, who have no further treatment, are at high risk for invasive carcinoma (8 to 10 times) relative to comparable women who have had no breast biopsy.
6. It should be noted that while the consensus statement defines relative risks for invasive carcinoma, the women who are at risk for invasive carcinoma are also at risk for in situ carcinoma.
7. The *radial scar* and the *lactiferous sinus solitary papilloma* have not been included in the risk categories because of the lack of specific data. Until data are available for these entities, they should be categorized by the characteristics of their epithelial components.

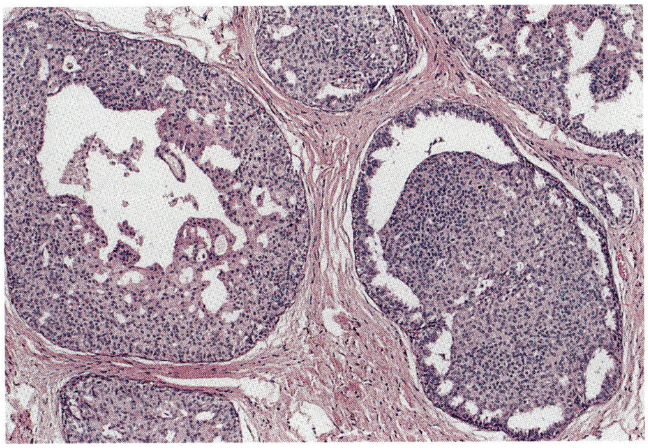

8.8 Florid hyperplasia of the breast containing residual lumina in the duct.

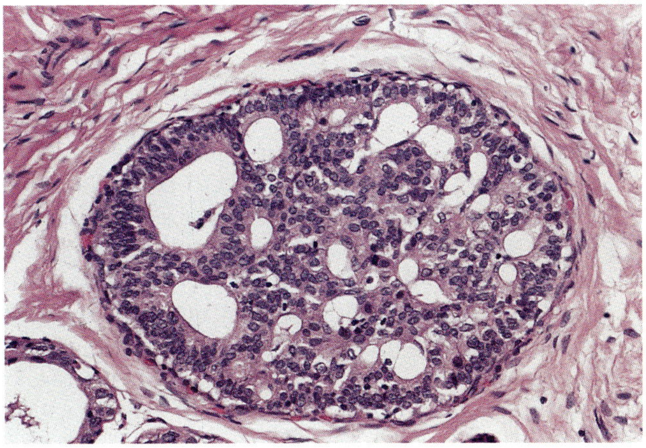

8.9 Atypical ductal hyperplasia in a single duct with secondary lumina of varying size.

CARCINOMA IN SITU

DCIS includes lesions that are similar to atypical ductal hyperplasia but encompasses one or more ducts that measure 2 mm or more in their aggregate cross-sectional diameter.[29,45] Low-grade or noncomedo DCIS may have a variety of patterns, including solid, cribriform (Figure 8-10), and micropapillary (Figure 8-11). An intermediate grade includes lesions that have either central necrosis without significant nuclear atypia or a cribriform DCIS with nuclear atypia but without central necrosis (Figure 8-12). High-grade DCIS consists of comedo carcinoma in situ with both central necrosis and nuclear atypia (Figures 8-13 and 8-14).

The distinction between atypical lobular hyperplasia and lobular carcinoma in situ (LCIS) has been more controversial than that between atypical ductal hyperplasia and DCIS. Because of this controversy, the term lobular neoplasia was introduced as a phrase to encompass both terms. Traditionally, atypical lobular hyperplasia refers to a proliferation of the lobular units with cells that distend the lobular unit but involving less than one half of the lobular structure. LCIS refers to lesions that involve over one half of the acini in a lobular unit (Figures 8-15 and 8-16).

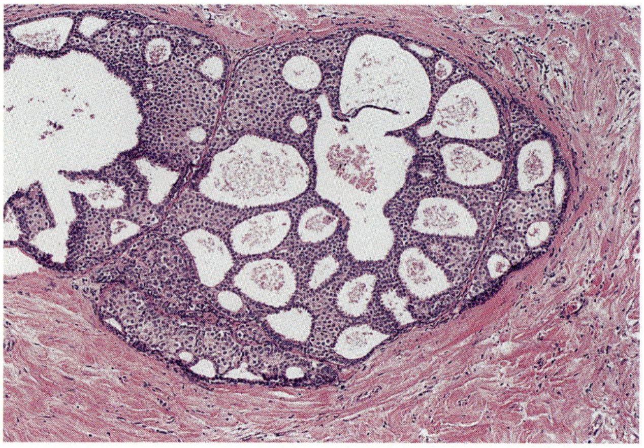

8.10 Low-grade ductal carcinoma in situ (DCIS) with a cribriform pattern.

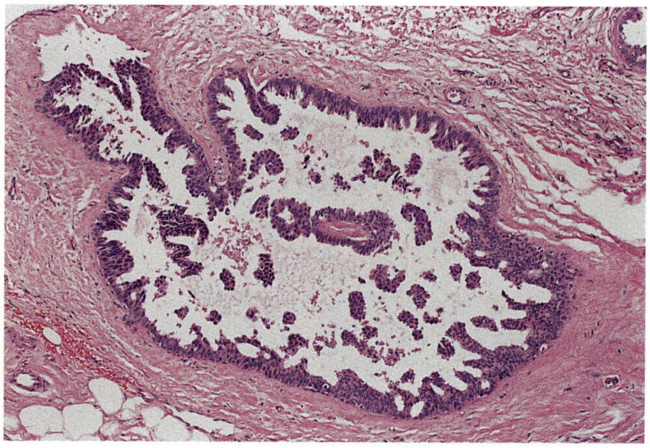

8.11 Low-grade DCIS with a micropapillary pattern.

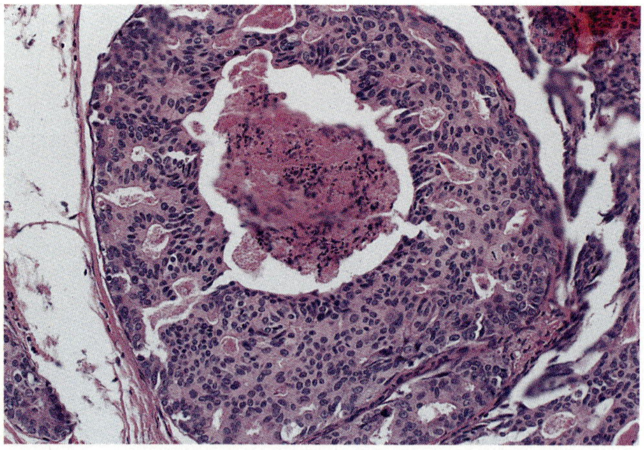

8.12 Intermediate-grade DCIS with a cribriform pattern and early central necrosis.

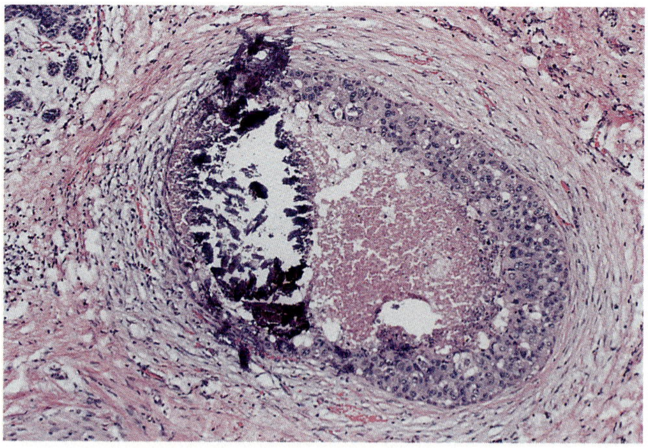

8.13 High-grade DCIS showing comedo necrosis and calcification.

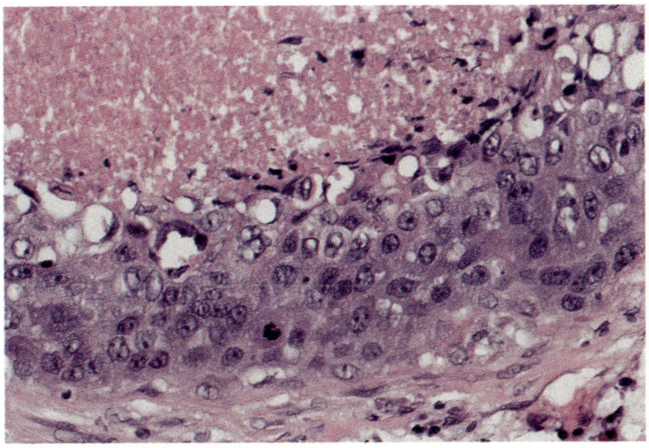

8.14 High-grade DCIS showing comedo necrosis and marked nuclear atypia in the ductal epithelium.

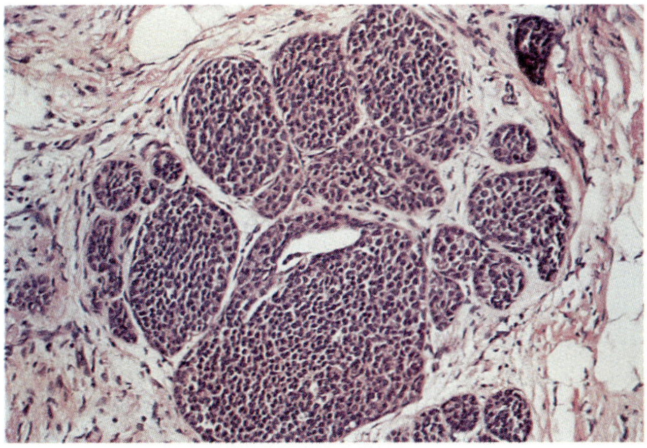

8.15 Lobular carcinoma in situ (LCIS) showing involvement of over 50% of the lobular unit.

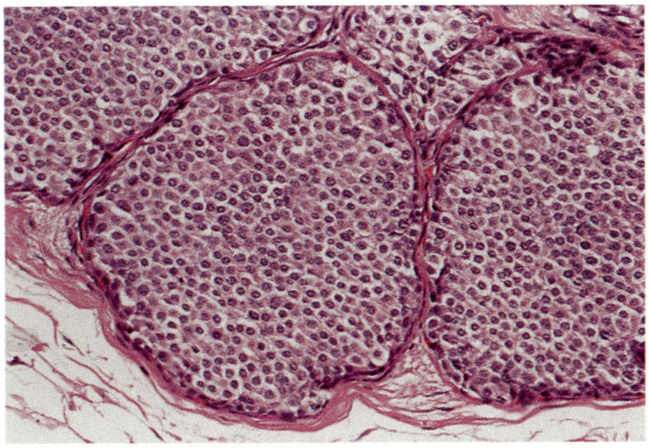

8.16 LCIS showing distended lobules replaced by a uniform proliferation of atypical lobular cells.

PAPILLARY LESIONS

A variety of papillary lesions may occur in the breast. True papillary lesions are distinguished from intraductal hyperplasias forming micropapillae by the presence of a fibrovascular connective tissue stalk. Solitary papillomas are usually in the subareolar region or involving a major duct (Figures 8-17 and 8-18). The papillary fibrovascular stalks are lined by a double layer of epithelial and myoepithelial cells (Figure 8-19). Intraductal papillomatosis or multiple papillomas may develop in the duct system and have a histologic appearance similar to a solid papilloma (Figure 8-20). Papillary carcinoma without invasion is a variant of intraductal carcinoma that lacks definitive stromal invasion. These tumors vary in size and may protrude into a cystic space (Figures 8-21 and 8-22). The hallmark that distinguishes this lesion from a papilloma is the loss of the myoepithelial cell layer. When invasion is observed, the lesion is termed invasive papillary carcinoma. Careful evaluation is necessary to distinguish these tumors from sclerosing papillomas.

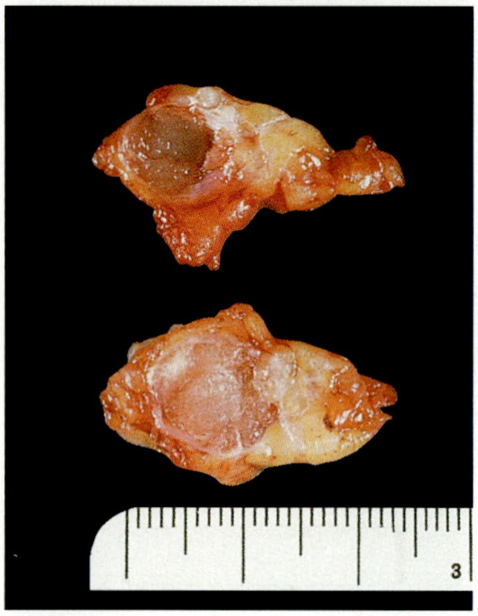

8.17 Solitary intraductal papilloma expanding a duct.

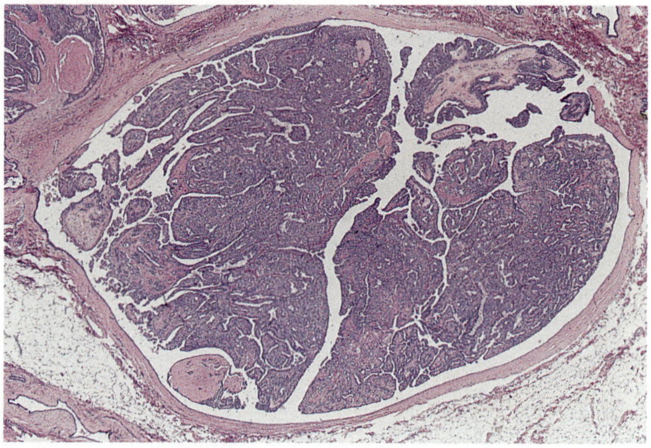

8.18 Solitary intraductal papilloma expanding a single duct.

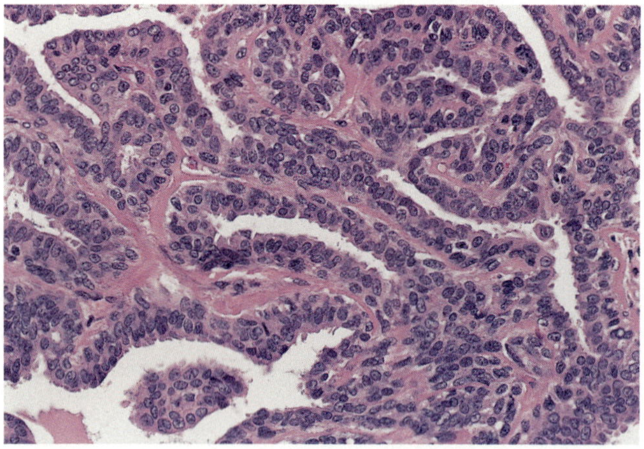

8.19 Solitary intraductal papilloma demonstrating fibrovascular cores lined with a double cell layer.

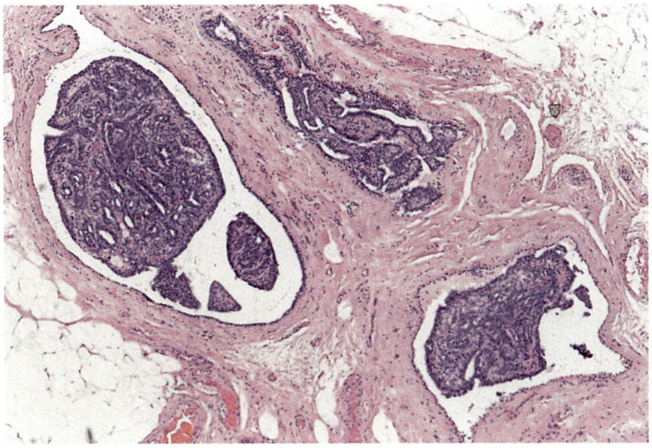

8.20 Multiple intraductal papillomas (papillomatosis).

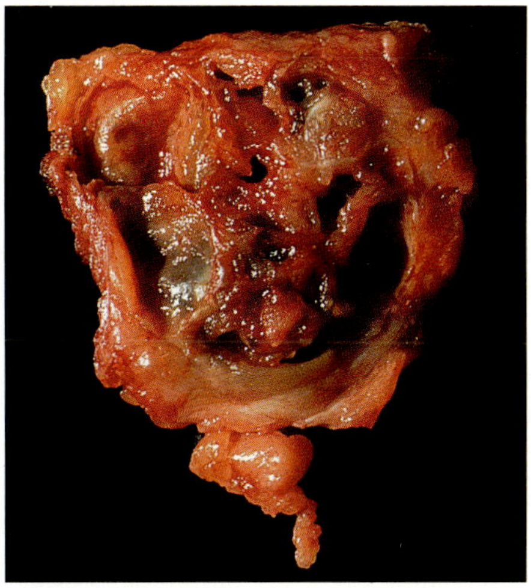

8.21 Intracystic papillary carcinoma.

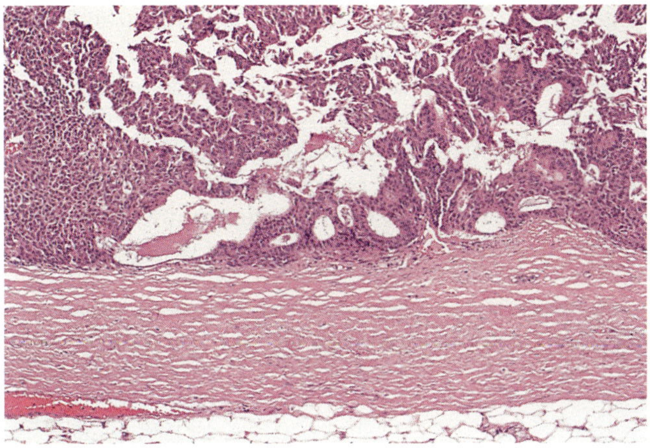

8.22 Noninvasive papillary carcinoma confined by a dense fibrous capsule.

INFILTRATING CARCINOMA

Infiltrating ductal carcinoma is the most common cell type seen in the breast. The tumor usually forms an irregular mass that is often calcified and extending with irregular, infiltrating margins into the surrounding fat (Figure 8-23). Histologically, the tumor is usually seen to be composed of infiltrating glands forming acinar structures with surrounding fibrosis (Figures 8-24 and 8-25). The grade of tumor is important as a prognostic indicator for infiltrating ductal carcinoma (Table 8-2).[16,18,19] Infiltrating lobular carcinoma is composed of smaller cells that often form a single row of infiltrating cells, some of which appear in a targetoid arrangement (Figure 8-26). Cytoplasmic vacuoles that indent the nucleus (signet ring cells) are often seen in infiltrating lobular carcinoma. Both infiltrating lobular carcinoma and lobular neoplasia often proliferate in a diffuse pattern without formation of a prominent mass. Medullary carcinoma forms a well-circumscribed solid mass (Figure 8-27). Histologically, it is characterized by a well-defined pushing margin composed of pleomorphic cells growing in solid sheets with prominent nucleoli and admixed with a dense lymphoplasmacytic infiltrate (Figures 8-28 and 8-29). The classic form of medullary carcinoma has a more favorable prognosis than the typical ductal carcinoma.

Mucinous or colloid carcinoma of the breast is usually seen in elderly patients and also has a more favorable prognosis.[38] The tumor has a gelatinous appearance grossly (Figure 8-30) and histologically is seen to consist of clusters of well-differentiated ductal cells embedded in abundant extracellular mucin (Figure 8-31). Tubular carcinoma is an extremely well differentiated variant (similar to minimum deviation adenocarcinoma of the cervix) that has a favorable prognosis. The tumor consists of open tubules with irregular angular outlines lined by a single layer of cells with minimal pleomorphism (Figure 8-32). Metaplastic carcinoma of the breast may show extensive squamous differentiation or contains a biphasic pattern with sarcomatous differentiation (figure 8-33). The term spindle cell carcinoma refers to a spindle cell variant of carcinoma having a uniform proliferation of spindle cells. The distinction between metaplastic carcinoma and spindle cell carcinoma is useful, since metaplastic carcinomas appear to have a less favorable prognosis. Paget disease of the breast usually presents with an excoriated, crusted lesion of the nipple having an eczematoid appearance (Figure 8-34). Histologically, the overlying epithelium is seen to be infiltrated with cells containing pale cytoplasm, irregular nuclei, and prominent nucleoli (Figure 8-35). Paget disease of the breast is almost always associated with an underlying infiltrating ductal carcinoma.

TABLE 8-2 Microscopic Grading of Breast Carcinoma *Modified Bloom-Richardson System*[16,18]

GRADE 1	
Low grade (well-differentiated)	3-5 points
GRADE 2	
Intermediate grade (moderately differentiated)	6-7 points
GRADE 3	
High grade (poorly differentiated)	8-9 points
Tubule formation	
1 point: Tubule formation in >75% of the tumor	
2 points: Tubule formation in 10% - 75% of the tumor	
3 points: Tubule formation in <10% of the tumor	
Nuclear pleomorphism	
1 point: Nuclei are uniform in size and shape, are relatively small, have dispersed chromatin patterns, and are without prominent nucleoli	
2 points: Nuclei are somewhat pleomorphic, have nucleoli, and are of intermediate size	
3 points: Nuclei are relatively large, have prominent nucleoli or multiple nucleoli, have coarse chromatin patterns, and vary in size and shape	
Mitotic count*	
1 point: 0-9 mitoses in 10 high-power fields (HPF)	
2 points: 10-19 mitoses in 10 HPF	
3 points: >20 mitoses in 10 HPF	
NOTTINGHAM PROGNOSTIC INDEX (NPI)	
NPI = 0.2 × tumor size (cm) + lymph node stage (1, 2, 3) + tumor grade (1, 2, 3)	

**Field diameter 0.59 mm/area 0.274 mm²$^{}$.*

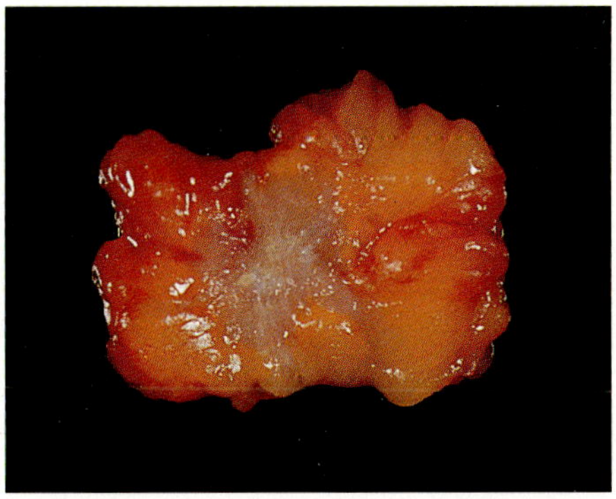

8.23 Infiltrating ductal carcinoma demonstrating an irregular fibrotic mass infiltrating the surrounding fat.

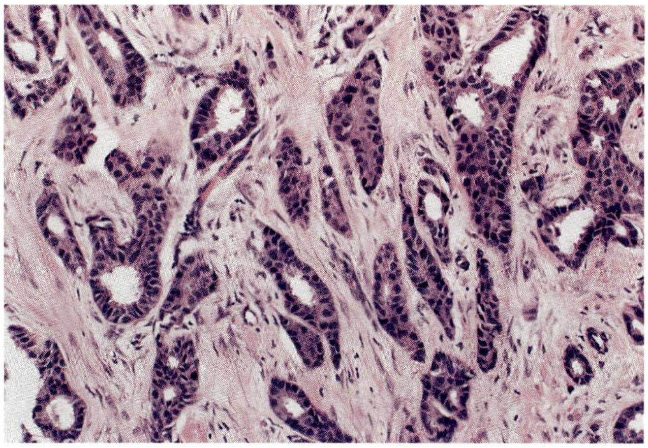

8.24 Well-differentiated (Grade I) infiltrating ductal carcinoma showing a predominance of tubular formation.

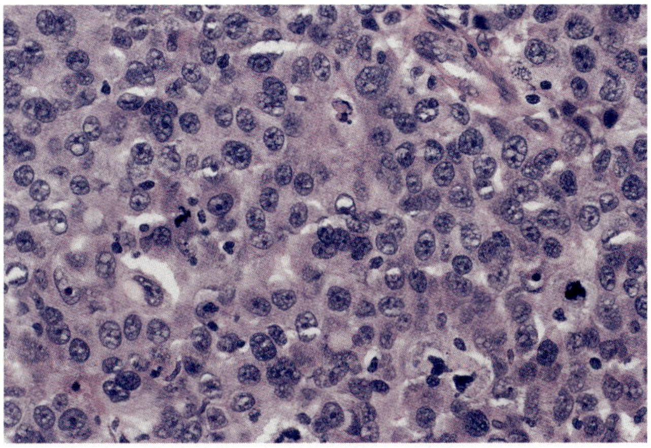

8.25 Poorly differentiated (Grade III) infiltrating ductal carcinoma showing a predominant solid proliferation of pleomorphic cells with numerous mitotic figures.

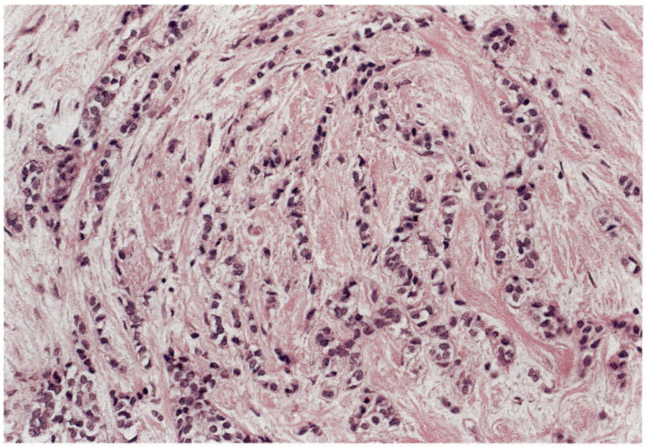

8.26 Infiltrating lobular carcinoma containing a proliferation of cells arranged in single-file fashion.

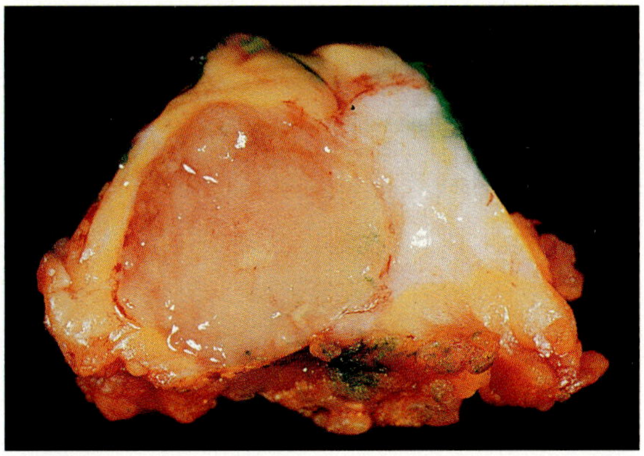

8.27 Medullary carcinoma of the breast demonstrating a well-circumscribed soft, fleshy mass.

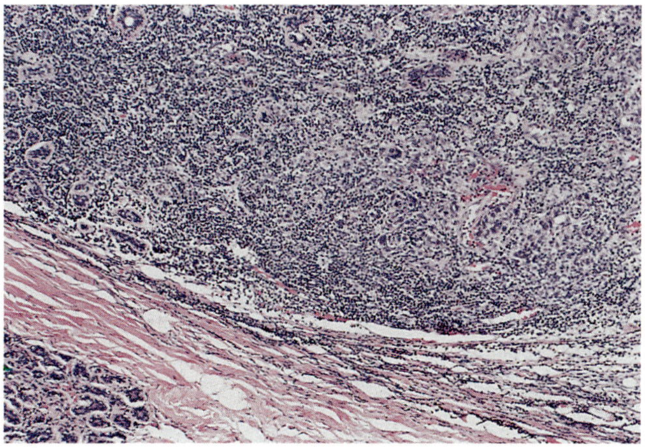

8.28 Medullary carcinoma of the breast demonstrating a pushing margin.

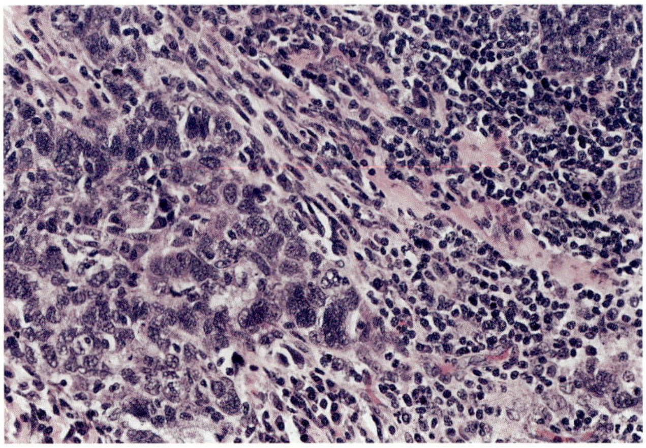

8.29 Medullary carcinoma of the breast showing pleomorphic epithelial cells surrounded by lymphoplasmacytic infiltrate.

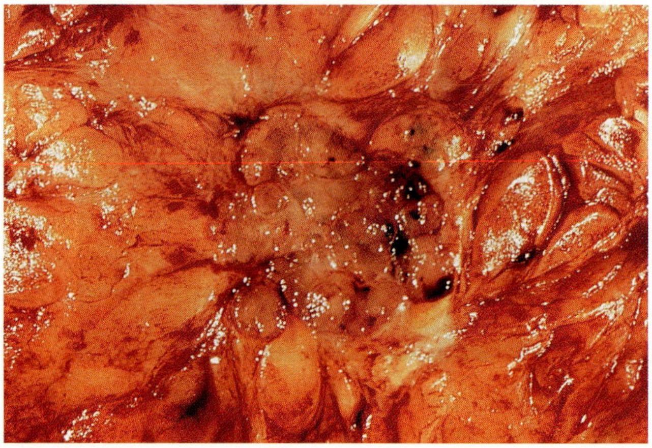

8.30 Mucinous (colloid) carcinoma of the breast having a gelatinous appearance.

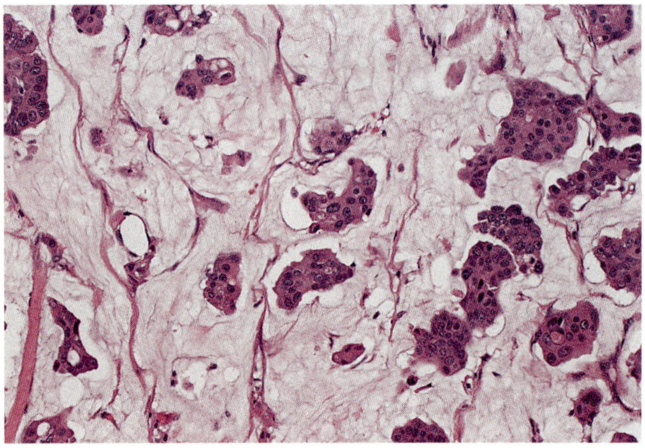

8.31 Mucinous (colloid) carcinoma of the breast containing clusters of well-differentiated ductal carcinoma embedded in a pool of extracellular mucin.

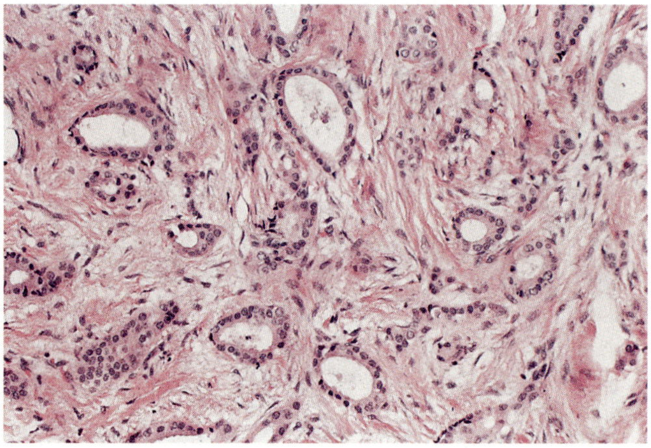

8.32 Tubular carcinoma with very well differentiated tubular glands embedded in a dense fibrous stroma.

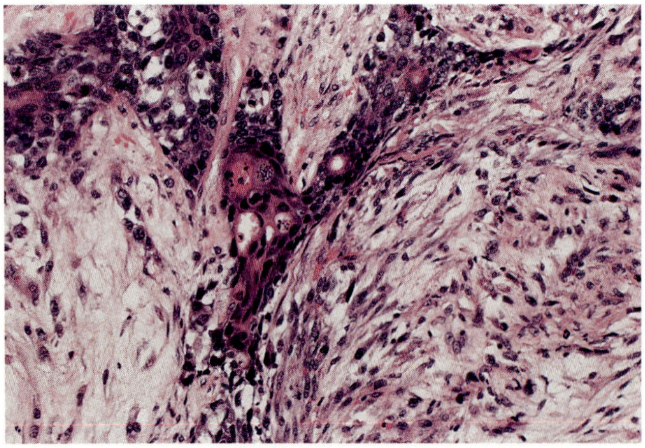

8.33 Metaplastic carcinoma showing a biphasic pattern of poorly differentiated carcinoma with a sarcomatoid stroma.

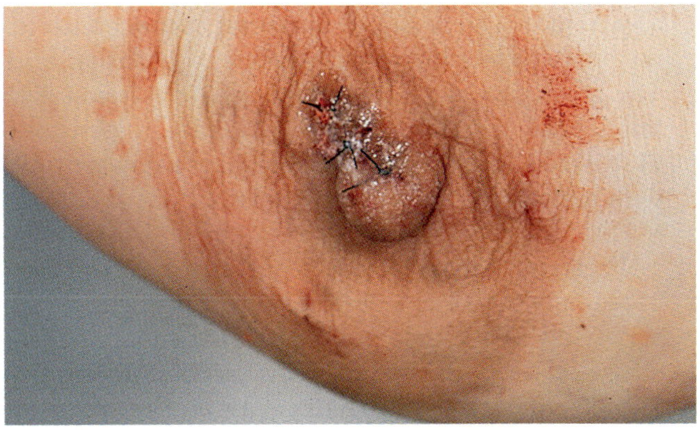

8.34 Paget disease of the breast demonstrating an excoriated, scaly lesion of the nipple.

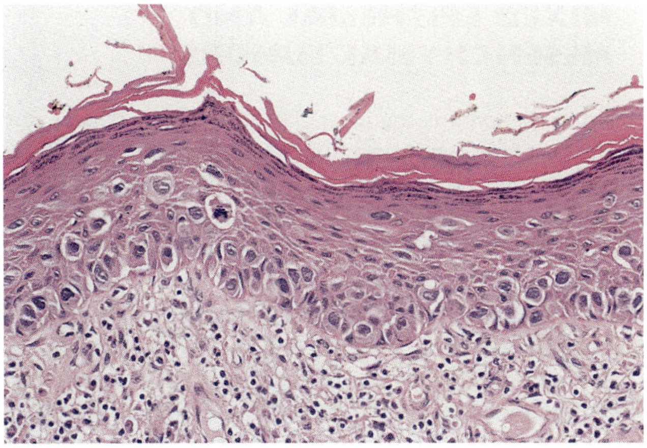

8.35 Paget disease of the breast demonstrating the squamous epithelium infiltrated with Paget cells containing pleomorphic nuclei and abundant cytoplasm.

MIXED EPITHELIAL AND MESENCHYMAL TUMORS

Fibroadenoma is the most common benign tumor of the breast. This lesion usually presents in the reproductive age group and is characterized by a well-circumscribed nodule that is uniform on cross-section (Figure 8-36). The histologic view is of a proliferation of epithelial and myoepithelial cells often seen in an intracanalicular pattern combined with a mesenchymal proliferation of bland fibroblastic cells (Figure 8-37). The tumors occasionally contain a mixture of fibrocystic changes with ductal dilatation and apocrine metaplasia. Intraductal and invasive carcinoma have been reported to arise in fibroadenoma, and most cases occur in women over the age of 40.[41] Juvenile fibroadenoma (Figure 8-38) is the most common breast mass in the adolescent female.[23] The tumor may rapidly enlarge over a short time. Histologically, it is usually characterized by a pericanalicular growth pattern, having a more adenomatous appearance (Figure 8-39). Lactating adenomas are solitary masses found in the pregnant or lactating breast. The gross view is of a well-circumscribed lesion with a tan lobular appearance on cut surface (Figure 8-40). Histologically, gestational changes are seen in the tubules with luminal secretion and vacuolated cytoplasm (Figure 8-41).

Phyllodes tumors of the breast grossly may have an appearance similar to a fibroadenoma, but in addition they are usually larger tumors and have a softer appearance on cross-section, often with cystic areas (Figure 8-42). Histologically, the tumor shares many of the features of an intracanalicular fibroadenoma. The mesenchymal component is more cellular, with broad, leaflike areas protruding into cystic spaces (Figure 8-43). The distinction between a benign phyllodes tumor and a malignant cystosarcoma phyllodes has been controversial. Stromal atypia, mitotic activity, abnormal mitotic figures, and stromal overgrowth (Figure 8-44) are useful features in predicting the behavior of cystosarcoma phyllodes.[34,37]

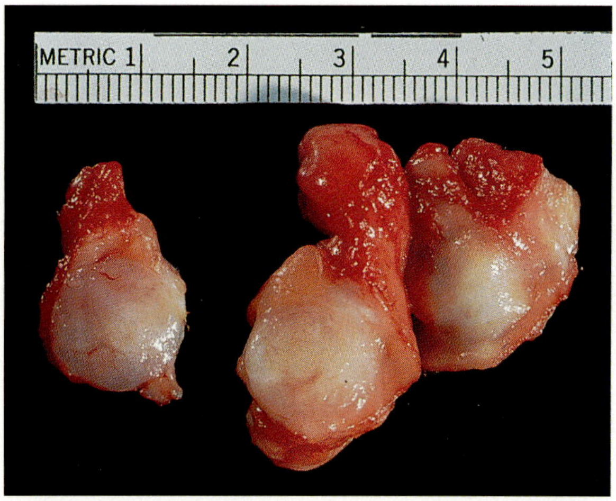

8.36 Fibroadenoma characterized by a well-circumscribed, light tan solid nodule.

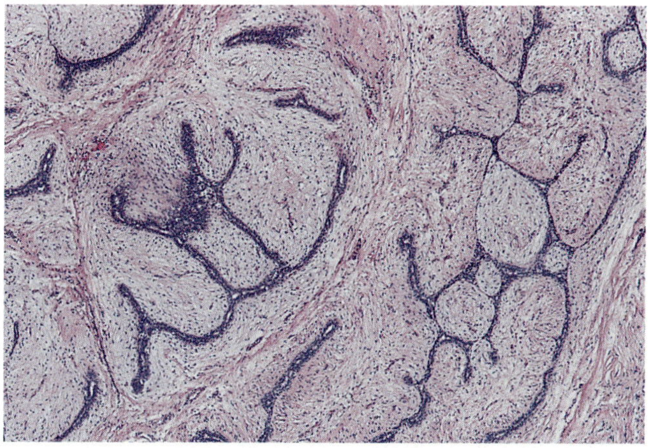

8.37 Fibroadenoma showing an intracanalicular pattern of epithelial cells surrounded by loose mesenchymal fibrous stroma.

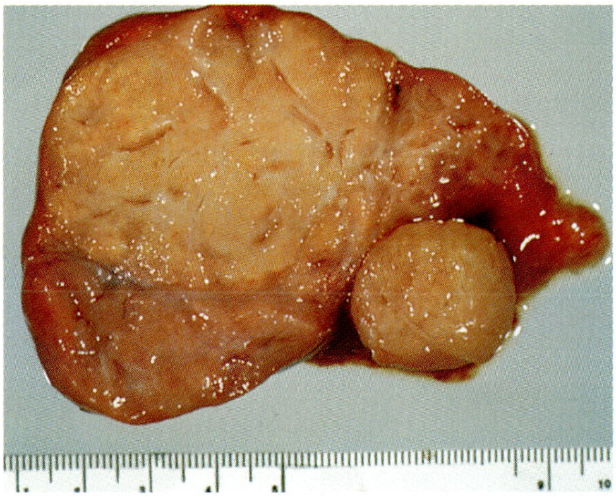

8.38 Juvenile fibroadenoma of the breast having a lobulated, tan-yellow appearance.

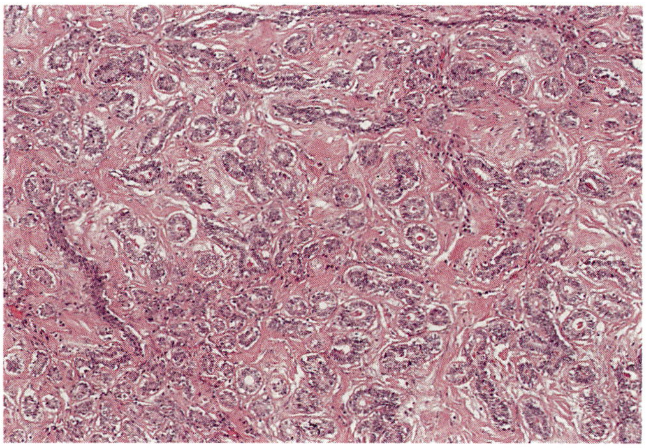

8.39 Juvenile fibroadenoma of the breast with a pericanalicular pattern.

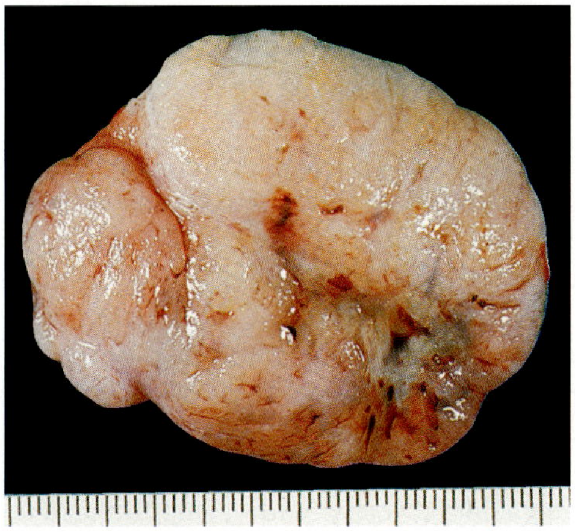

8.40 Lactating adenoma of the breast.

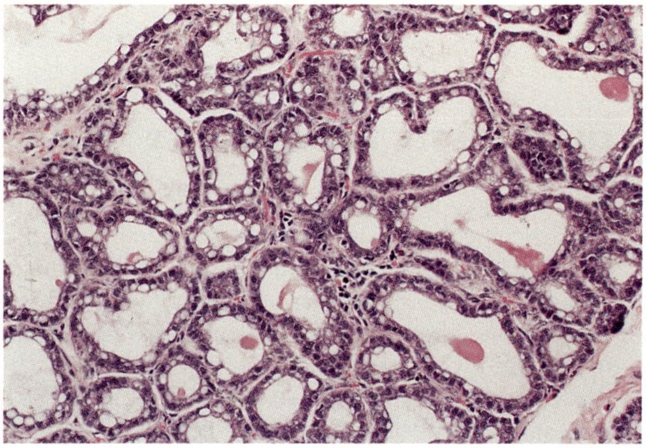

8.41 Lactating adenoma of the breast demonstrating secretory material in the lumen and a vacuolated cytoplasm.

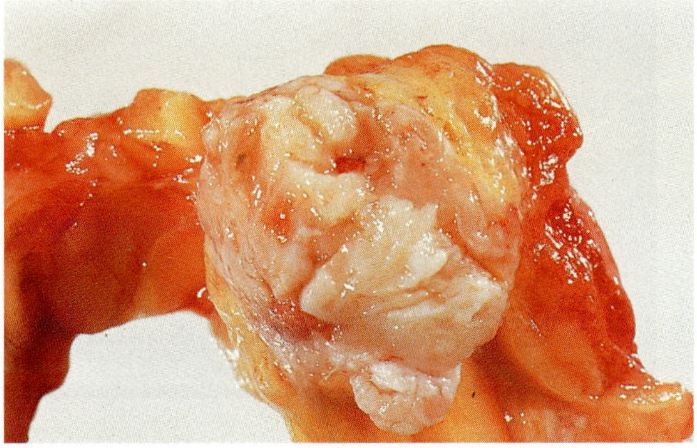

8.42 Phyllodes tumor of the breast demonstrating a fleshy mass with a leaflike proliferation.

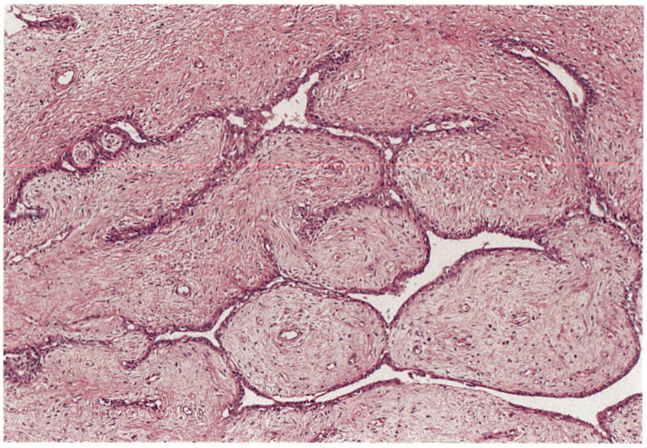

8.43 Phyllodes tumor of the breast showing an intracanalicular proliferation with broad, leaflike structures protruding into cystic space.

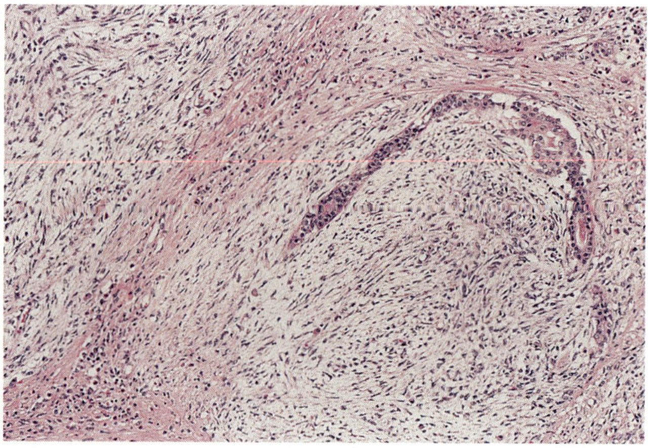

8.44 Cystosarcoma phyllodes demonstrating stromal overgrowth.

DIAGNOSTIC PROCEDURES

Screening mammograms are very useful for detecting early occult carcinomas of the breast. Mammograms are especially useful in the detection of early calcified tumors. The calcified area is localized by the radiologist with a wire probe. After surgical excision of the area around the needle, a specimen radiograph is performed to verify the presence of the area in question (Figure 8-45). Stereotactic core biopsies[32] and fine needle aspiration biopsies may be performed on mammographically detected lesions. Practice parameters have been defined for the use of frozen sections on breast biopsies.[20]

A useful and cost-effective[30,40] diagnostic tool for palpable breast masses is fine needle aspiration (FNA) biopsy.* If there is clinical or mammographic evidence of malignancy, an excisional biopsy should always be performed, regardless of the FNA findings. This has been referred to as the "triple test" (physical examination, mammography, and FNA) in the evaluation of breast lumps.[13,26,36] FNA complements the increase in the use of limited surgery (lumpectomy) for breast carcinoma.[21,31] It provides information that allows the patient to be counseled about various treatment options before surgery. FNA also permits definitive surgery to be performed in a one-stage procedure with wide margins taken at the time of surgery. Techniques are available for hormone receptor and DNA analysis on FNA specimens.[11,35]

*References 12, 14, 15, 22, 24, 39, 42, 44, 46, 47.

Fibrocystic masses usually contain apocrine metaplastic cells (Figure 8-46). Fibroadenomas have a characteristic finding on FNA biopsy with cellular clusters of bland ductal epithelium in a background of bipolar "naked" nuclei (Figure 8-47). A cystosarcoma phyllodes, in contrast, demonstrates a cellular spindle cell stromal component (Figure 8-48). Infiltrating ductal carcinoma is usually cellular with nuclear pleomorphism (Figure 8-49). Medullary carcinoma contains a mixture of pleomorphic ductal cells with lymphoplasmacytic cells (Figure 8-50).

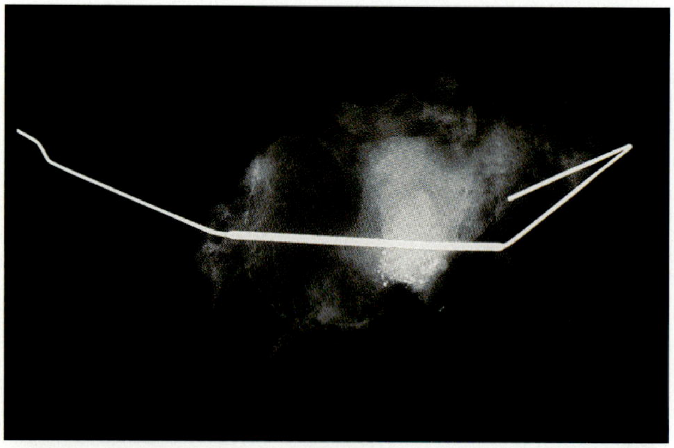

8.45 Specimen radiograph from a needle-localized breast specimen demonstrating microcalcification.

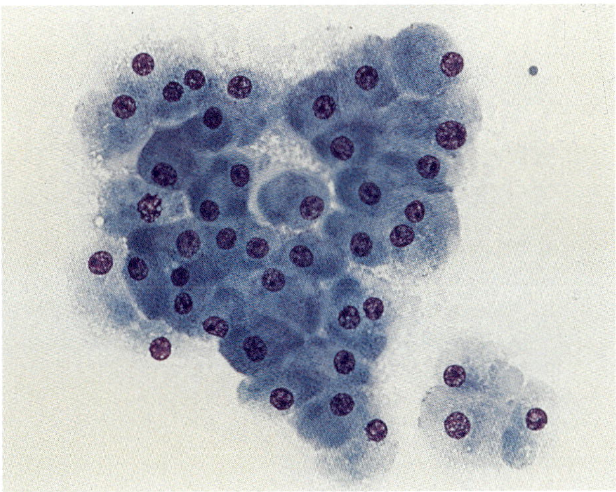

8.46 Fine needle aspiration (FNA) biopsy of the breast demonstrating apocrine metaplastic cells seen on a modified Wright-Giemsa stain.

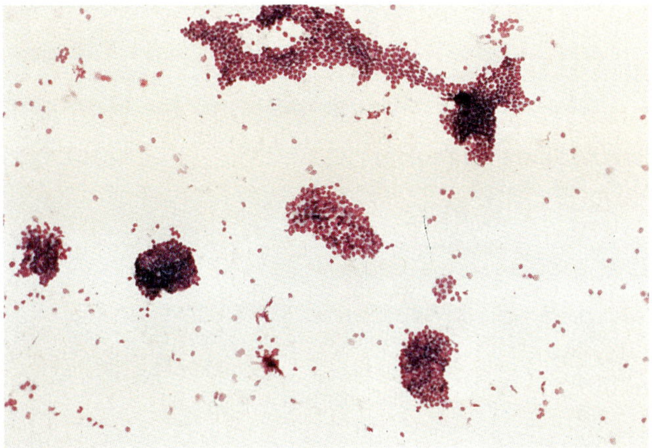

8.47 FNA biopsy of a fibroadenoma demonstrating clusters of epithelial cells surrounded by individual bipolar "naked" nuclei.

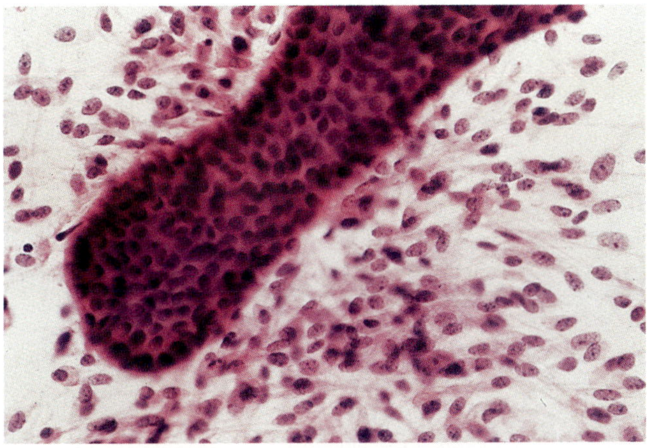

8.48 FNA biopsy of a cystosarcoma demonstrating bland ductal epithelium surrounded by proliferation of cellular spindle cells.

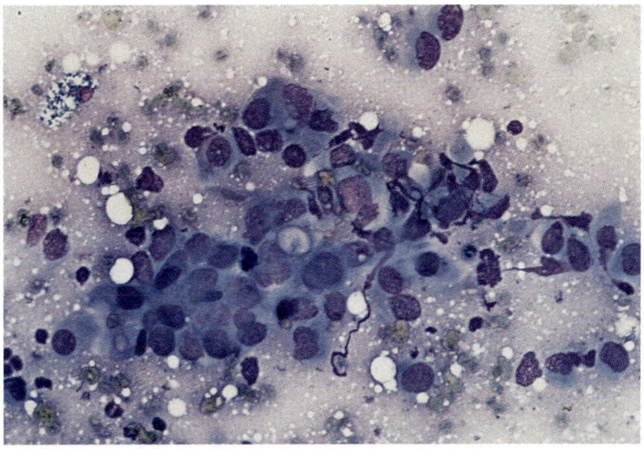

8.49 FNA biopsy of an infiltrating ductal carcinoma demonstrating pleomorphic ductal cells with atypical nuclei seen on a modified Wright-Giemsa stain.

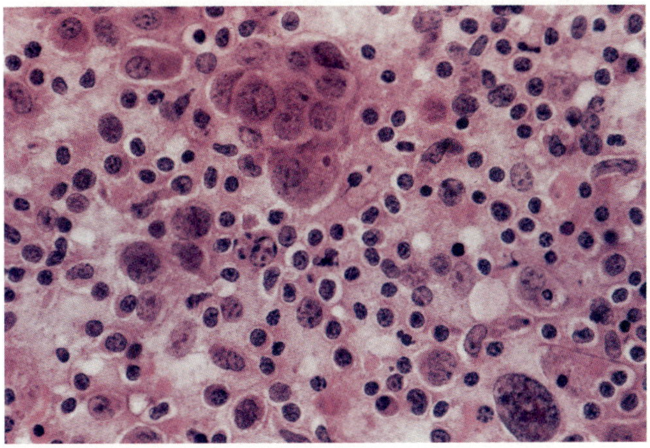

8.50 FNA biopsy of a medullary carcinoma demonstrating pleomorphic epithelial cells surrounded by a lymphoplasmacytic infiltrate.

Histologic Classification of Breast Tumors

AFIP modification (in italics) of the WHO Classification[6]

I. Epithelial Tumors
- A. Benign
  - 1. Papilloma
  - 2. *Papilloma variants*
    - a. *Adenomyoepithelioma*
    - b. *Mixed tumor (pleomorphic adenoma)*
    - c. *Ductal adenoma*
  - 3. Florid papillomatosis (adenoma) of nipple
  - 4. *Syringomatous adenoma of nipple*
  - 5. Adenoma
    - a. Tubular
    - b. Lactating
    - c. *Apocrine*
- B. Malignant
  - 1. Noninvasive
    - a. Intraductal carcinoma
      - (1) With Paget disease
    - b. Lobular carcinoma in situ
  - 2. Invasive
    - a. Invasive ductal carcinoma
      - (1) With Paget disease
    - b. Invasive ductal carcinoma with predominant intraductal component
    - c. Invasive lobular carcinoma
    - d. Medullary carcinoma
    - e. Mucinous carcinoma
    - f. Invasive papillary carcinoma
    - g. Tubular carcinoma
    - h. Adenoid cystic carcinoma
    - i. Secretory (juvenile) carcinoma
    - j. Apocrine carcinoma
    - k. Carcinoma with metaplasia
    - l. *Carcinoma with osteoclast-like giant cells*
    - m. *Cystic hypersecretory carcinoma with invasion*
    - n. *Carcinoma with endocrine differentiation*
    - o. *Glycogen-rich carcinoma*
    - p. *Lipid-rich* (lipid-secreting) *carcinoma*
    - q. *Invasive cribriform carcinoma*

II. Unusual Clinical Presentation of Carcinoma
- A. Inflammatory carcinoma
- B. *Carcinoma in pregnancy and lactation*
- C. *Occult carcinoma presenting with axillary lymph node metastases*
- D. *Carcinoma in ectopic breast*
- E. *Carcinoma in males*
- F. *Carcinoma in children*

III. Mixed Connective Tissue and Epithelial (Fibroepithelial) Neoplasms
- A. Benign
  - 1. Fibroadenoma
    - a. not otherwise specified
    - b. *Juvenile fibroadenoma*
  - 2. Benign cystosarcoma phyllodes (phyllodes tumor)
- B. Malignant
  - 1. Malignant cystosarcoma phyllodes

IV. Miscellaneous Tumors
- A. Mesenchymal tumors
  - 1. Benign
    - a. Hemangioma
      - (1) Perilobular hemangioma
      - (2) Hemangioma not otherwise specified
      - (3) *Venous hemangioma*
      - (4) *Nonparenchymal subcutaneous hemangioma*
    - b. *Angiomatosis*
    - c. *Fibromatosis*
    - d. *Myofibroblastoma*
    - e. *Neurofibroma*
    - f. *Leiomyoma*
    - g. *Lipoma*
      - (1) *Adenolipoma*
      - (2) *Angiolipoma*
    - h. *Chondroma*
    - i. Granular cell tumor
  - 2. Malignant
    - a. Angiosarcoma
    - b. *Fibrosarcoma*
    - c. *Leiomyosarcoma*
    - d. *Chondrosarcoma*
    - e. *Osteosarcoma*
    - f. *Hemangiopericytoma*
    - g. *Dermatofibrosarcoma protuberans*
- B. Skin tumors
  - 1. *Malignant melanoma of the nipple*
  - 2. *Squamous cell carcinoma of nipple*
  - 3. *Basal cell carcinoma of nipple*
  - 4. *Neoplasms of mammary skin*
- C. Lymphoid and hematopoietic tumors
  - 1. *Non-Hodgkin lymphoma*
  - 2. *Plasmacytoma*
  - 3. *Leukemic infiltration*
  - 4. *Hodgkin disease*

Histologic Classification of Breast Tumors—Cont'd

AFIP modification (in italics) of the WHO Classification[6]

V. Mammary Dysplasia/Fibrocystic Changes

- A. Ductal hyperplasia
  - 1. Atypical ductal hyperplasia
- B. Lobular hyperplasia
  - 1. Atypical lobular hyperplasia
- C. Adenosis
  - 1. *Sclerosing adenosis*
  - 2. *Adenosis tumor*
  - 3. *Microglandular adenosis*
  - 4. *Tubular adenosis*
- D. Cysts
- E. Fibroadenomatoid hyperplasia
- F. *Radial sclerosing lesion (radial scar)*

VI. Tumor-Like Lesions

- A. Duct ectasia
- B. Inflammatory pseudotumors
  - 1. Foreign body reaction
  - 2. Fat necrosis
  - 3. *Infarct*
  - 4. Infection
- C. Hamartoma
- D. Gynecomastia
- E. *Juvenile papillomatosis*
- F. *Fibrous tumor*
- G. *Diabetic mastopathy*
- H. *Amyloid tumor*
- I. *Pseudoangiomatous stromal hyperplasia*
- J. Other
  - 1. Asynchronous involution
  - 2. Vaginal hyperplasia

TNM Staging of Breast Carcinoma

I. Regional Lymph Nodes

A. Axillary (ipsilateral) and interpectoral (Rotter) nodes: lymph nodes along the axillary vein and its tributaries, which may be divided into the following levels:

1. Level I (low-axilla): lymph nodes lateral to the lateral border of the pectoralis minor muscle.
2. Level II (mid-axilla): lymph nodes between the medial and lateral borders of the pectoralis minor muscle and the interpectoral (Rotter) lymph nodes
3. Level III (apical axilla): lymph nodes medial to the medial margin of the pectoralis minor muscle including those designated as subclavicular, infraclavicular, or apical

Note: Intramammary lymph nodes are coded as axillary lymph nodes

B. Internal mammary (ipsilateral): lymph nodes in the intercostal spaces along the edge of the sternum in the endothoracic fascia

Any other lymph node metastasis is coded as a distant metastasis (M1), including supraclavicular, cervical, and contralateral internal mammary lymph nodes

II. TNM Clinical Classification

T—Primary Tumor

TX Primary tumor cannot be assessed

T0 No evidence of primary tumor

Tis Carcinoma in situ: intraductal carcinoma, or lobular carcinoma in situ, or Paget disease of the nipple with no tumor

Note: Paget disease associated with a tumor is classified according to the size of the tumor

T1 Tumor 2 cm or less in greatest dimension

T1a 0.5 cm or less in greatest dimension

T1b More than 0.5 cm but not more than 1 cm in greatest dimension

T1c More than 1 cm but not more than 2 cm in greatest dimension

T2 Tumor more than 2 cm but not more than 5 cm in greatest dimension

T3 Tumor more than 5 cm in greatest dimension

T4 Tumor of any size with direct extension to chest wall or skin

Note: Chest wall includes ribs, intercostal muscles, and serratus anterior muscle but not pectoral muscle

T4a Extension to chest wall

T4b Edema (including peau d'orange), or ulceration of the skin of the breast, or satellite skin nodules confined to the same breast

T4c Both 4a and 4b above

T4d Inflammatory carcinoma

Notes: Inflammatory carcinoma of the breast is characterized by diffuse, brawny induration of the skin with an erysipeloid edge, usually with no underlying palpable mass. If the skin biopsy is negative and there is no localized, measurable primary cancer, the T category is pTX when pathologically staging a clinical inflammatory carcinoma (T4d). Dimpling of the skin, nipple retraction, or other skin changes, except those in T4, may occur in T1, T2, or T3 without affecting the classification.

N—Regional Lymph Nodes

NX Regional lymph nodes cannot be assessed (e.g., previously removed)

N0 No regional lymph node metastasis

N1 Metastasis to movable ipsilateral axillary node(s)

N2 Metastasis to ipsilateral axillary node(s) fixed to one another or to other structures

N3 Metastasis to ipsilateral internal mammary lymph node(s)

M—Distant Metastasis

MX Presence of distant metastasis cannot be assessed

M0 No distant metastasis

M1 Distant metastasis (includes metastasis to supraclavicular lymph nodes)

The category M1 may be further specified according to the following notation:

Pulmonary	PUL	Bone marrow	MAR
Osseous	OSS	Pleura	PLE
Hepatic	HEP	Peritoneum	PER
Brain	BRA	Skin	SKI
Lymph nodes	LYM	Other	OTH

III. pTNM Pathologic Classification

pT—Primary Tumor

The pathologic classification requires examination of the primary carcinoma with no gross tumor at the margins of resection. A case can be classified pT is there is only microscopic tumor in a margin.

The pT categories correspond to the T categories.

pN—Regional Lymph Nodes

The pathologic classification requires resection and examination of at least the low axillary lymph nodes (level II). Such a resection will ordinarily include six or more lymph nodes.

pNX Regional lymph nodes cannot be assessed (not removed for study or previously removed)

pN0 No regional lymph node metastasis

pN1 Metastasis to movable ipsilateral axillary node(s)

pN1a Only micrometastasis (none larger than 0.2 cm)

pN1b Metastasis to lymph node(s), any larger than 0.2 cm

pN1bi Metastasis in one to three lymph nodes, any more than 0.2 cm and all less than 2.0 cm in greatest dimension

TNM Staging of Breast Carcinoma—Cont'd

pN1bii Metastasis to four or more lymph nodes, any more than 0.2 cm and all less than 2.0 cm in greatest dimension

pN1biii Extension to tumor beyond the capsule of a lymph node, metastasis less than 2.0 cm in greatest dimension

pN1biv Metastasis to a lymph node 2.0 cm or more in greatest dimension

pN2 Metastasis to ipsilateral axillary lymph nodes that are fixed to one another or to other structures

pN3 Metastasis to ipsilateral internal mammary lymph node(s)

pM—Distant Metastasis

The pM categories correspond to the M categories.

IV. G Histopathologic Grading

GX Grade of differentiation cannot be assessed

G1 Well differentiated

G2 Moderately differentiated

G3 Poorly differentiated

G4 Undifferentiated

V. R Classification

The absence or presence of residual tumor after treatment may be described by the symbol R.

RX Presence of residual tumor cannot be assessed

R0 No residual tumor

R1 Microscopic residual tumor

R2 Macroscopic residual tumor

VI. Stage Grouping

Stage 0	Tis	N0	M0
Stage I	T1	N0	M0
Stage IIA	T0	N1	M0
	T1	N1	M0
	T2	N0	M0
Stage IIB	T2	N1	M0
	T3	N0	M0
Stage IIIA	T0	N2	M0
	T1	N2	M0
	T2	N2	M0
	T3	N1, N2	M0
Stage IIIB	T4	Any N	M0
	Any T	N3	M0
Stage IV	Any T	Any N	M1

BIBLIOGRAPHY

General Reading

1. Association of Directors of Anatomic and Surgical Pathology: Recommendations for the reporting of breast carcinoma, *Mod Pathol* 9:77-81, 1996.
2. Association of Directors of Anatomic and Surgical Pathology: Immediate management of mammographically detected breast lesions, *Am J Surg Pathol* 17:850-851, 1993.
3. Bears OH, Henson DE, Hutter RVP, Kennedy BJ, editors: *AJCC manual for staging of cancer,* ed 4, Philadelphia, 1992, JB Lippincott.
4. Fechner RE, Mills SE: *Breast pathology: benign proliferations, atypias and in situ carcinomas,* Chicago, 1990, ASCP Press.
5. Oertel YC: *Fine needle aspiration of the breast,* Boston, 1987, Butterworths.
6. Page DL, Anderson TJ: *Diagnostic histopathology of the breast,* New York, 1987, Churchill Livingstone.
7. Powell DE, Stelling CB: *The diagnosis and detection of breast disease,* St Louis, 1994, Mosby-Year Book.
8. Rosen PP, Oberman HA: *Tumors of the mammary gland. Atlas of tumor pathology,* 3rd series, fascicle 7, Washington, DC, 1993, Armed Forces Institute of Pathology.
9. Spiessl B, editor: International Union Against Cancer. *TMN atlas: illustrated guide to the TNM/pTMN classification of malignant tumours,* ed 3, 2nd revision, Berlin, 1992, Springer-Verlag.
10. Tavassoli FA: *Pathology of the breast,* Norwalk, CT, 1992, Appleton & Lange.

References

11. Azavedo E, Baral E, Skoog L: Immunohistochemical analysis of estrogen receptors in cells obtained by fine needle aspiration from human mammary carcinomas, *Anticancer Res* 6:263-266, 1986.
12. Bottles K, Taylor RN: Diagnosis of breast masses in pregnant and lactating women by aspiration cytology, *Obstet Gynecol* 66:76S-78S, 1985.
13. Casey TT, Rodgers WH, Baxter JW, Sawyers JL, Reynolds VH, Page DL: Stratified diagnostic approach to fine needle aspiration of the breast, *Am J Surg* 163:305-311, 1992.
14. Ciatto S, Cariaggi P, Bulgaresi P: The value of routine cytologic examination of breast cyst fluids, *Acta Cytol* 31:301-304, 1987.
15. Cohen MB, Rodgers RPC, Hales MS, Gonzales JM, Ljung B-M, Beckstead JH, Bottles K, Miller TR: Influence of training and experience in fine-needle aspiration biopsy of breast, *Arch Pathol Lab Med* 111:518-520,1987.
16. Dalton LW, Page DL, Dupont WD: Histologic grading of breast carcinoma. A reproducibility study, *Cancer* 73:2765-2770, 1994.
17. DuPont WD, Page DL: Risk factors for breast cancer in women with proliferative breast disease, *N Engl J Med* 312:146-151, 1985.
18. Ellis IO, Elston CW, Blamey RW: The Nottingham prognostic index (NPI): a combination of multiple prognostic factors derived from the Nottingham Tenovus primary cancer study, *Mod Pathol* 4:11A, 1991.
19. Elston CW, Ellis IO: Pathological prognostic factors in breast cancer. I. The value of histological grade in breast cancer: experience from a large study with long-term follow-up, *Histopathology* 19:410-430, 1991.
20. Fechner RE: Frozen section examination of breast biopsies. Practice parameters, *Am J Clin Pathol* 103:6-7, 1994.
21. Fisher B: Reappraisal of breast biopsy prompted by the use of lumpectomy. Surgical strategy, *JAMA* 253:3585-3588, 1985.
22. Giard RWM, Hermans J: The value of aspiration cytologic examination of the breast, *Cancer* 69:2104-2110, 1992.
23. Goldstein DP, Miler V: Breast masses in adolescent females, *Clin Pediatr* 21:17-19, 1982.
24. Gupta RK, McHutchison AG, Dowle CS, Simpson JS: Fine-needle aspiration cytodiagnosis of breast masses in pregnant and lactating women and its impact on management, *Diagn Cytopathol* 9:156-159, 1993.
25. Heland KV, Rutledge P: Medicolegal issues, *Obstet Gynecol Clin* 21:781-788, 1994.
26. Hermansen C, Poulsen HS, Jensen J, Langfelt B, Sreenskov V, Frederiksen P, Jensen OM: Diagnostic reliability of combined physical examination, mammography, and fine-needle puncture ("triple-test") in breast tumors, *Cancer* 60:1866-1871, 1987.
27. Hutter RVP: Consensus meeting: Cancer Committee of the College of American Pathologists: is "fibrocystic disease" of the breast precancerous?, *Arch Pathol Lab Med* 110:171-173, 1986.

28. Hutter RVP: The role of the pathologist in breast cancer management, *Cancer* 66:1363-1372, 1990.
29. Lagios MD, Margolin FR, Westdahl, Rose MR: Mammographically detected duct carcinoma in situ: frequency of local recurrence following tylectomy and prognostic effect of nuclear grade on local recurrence, *Cancer* 63:618-624, 1989.
30. Layfield LJ, Chrischilles EA, Cohen MB, Bottles K: The palpable breast nodule. A cost-effective analysis of alternate diagnostic approaches, *Cancer* 72:1642-1651, 1993.
31. Margoless R, Poisson R, Shibata H, Pilch Y, Lerner H, Fisher B: The technique of segmental mastectomy (lumpectomy) and axillary dissection: a syllabus from the National Surgical Adjuvant Breast Project workshops, *Surgery* 102:828-834, 1987.
32. McCombs MM, Bassett LW, Jahan R, Fu YS: Imaging-guided core biopsy of the breast, *Breast J* 1:9-16, 1995.
33. Page DL, Dupont WD: Anatomic markers of premalignancy and risk of breast cancer, *Cancer* 6:1326-1335, 1990.
34. Reinfuss M, Mitus J, Duda K, Steimach A, Rys J, Smolak K: The treatment and prognosis of patients with phyllodes tumors of the breast. An analysis of 170 cases, *Cancer* 77:910-916, 1996.
35. Remvikos Y, Magdelenat H, Zajdel A: DNA flow cytometry applied to fine needle sampling of human breast cancer, *Cancer* 61:1629-1634, 1988.
36. Rogers LA, Lee KR: Breast carcinoma simulating fibroadenoma or fibrocystic change by fine-needle aspiration, *Anat Pathol* 98:155-160, 1992.
37. Sahin AA, Sneige N, Singletary SE: Phyllodes tumors of the breast, *Cancer Bull* 47:392-395, 1995.
38. Scopsi L, Andreola S, Pilotti S, Bufalino R, Baldini MT, Testori A, Rilke F: Mucinous carcinoma of the breast. A clinicopathologic, histochemical and immunocytochemical study with special reference to neuroendocrine differentiation, *Am J Surg Pathol* 18:702-711, 1994.
39. Shabot MM, Goldberg IM, Schick P, Nieberg R, Pilch YH: Aspiration cytology is superior to Tru-Cut needle biopsy in establishing the diagnosis of clinically suspicious breast masses, *Ann Surg* 196:122-126, 1981.
40. Silverman JF: Diagnostic accuracy, cost-effectiveness, and triage role of fine-needle aspiration biopsy in the diagnosis of palpable breast lesions, *Breast J* 1:3-8, 1995.
41. Simpson RH, James KA, Holdstock JB, Kelly RM, Yankah DHT: Carcinoma of the breast fibroadenoma, *Acta Cytol* 31:313-316, 1987.
42. Sneige N: Fine-needle aspiration of the breast: a review of 1,995 cases with emphasis on diagnostic pitfalls, *Diagn Cytopathol* 9:106-112, 1993.
43. Sneige N, Fornage BD, Saleh G: Ultrasound-guided fine-needle aspiration of nonpalpable breast lesions. Cytologic and histologic findings, *Am J Clin Pathol* 102:98-101, 1994.
44. Stanley MW, Abele J, Kline T, Silverman JF, Skoog L: What constitutes adequate sampling of palpable breast lesions that appear benign by clinical and mammographic criteria?, *Diagn Cytopathol* 13:473-485, 1995.
45. Tavassoli FA, Norris HJ: A comparison of the results of long-term follow-up for atypical intraductal hyperplasia and intraductal hyperplasia of the breast, *Cancer* 65:518-529, 1990.
46. Thomas PA, Cangiarella J, Raab SS, Waisman J: Fine needle aspiration biopsy of proliferative breast disease, *Mod Pathol* 8:130-136, 1995.
47. Willis SL, Ramzy I: Analysis of false results in a series of 835 fine needle aspirates of breast lesions, *Acta Cytol* 39:858-864, 1994.
48. Zylstra S, Bors-Koefoed R, Mondor M, Anti D, Giordano K, Resseguie LJ: A statistical model for predicting the outcome in breast cancer malpractice lawsuits, *Obstet Gynecol* 84:392-398, 1994.

Index

A

Abruptio placentae, 176
Absceses
 Bartholin gland, 13
 subareolar, 192
 tubo-ovarian, 106, 108
Actinomycosis
 of endometrium, 72
 tubo-ovarian abscess and, 106, 108
Acute atherosis, 176, 179
Acute cervicitis, 42, 43
Acute chorioamnionitis, 173
Acute endometritis, 72
Acute salpingitis, 106-107
Acute villitis, 176, 178
Adenocarcinomas
 of Bartholin gland, 14, 15-16
 of cervix, 51, 53, 54-56
 of colon, metastatic to ovary, 158
 endometrial, 79, 81-82
  with squamous differentiation, 79, 80, 82
  with villoglandular pattern, 80, 82
 of fallopian tube, 110, 111-112
 of ovary
  clear cell, 141-142
  endometrioid, 139
  mucinous, 135, 137
 of peritoneum, 115, 119
 of vagina, 29, 33
Adenofibromas
 of cervix, 60
 of ovary, 139, 140, 141
 paratubal, 114
 of uterus, 93
Adenoid basal carcinoma of cervix, 56, 57
Adenoid cystic carcinoma
 of Bartholin gland, 14, 16
 of cervix, 56
Adenoma malignum, 51, 54
Adenomas, lactating, of breast, 204, 205
Adenomatoid tumor of fallopian tube, 115, 116
Adenomatous hyperplasia of endometrium, 77
Adenomyoepithelioma of Bartholin gland, 14, 16
Adenomyosis, 75
Adenosarcomas of uterus, 93, 94
Adenosis
 breast, 193
 vagina, 28, 29
Adenosquamous carcinoma, endometrial, 79, 82
Aggressive angiomyxoma of vulva, 16, 17
Allantoic duct remnants, 170
Alpha-fetoprotein, 151, 152
Amnion
 bands, 173, 174
 reactive hyperplasia in, 173, 174
 squamous metaplasia of, 173, 174
Amnion nodosum, 173-174
Androblastomas (Sertoli-Leydig cell tumors), 146, 148-149
Androgen insensitivity syndrome, 128, 130
Angiomyxomas, aggressive, of vulva, 16, 17
Apocrine metaplasia, in breast, 193, 207
Appendix, mucinous tumor of, 115, 119
Arias-Stella reaction, 51, 53, 74, 76
Atherosis, 176, 179
Atrophic endometrium, 77
Atypical hyperplasia of endometrium, 77, 78
Atypical polypoid adenomyoma of uterus, 93, 94

B

Bartholin gland, 13-16
Basal cell carcinoma
 pseudoadenomatous, of Bartholin gland, 14, 16
 of vulva, 6, 10
Battledore placenta, 170, 171
Benign metastasizing leiomyoma of uterus, 87
Bethesda System, 65-66
Biopsy, breast, 206
Bizarre cellular leiomyoma of uterus, 86-87, 90
Bowen disease, 5
Bowenoid papulosis, 6
Breast, 192-213
 carcinoma
  infiltrating, 200-203
  in situ, 196-197
  metastatic, 61, 158
  microscopic grading, 200
  relative risk based on pathologic examination of benign breast tissue, 194
  staging, 210-211
 diagnostic procedures, 206-207
 histologic classification of tumors of, 208-209
 mixed epithelial mesenchymal tumors, 204-206
 papillary lesions, 198-199
 proliferative changes, 193-195
 reactive and inflammatory lesions, 192
Brenner tumor of ovary, 140, 142-143
Broad ligament
 histologic classification of tumors and tumor-like lesions of, 121
 tumors, 113, 114
Burkitt lymphoma of ovary, 158

C

Calcification
in breast tumors, 196, 206
in gonadoblastoma of ovary, 155, 157
Call-Exner bodies, 144
Calymmatobacterium granulomatis, 2
Candida albicans, 42, 43
Candidiasis, 28
Carcinoid syndrome, 155
Carcinoid tumor
of cervix, 56, 57
of ovary, 155, 156
Carcinoma in situ
of breast, 196-197
of cervix, 46
of fallopian tube, 112
Carcinosarcomas
of cervix, 60
of ovary, 140
of uterus, 93, 94-95
Cavernous hemangioma of vulva, 18
Cellular fibroma of ovary, 147
Cellular leiomyoma of uterus, 86, 90
bizarre, 86-87, 90
definition, 88
endometrial stromal nodules vs., 86
Cervical dysplasia, 46, 47, 48
Cervical intraepithelial neoplasia (CIN), 44, 46, 47-48
Cervical vaginitis emphysematosa, 42
Cervicitis, 42-43
Cervix, uterine; *see* Uterine cervix
Chancroid, 2
Chlamydia trachomatis
cervical infection, 42, 43
in salpingitis, 106
vaginal infection, 28
Chondroid differentiation, carcinosarcoma of uterus with, 93, 95
Chorangiosis, 176, 180
Chorioamnionitis, 173, 178
Chorioangiomas, 176, 180
Choriocarcinomas
gestational, 183
of ovary, 152, 154
Chorionic villi, 176, 178, 179, 181
Chronic cervicitis, 42, 43
Chronic endometritis, 72
Chronic salpingitis, 106
Chronic villitis, 176
Circummarginate placenta, 173
Circumvallate placenta, 173
Clear cell adenocarcinoma
of cervix, 51, 55
of ovary, 141-142
of vagina, 29, 32
Clear cell carcinoma
of endometrium, 80, 83
of fallopian tube, 111-112
of ovary, 140, 141-142
Clitoris
endodermal sinus tumor of, 18
hemangioma of, 18
Colloid carcinoma of breast, 200, 202
Colon carcinoma, metastatic, 158
Comedo necrosis, in ductal carcinoma in situ, 196-197
Complete hydatidiform mole, 181-182
Complex hyperplasia of endometrium, 77, 78
Condyloma acuminatum
of cervix, 44
of vulva, 2-3, 4
Condyloma latum, 2
Contraceptives, oral, endometrium and, 74, 76
Corpus luteum cysts, 128, 129
Cribiform pattern, in ductal carcinoma in situ, 196
Crystals of Reinke, 149, 150
Cylindroma, malignant, of Bartholin gland, 14, 16
Cystadenocarcinoma of ovary
mucinous, 135, 137
serous, 132, 134
Cystadenoma of ovary
mucinous, 136
serous, 132-133
Cystic follicles, 128, 129, 130
Cystic hyperplasia of endometrium, 77
Cystic teratoma, mature, 155-156
Cystosarcoma phyllodes, 204, 206, 207
Cysts
Bartholin gland, 13-14, 15
breast, 193
dermoid, 155-156
epidermal inclusion
of vagina, 28, 31
of vulva, 5, 7
epidermoid, of ovary, 155, 157
mucinous, of vulva, 12
multiloculated mesothelial, 115, 116
nabothian, 51
ovarian, 128-130
paratubal, 113-114
of rete ovarii, 158
of vagina, 28, 31
Cytomegalovirus infection of placenta, 176
Cytotrophoblasts
in choriocarcinoma
gestational, 183
of ovary, 154
in complete hydatidiform mole, 182

D

Decidual cast from endometrium, 74, 76
Decidual change of fallopian tube, 104
Decidual reaction of cervix, 58

Decidual vasculopathy, in pregnancy-induced hypertension, 176, 179
Dermoid cysts, 155-156
DES, 28, 29, 51
Diabetes mellitus, placenta in, 176
Diethylstilbestrol, 28, 29, 51
Diffuse granulosa cell tumor of ovary, 144, 145
Disordered proliferative endometrium, 77
Disseminated peritoneal leiomyomatosis, 87
Ductal carcinoma in situ, 196-197
Ductal carcinoma of breast, infiltrating, 200, 201
 biopsy, 206, 207
Ductal dilatation, in breast, 193
Ductal hyperplasia of breast, 193, 195
Dysgerminomas of ovary, 151, 152-153
Dyskeratosis, in condyloma acuminatum, 44, 45
Dysplasia, cervical, 46

E

Ectopic pregnancy
 in fallopian tube, 104-105
 ovarian, 128, 131
Ectropion of cervix, 28, 29
Edema
 ovarian, from torsion, 128, 131
 umbilical cord, 170, 171
 villous, 176, 178
Embryonal carcinoma of ovary, 152, 154
Embryonal rhabdomyosarcoma
 of cervix, 58, 59
 of vagina, 29, 34-35
Emdometrioid variant of yolk sac tumor, 152, 154
Endocervical adenocarcinoma, 51, 54
Endocervical cells, 51
Endocervical glandular dysplasia, 51
Endocervical polyps, 51, 53
Endocervical stromal sarcoma, 58-59
Endocervical tunnel clusters, 51, 52
Endodermal sinus tumor of vulva, 18
Endodermal sinus (yolk sac) tumor, 151-152, 153-154
Endolymphatic stromal myosis, 84, 85
Endometrial carcinoma, 79-83, 97
Endometrial dating criteria, 73
Endometrial stromal tumors, 84-86
 highly cellular leiomyomas vs., 86
Endometrioid tumors, of ovary, 138-140, 141
Endometriomas of ovary, 138
Endometriosis
 of cervix, 51, 53
 of ovary, 138
 of peritoneum, 115, 117
 of vagina, 28, 30
Endometritis, 72
Endometrium
 actinomycosis, 72
 atrophic, 77
 disordered proliferative, 77
 functional states, 73-76
 hyperplasia, 77, 79
 hypersecretory, 75, 76
 metaplasia, 77, 78-79
 mixed carcinoma, 80
 oral contraceptives and, 74, 76
 polyps, 77, 78
 proliferative, 73, 74
 secretory, 73-74, 75
Endosalpingiosis, 115, 117
Epidermal inclusion cysts
 of vagina, 28, 31
 of vulva, 5, 7
Epidermoid cysts of ovary, 155, 157
Epidermoid metaplasia of cervix, 51, 52
Epithelial tumors
 of cervix, 42-57, 62
 of uterus, 96
 of vagina, 36
 of vulva, 19
Epithelioid leiomyosarcoma of cervix, 58
Epithelioid smooth muscle tumors of uterine corpus, 86, 88, 89-90
Erythroblastosis fetalis, 176, 178
Erythroplasia of Queyrat, 5
Escherichia coli, 28
Estrogen, in disordered proliferative endometrium, 77

F

Fallopian tube
 adenomatoid tumor, 115, 116
 ectopic pregnancy in, 104-105
 histologic classification of tumors and tumor-like lesions of, 120
 hyperplasia, 110
 paratubal cysts and tumors, 113-114
 primary carcinoma
  criteria for, 110
  FIGO staging, 121
 prolapsed, 28, 29
 salpingitis, 106-109
 tumor-like lesions, 104-105, 120
 tumors, 110-112, 120
Fat, infiltrating ductal carcinoma and, 200, 201
Fat necrosis of breast, 192
Female adnexal tumor of probable wolffian origin, 113, 114
Fibroadenomas of breast, 204, 206, 207
Fibrocystic changes of breast, 193-195
Fibroepithelial polyps
 of vagina, 28, 31
 of vulva, 5, 6-7
Fibromas of ovary, 146, 147
Fibrosis, in dysgerminoma of ovary 151, 152

Fibrothecomas of ovary, 146, 147-148
Fibrous stroma in breast, 193, 202, 204
FIGO staging
of cervical carcinoma, 64
of endometrial carcinoma, 20
of fallopian tube carcinoma, 121
of gestational trophoblastic disease, 185
of ovarian tumors, 162
Filamentous bacteria, in actinomycosis of endometrium, 72
Fine needle aspiration biopsy of breast, 206, 207
Florid hyperplasia of breast, 193, 195
5-Fluorouracil, for condyloma acuminatum, 44
Foamy histiocystes, 77, 179, 192
Follicular cervicitis, 42
Follicular cysts, 128-129, 130
Follicular hyperthecosis, 128
Follicular salpingitis, 42
Funisitis, 170, 172
Furcate insertion of umbilical cord, 170, 171

G

Gardnerella vaginalis, 28, 42
Gartner's duct cyst, 28, 31
Germ cell tumors, 151-157, 161
Gestational trophoblastic disease
histologic classification, 184
miscellaneous lesions, 184
molar lesions, 181-182
nonmolar lesions, 183
staging, 185
Giant cells
multinucleated; see Multinucleated giant cells
osteoclastic-like, leiomyosarcoma of uterus with, 87, 92
syncytiotrophoblastic, in dysgerminoma of ovary, 153
Glandular differentiation, in yolk sac tumor, 153-154
Glandular lesions
of cervix, 51-55
of vulva, 12-13
Glassy cell carcinoma of cervix, 56
Glial implants, in immature teratoma of ovary, 152
Gliomatosis peritonei, 115, 118
Gonadal dysgenesis, 128
Gonadal stromal tumors of ovary, 144-151
Gonadoblastomas of ovary, 155, 157
Granular cell tumors of vulva, 16, 17
Granulation tissue, in vagina, 28, 29
Granuloma inguinale, 2, 4
Granuloma, in dysgerminoma of ovary, 151, 153
Granulomatous inflammation
in syphilis of cervix, 42, 43
in tuberculous salpingitis, 108
Granulomatous mastitis, 192
Granulosa cell tumors of ovary, 144-146
Granulosa cells, follicular cyst and, 129
Gynandroblastomas of ovary, 149, 150

H

Hamartomas, Sertoli cell, 128, 130
Hemangiomas
of cervix, 58
of vulva, 16, 18
Hematomas, retroplacental, 176, 177
Hematosalpinx, 106, 107
Hemorrhage, ovarian, from torsion, 128, 131
Hemorrhagic cornual pregnancy, 105
Hemorrhagic corpus luteum, 128, 129
Hemorrhagic cyst, 128
Hepatoid pattern, in yolk sac tumor, 152, 153
Hermaphroditism, true, 128
Herpes genitalis, 2, 3
Herpesvirus, cervical infection, 42
Hidradenitis suppurativa, 3, 4
Hidradenoma papilliferum of vulva, 12
High-grade stromal sarcoma, endometrial, 84, 86
Hilus cells, in rete ovarii cysts, 158
Hilus cell tumors of ovary, 149
Histiocytes
in acute atherosis, 179
in mamary duct ectasia, 192
in xanthogranulomatous oophoritis, 131
Hobnail cells, 74, 76, 142
HPV infection
cervical, 44-45, 46, 47, 50
vaginal, 28
vulvar, 2-3, 4
Human chorionic gonadotropin, 151, 152
Human papillomavirus infection
cervical, 44-45, 46, 47, 50
vaginal, 2-3, 4
vulvar, 28
Hyaline necrosis, leiomyoma with, 87, 92
Hydatidiform mole, 181-182
Hydropic abortus, 181
Hydrosalpinx, 106, 107
Hyperplasia
breast, 193, 195, 196
endometrial, 77, 79
mesothelial, 115
Hyperreactio luteinalis, 128
Hypersecretory endometrium, 75, 76
Hypertension, pregnancy-induced, 176, 179

I

Immature teratoma of ovary, 152, 154
Infarction, placental, 176, 179

Infections
of cervix, 42
placental, 176
in salpingitis, 106
of vagina, 28, 30
of vulva, 2-4
Infiltrating carcinoma of breast, 200-203
biopsy, 206, 207
Infiltrating leiomyoma of uterus, 87
Inflammation
Bartholin gland, 13
breast, 192
cervix, 42-43
ovary, 128
salpingitis, 106-109
uterine corpus, 72
vagina, 28, 30
Insular granulosa cell tumor of ovary, 144, 145
Insular pattern, in carcinoid tumor of ovary, 155, 156
Interferon, for condyloma acuminatum, 44
International Federation of Gynecology and Obstetrics; *see* FIGO staging
International Society for the Study of Vulvar Disease, 5
Intraductal papillomatosis, 198, 199
Intrauterine devices, 72, 106, 108
Intravascular leiomyoma of uterus, 87, 91
Intravenous leiomyomatosis of uterus, 87, 91
Invasive hydatidiform mole, 181, 182

J

Juvenile fibroadenoma of breast, 204, 205
Juvenile granulosa cell tumor of ovary, 144, 146, 150

K

Keratinizing squamous cell carcinoma of cervix, 46, 50
Keratoacanthomas of vulva, 5, 7
Knots in umbilical cord, 170, 171-172, 174
Koilocytosis
in cervical dysplasia, 47
in condyloma acuminatum, 44, 45
Krukenberg tumor, 158, 159

L

Lactating adenoma of breast, 204, 205
Laminated intervillous thrombi, 176, 178
Leiomyomablatomas of uterine corpus, 89-90
Leiomyomas
of uterine corpus, 86-92
of vagina, 33
of vulva, 17
Leiomyomatosis peritonealis disseminata, 115, 118
Leiomyosarcomas
of cervix, 58
of uterus, 87, 88, 91-92
of vulva, 16
Lentigo maligna of vulva, 11
Lentigo simplex of vulva, 11
Leukocytes, in acute funisitis of umbilical cord, 172
Leydig cells, 148-149
Leydig cell tumor of ovary, 150
Lichen sclerosus, 5 8
Lipid-laden macrophages, in endometrium, 77
Lipoleiomyoma of uterus, 91
Lipomas of broad ligament, 113, 114
Listeria *monocytogenes,* 176, 178
Lobular carcinoma in situ, 196, 197
Lobular carcinoma of breast, infiltrating, 200, 201
Low-grade stromal sarcoma, endometrial, 84, 85
Luteinized follicle cyst, 128, 130
Luteomas, in pregnancy, 128, 129-130
Lymph nodes, breast carcinoma and, 210
Lymphocytes
in dysgerminoma of ovary, 151, 152
in xanthogranulomatous oophoritis, 131
Lymphoepithelioma-like squamous carcinoma of cervix, 46, 50
Lymphogranuloma venereum, 2
Lymphomas
of cervix, 60, 61
of ovary, 158

M

Macrofollicular granulosa cell tumor of ovary, 144, 145
Macrophages
lipid-laden, in endometrium, 77
meconium and, 173, 174
Macroscopic cysts of breast, 193
Malakoplakia of vagina, 28, 30
Malignant cylindroma of Bartholin gland, 14, 16
Malignant melanoma
of cervix, 60
of uterus, 93, 94-95
Mammary duct ectasia, 192
Mammograms, 206
Mastitis, 192
Mature teratoma of ovary, 155
Meconium-stained placenta, 173, 174
Medullary carcinoma of breast, 200, 201-202
biopsy, 206, 207
Meigs syndrome, 146
Melanoma, malignant
of cervix, 60
of vulva, 11
Merkel cell carcinoma of vulva, 18
Mesonephric duct remnants, 51, 52

Mesotheliomas, 115, 116-117
Metaplastic carcinoma of breast, 200, 202
Metaplastic papillary tumor of fallopian tube, 105
Metastatic carcinoma
 to cervix, 61
 to ovary, 158, 159
 to umbilicus, 115, 119
Michaelis-Gutmann bodies, in malakoplakia of vagina, 28, 30
Microcystic pattern, in yolk sac tumor, 151
Microfollicular granulosa cell tumor of ovary, 144, 145
Microglandular hyperplasia of cervix, 51, 52
Microinvasive squamous carcinoma, 46, 48
Micropapillary pattern, in ductal carcinoma in situ, 196
Minimum deviation adenocarcinoma, 51, 54
Mitotic activity, in smooth muscle tumors of uncertain malignant potential, 87
Moles, hydatidiform, 181-182
Molluscum contagiosum, 2, 3
Mucin, inspissated, in Bartholin gland, 14, 15
Mucinous adenocarcinoma of endocervix, 51, 54
Mucinous carcinoma
 of breast, 200, 202
 of endometrium, 80, 83
Mucinous cyst of vulva, 12
Mucinous tumors, ovarian, 135-137, 141
Müllerian tumors
 malignant mixed
  of cervix, 60
  of uterus, 93, 94-95
 papilloma of cervix, 51, 53
 of peritoneum, 115
Multiloculated cystic mesothelioma, 115, 116
Multiloculated mucinous tumor of ovary, 135, 136
Multinucleated giant cells
 in granulomatous mastitis, 192
 in leiomyoma of uterus, 86-87, 90
 in mucinous ovarian tumor, 140
 in syphilis of cervix, 43
 in tuberculous salpingitis, 108
 in xanthogranulomatous oophoritis, 131
Multinucleation, in condyloma acuminatum, 44, 45
Multiple intraductal papillomas, 198, 199
Mural nodules, in mucinous tumor of ovary, 135, 137, 140
Myometrium
 invasive hydatidiform mole infiltrating, 181, 182
 placental site trophoblastic tumor in, 183, 184
Myxoid degeneration, in leiomyomas of uterine corpus, 89
Myxoid leiomyosarcoma of uterus, 87, 92

N

Nabothian cysts, 51
Neisseria gonorrhoeae, 13, 28, 106
Neurilemomas, leiomyomas resembling, 87, 90
Neutrophils, in acute chorioamnionitis, 173
Nevi of vulva, 11
Nipples, excoriated scaly lesions of, 200, 203
Nonkeratinizing squamous cell carcinoma of cervix, 46, 49
Nottingham Prognostic Index, 200
Nuclear-cytoplasmic ratio
 in cellular leiomyoma of uterus, 90
 in cervical squamous lesions, 47
Nuclear grooves, coffee bean-type, 144, 145

O

Omphalomesenteric vitelline duct remnants, 170
Oophoritis, xanthogranulomatous, 128, 131
Oral contraceptives, endometrium and, 74, 76
Osteoid differentiation, carcinosarcoma of uterus with, 93, 95
Oval nuclei
 in leiomyomas of uterine corpus, 89
 in proliferative endometrium, 73, 74
Ovarian sex cord tumor, uterine tumor resembling, 84, 86
Ovary, 128-166
 germ cell tumors, 151-157
 gonadal stromal tumors, 144-151
 histologic classification of tumors of, 160-161
 miscellaneous tumors, 158-159
 nonneoplastic lesions, 128-131
 staging and stage grouping of tumors, 162-163
 surface epithelial tumors
  Brenner, 140, 142-143
  endometrioid, 138-140, 141
  mucinous, 135-137, 141
  serous, 132-134, 141
Ovotestes, 128, 130

P

Paget disease
 of breast, 200, 203
 of vulva, 11, 12, 13
Papillary adenocarcinoma of fallopian tube, 110
Papillary adenofibroma of uterus, 93
Papillary carcinoma of breast, 198, 199
Papillary hidradenoma of vulva, 12
Papillary mesothelioma, 115, 116
Papillary metaplasia of endometrium, 77, 79
Papillary serous tumors
 cystadenofibromas, 113, 114
 endometrial, 80, 83
 ovarian, 132, 133-134
 peritoneal, 115, 118
Papillary squamous carcinoma of cervix, 46, 50
Papillary tumor, metaplastic, of fallopian tube, 105
Papillomas, 44
 of breast, 198-199
 of cervix, müllerian, 51, 53

Papillomatosis, intraductal, 198, 199
Papillomaviral infection
cervical, 44-45, 46, 47, 50
vaginal, 28
vulvar, 2-3, 4
Parasitic leiomyoma of uterus, 87
Paratubal cysts and tumors, 113-114
Partial hydatidiform mole, 181-182
Peritoneal leiomyomatosis, 115, 118
Peritoneum, tumors and tumor-like lesions of, 115-119, 122
Peutz-Jeghers syndrome, 149
Phyllodes tumor of breast, 204, 205-206
Pigmented lesions of vulva, 11
Placenta
disk, 176-180
examination, indications for, 170
membranes, 173-175
umbilical cord, 170-172
Placenta accreta, 176
Placenta increta, 176
Placental site trophoblastic tumor and reaction, 183, 184
Placenta membranacea, 173
Placenta percreta, 176
Placenta previa, 176
Plaque, placental site, 183, 184
Plasma cells
in chronic endometritis, 72
in syphilis of cervix, 43
in xanthogranulomatous oophoritis, 131
Pleomorphic cells
in bizarre cellular leiomyoma of uterus, 86, 90
in infiltrating ductal carcinoma, 200, 202, 207
in malignant melanoma of cervix, 60
in medullary carcinoma of breast, 207
in Paget disease of breast, 203
Plexiform tumor of uterus, 90
Polycystic ovaries, 128
Polyembryoma of ovary, 152
Polyps
endocervical, 51, 53
endometrial, 77, 78
fibroepithelial
of vagina, 28, 31
of vulva, 5, 6
Pregnancy
ectopic
in fallopian tube, 104-105
ovarian, 128, 131
hemorrhagic cornual, 105
luteomas in, 128, 129-130
Pregnancy-induced hypertension, 176, 179
Premenstrual endometrium, 76
Progesterone secretion, 73-74
Progesterone therapy, 74, 76
Proliferative endometrium, 73, 74
Psammoma bodies, 104, 118, 132, 134
Pseudoadenomatous basal cell carcinoma of Bartholin gland, 14, 16
Pseudocysts, umbilical cord edema forming, 170, 171
Pseudomyxoma peritonei, 115, 119
Pyosalpinx, 106-107

Q

Queyrat erythroplasia, 5

R

Reinke crystals, 149, 150
Rete ovarii cysts, 158
Reticular pattern, in yolk sac tumor, 151
Retroperitoneum tumors and tumor-like lesions, histologic classification of, 122
Retroplacental hematoma, 176
Rhabdomyoblastic differentiation, carcinosarcoma of uterus with, 93, 95
Rhabdomyomas of vagina, 29, 33-34
Rhabdomyosarcomas, embryonal
of cervix, 58, 59
of vagina, 29, 34-35
Rokitansky protuberance, 155

S

Salpingitis, 106-109
Salpingitis follicularis, 42, 106, 107
Salpingitis isthmica nodosa, 106, 109
Sarcoma botryoides
of cervix, 58, 59
of vagina, 29, 34-35
Sarcomas
of cervix, 58-59
endometrioid, 140
of uterine corpus, 93, 94
Sarcomatoid granulosa cell tumor of ovary, 144, 145
Sarcomatoid stroma, in metaplastic carcinoma of breast, 202
Schiller-Duval bodies, 151, 153
Sclerosing adenosis, in breast, 193
Sclerosing scromal tumor of ovary, 146, 148
Seborrheic keratosis of vulva, 5, 7
Secretory endometrium, 73-74, 75
Serous papillary adenocarcinoma of cervix, 56
Serous tumors, papillary
cystadenofibromas, 113, 114
of endometrium, 80, 83
of ovary, 132-134, 141
of peritoneum, 115, 118
Sertoli cell nodules, 128, 130
Sertoli-Leydig cell tumors, 146, 148-149
Sex cord—stromal tumors of ovary, 160-161

Sex cord tumor with annular tubules, 149, 151
Signet ring cells
 in infiltrating lobular carcinoma, 200
 in Krukenberg tumor, 158, 159
Simple cyst, 128
Simple hyperplasia of endometrium, 77, 78
Sister Mary-Jospeh nodule, 115, 119
Small cell carcinoma
 of cervix, 56, 57
 of ovary, 158, 159
Smooth muscle tumors
 of cervix, 58
 of uncertain malignant potential, 87, 88
 of uterine corpus, 86-92
 of vagina, 29, 33
 of vulva, 16, 17
Soft tissue lesions
 of cervix, 58-59
 of vulva, 16-18, 19
Solitary intraductal papilloma, 198
Spiked surface, in condyloma acuminatum, 44, 45
Spindle cell carcinoma of breast, 200
Spindle cells
 in cystosarcoma phyllodes, 206, 207
 in endocervical stromal sarcoma, 59
Spirochetes, in syphilis of cervix, 43
Squamous atypia, 46
Squamous cell carcinoma
 of cervix, 46, 49-40
 of fallopian tube, 110, 112
 of ovary, 155, 156
 of vagina, 29, 32
 of vulva, 6, 9
  Bartholin gland, 14, 15
Squamous epithelium, in Paget disease of breast, 203
Squamous intraepithelial lesion, 46
Squamous lesions
 of cervix, 46-50
 of endometrium, 79-80, 82
 of vagina, 28-29, 32
 of vulva, 5-10
  Bartholin's gland, 14, 15
Squamous metaplasia
 of amnion, 173, 174
 of endometrium, 77, 78
Staging
 cervical carcinoma, 63-64
 endometrial carcinoma, 97
 ovarian tumors, 162-163
 vulvar carcinoma, 20
 vulvar malignant melanoma, 21
Steroid cell tumor of ovary, 149, 150
Streak gonads, 128, 129
Stromal nodule, endometrial, 84, 85
Stromal overgrowth, in cystosarcoma phyllodes, 204, 206
Stromal sarcoma
 of cervix, 58-59
 endometrioid, 140
 of uterine corpus, 93, 94
Stromal tumors
 endometrial, 84-86
 gonadal, of ovary, 144-151
Struma carcinoid tumors, 155, 157
Struma ovarii, 155, 156
Succenturiate lobes, 173
Sulfur granules
 in actinomycosis of endometrium, 72
 in tuberculous salpingitis, 106
Surface epithelial-stromal tumors of ovary, 132-143, 160
Symplastic leiomyoma of uterus, 86-87, 88, 90
Syncytial cells
 in choriocarcinoma
  gestational, 183
  of ovary, 154
 in complete hydatidiform mole, 182
Syncytial knots, 176, 179
Syncytial membranes, vascular, 179
Syncytiotrophoblastic giant cells, in dysgerminoma of ovary, 151, 153
Syphilitic cervicitis, 42, 43
Syphilitic chancre, 2
Syphilitic placentitis, 176, 177-178

T

Tertomas of ovary, 152, 154-155
Testicular feminization, 128, 130
Theca cells, follicular cyst and, 129
Theca lutein cysts, 128
Thecomas of ovary, 146, 147
Thrombi, laminated intervillous, 176, 178
Thyroid follicles, in struma ovarii, 155, 156
TNM staging
 of breast carcinoma, 210-211
 of cervical carcinoma, 63
 of endometrial carcinoma, 20
 of ovarian tumors, 162
 of vulvar carcinoma, 20
 of vulvar malignant melanoma, 21
Torsion, ovarian, 128, 131
Trabecular granulosa cell tumor of ovary, 144, 145
Trabecular pattern, in carcinoid tumor of ovary, 155, 156
Transitional cell carcinoma
 of Bartholin gland, 14, 16
 of ovary, 140, 143
Treponema pallidium, 2
Trichomonas vaginalis, 28, 42
Triple test for breast lumps, 206
Trophoblastic lesions
 histologic classification, 184
 miscellaneous, 184

Trophoblastic lesions—cont'd
molar, 181-182
nonmolar, 183
staging, 185
True hermaphroditism, 128
Tubal metaplasia
of cervix, 51, 52
of endometrium, 77, 79
Tuberculosis of vulva, 2
Tuberculous cervicitis, 42
Tuberculous endometritis, 72
Tuberculous salpingitis, 106, 108
Tubo-ovarian abscess, 106, 108
Tubular carcinoma of breast, 200, 202
Tubular glands, in leiomyosarcoma of uterus, 87, 92
Tumor-nodes-metastases staging; see TNM staging
Turner syndrome, 128
Twin placenta, 173, 174-175

U

Umbilical artery, single, 170, 171
Umbilical cord, 170-172
constriction, 173, 174
Umbilicus, metastatic carcinoma to, 115, 119
Undifferentiated uterine sarcoma, 84, 85
Uterine cervix, 42-68
Bethesda System for reporting cytologic diagnoses, 65-66
carcinoma, 60-61
adenocarcinoma, 51, 53-56
squamous cell, 46, 49-50
TNM staging and stage grouping, 63-64
decidual reaction, 58
ectropion, 28, 29
embryonal rhabdomyosarcoma, 29, 34-35
epithelial tumors and related lesions
glandular lesions, 51-55
human papillomavirus, 44-45
inflammation, 42-43
miscellaneous epithelial tumors, 56-57
squamous lesions, 46-50
histologic classification of tumors of, 62
mesenchymal tumors, 58-59
miscellaneous tumors, 60-61
mixed epithelial and mesodermal tumors, 60
premalignant lesions, classification of, 46, 48
secondary tumors, 61
Uterine corpus, 72-100
abnormal proliferative states, 77-79
endometrial carcinoma, 79-83
TNM and FIGO staging, 97
functional states of endometrium, 73-76
histologic classification of endometrium, 73-76
hydatidiform mole, 181
inflammation, 72
mesenchymal tumors, 84-86
mixed epithelial and mesenchymal tumors, 93-95
smooth muscle tumors, 86-92
Uterine sarcoma, undifferentiated, 84, 85
Uterine tumor resembling ovarian sex cord tumor, 84, 86

V

Vagina, 28-39
adenosis, 28, 29
benign mixed tumor, 29, 35
Bethesda System for reporting cytologic diagnoses, 65-66
cysts, 28, 31
diethylstilbestrol and, 28, 29
endometriosis, 28, 31
fibroepithelial polyps, 28, 31
histologic classification of tumors of, 36
inflammatory and infectious diseases, 28, 30
malignant tumors, 29, 32-35
squamous lesions, 28-29, 32
Vaginal intraepithelial neoplasia (VAIN), 28-29, 32
Vaginitis, 28, 30
Vaginitis emphysematosa, cervical, 42
Vascular involvement of uterine leiomyoma, 87, 91
Vascular syncytial membranes, 179
Velamentous insertion of umbilical cord, 170, 171
Verrucous carcinoma
of cervix, 46
of vulva, 6, 9-10
Villitis, 176, 178
Villoglandular adenocarcinoma, of cervix, 51, 55
Villous edema, 176, 178
Vulva, 2-25
Bartholin gland, 13-16
carcinoma
basal cell, 6, 10
Merkel cell, 18
squamous cell, 6, 9
TNM staging and stage grouping, 20
verrucous, 6, 9-10
yolk sac, 18
epithelial hyperplasia with chronic inflammation, 8
glandular lesions, 12-13
histologic classification of tumors of, 19
infectious diseases, 2-4
malignant melanoma, TNM staging, 21
miscellaneous lesions, 18
nomenclature for disease, 5
pigmented lesions, 11
soft tissue lesions, 16-18
squamous lesions, 5-10
stromal invasion, 8
tumor measurement, 6, 9
vestibulitis, 3, 4
Vulvar intraepithelial neoplasia (VIN), 3, 8
classification, 5-6

W

Walthard rests, 112, 113
Warty squamous cell carcinoma of cervix, 46, 50
Well-differentiated papillary mesothelioma, 115, 117
World Health Organization (WHO), histologic classification of tumors
of breast (modified), 208-209
gestational trophoblastic disease, 184
of ovary (modified), 160-161
of uterine cervix, 62
of uterine corpus, 96
of vagina, 36
of vulva, 19

X

Xanthogranulomatous oophoritis, 128, 131

Y

Yolk sac carcinoma of vulva, 18
Yolk sac tumor, 151-152, 153-154

Other Pathology Titles Published By Mosby–Year Book, Inc.

Bostwick/Eble: Urologic Surgical Pathology (0-8016-7503-0)

Damjanov/Linder: Anderson's Pathology, 10/e (0-8016-7236-8)

Dorfman/Czerniak: Bone Tumors (0-8151-2746-4)

Enzinger/Weiss: Soft Tissue Tumors, 3/e (0-8151-3132-1)

Garcia/Budka/McKeever/Sarnat/Sima: Neuropathology: A Diagnostic Approach (0-8151-5562-X)

Gilbert-Barness: Potter's Pathology of the Fetus and Infant (0-8016-7870-6)

Meis-Kindblom/Enzinger: Color Atlas of Soft Tissue Tumors (0-8151-5895-5)

Rosai: Ackerman's Surgical Pathology, 8/e (0-8016-7004-7)